# Emergency Medicine and Critical Care

# Emergency Medicine and Critical Care

Edited by Abby Cusack

hayle medical
New York

Hayle Medical,
750 Third Avenue, 9th Floor,
New York, NY 10017, USA

Visit us on the World Wide Web at:
www.haylemedical.com



ISBN: 978-1-63241-477-9

The publisher's policy is to use permanent paper from mills that operate a sustainable forestry policy. Furthermore, the publisher ensures that the text paper and cover boards used have met acceptable environmental accreditation standards.



Printed in China.

**Cataloging-in-Publication Data**

Emergency medicine and critical care / edited by Abby Cusack.
p. cm.
Includes bibliographical references and index.
ISBN 978-1-63241-477-9
1. Emergency medicine. 2. Critical care medicine.
3. Emergency medical services. I. Cusack, Abby.
RC86.7 .E44 2018
616.025--dc23

# Table of Contents

# Preface

The world is advancing at a fast pace like never before. Therefore, the need is to keep up with the latest developments. This book was an idea that came to fruition when the specialists in the area realized the need to coordinate together and document essential themes in the subject. That's when I was requested to be the editor. Editing this book has been an honour as it brings together diverse authors researching on different streams of the field. The book collates essential materials contributed by veterans in the area which can be utilized by students and researchers alike.

Emergency medicine is an important part of medical studies and is treated as one of the most crucial divisions all across the globe. It refers to the practice of providing care and treatment of patients who require quick and immediate attention. It is mainly used in spontaneous and unplanned circumstances like earthquakes, building collapses, road accidents, etc. This book traces the progress of the field of emergency medicine and highlights some of its key concepts and applications. This text strives to provide a fair idea about this discipline to help develop a better understanding of the latest advances within this field. This book, with its detailed analyses and data, will prove immensely beneficial to professionals and students involved in this area at various levels.

Each chapter is a sole-standing publication that reflects each author´s interpretation. Thus, the book displays a multi-facetted picture of our current understanding of application, resources and aspects of the field. I would like to thank the contributors of this book and my family for their endless support.

**Editor**

1

# Morbidity and Mortality following Traditional Uvulectomy among Children Presenting to the Muhimbili National Hospital Emergency Department in Dar es Salaam, Tanzania

**H. R. Sawe,**[1,2] **J. A. Mfinanga,**[1,2] **F. H. Ringo,**[2] **V. Mwafongo,**[1,2] **T. A. Reynolds,**[2,3] **and M. S. Runyon**[1,4]

[1] *Muhimbili University of Health and Allied Sciences, Dar es Salaam, Tanzania*
[2] *Muhimbili National Hospital, Dar es Salaam, Tanzania*
[3] *University of California, San Francisco, CA, USA*
[4] *Carolinas Medical Center, Charlotte, NC, USA*

Correspondence should be addressed to M. S. Runyon; michael.runyon@carolinas.org

Academic Editor: Wen-Jone Chen

*Background.* Traditional uvulectomy is performed as a cultural ritual or purported medical remedy. We describe the associated emergency department (ED) presentations and outcomes. *Methods.* This was a subgroup analysis of a retrospective review of all pediatric visits to our ED in 2012. Trained abstracters recorded demographics, clinical presentations, and outcomes. *Results.* Complete data were available for 5540/5774 (96%) visits and 56 (1.0%, 95% CI: 0.7–1.3%) were related to recent uvulectomy, median age 1.3 years (interquartile range: 7 months–2 years) and 30 (54%) were male. Presenting complaints included cough (82%), fever (46%), and hematemesis (38%). Clinical findings included fever (54%), tachypnea (30%), and tachycardia (25%). 35 patients (63%, 95% CI: 49–75%) received intravenous antibiotics, 11 (20%, 95% CI: 10–32%) required blood transfusion, and 3 (5%, 95% CI: 1–15%) had surgical intervention. All were admitted to the hospital and 12 (21%, 95% CI: 12–34%) died. By comparison, 498 (9.1%, 95% CI: 8–10%) of the 5484 children presenting for reasons unrelated to uvulectomy died ($p = 0.003$). *Conclusion.* In our cohort, traditional uvulectomy was associated with significant morbidity and mortality. Emergency care providers should advocate for legal and public health interventions to eliminate this dangerous practice.

## 1. Introduction

Traditional uvulectomy is an excision of the uvula, usually performed by nonphysician healers. The procedure has been touted as a remedy for, or prevention of, infections associated with throat and chest and has also been completed as part of ritual practice [1–4]. Unlike the uvulopalatoplasty, which is typically performed by an otolaryngologist to treat snoring or obstructive sleep apnea [5–7], the traditional uvulectomy is performed by local healers who inherit the skills from their predecessors with no formal medical training. It is often completed without regard to recommended standards of good surgical practices [8].

In sub-Saharan Africa, traditional uvulectomy is largely driven by indigenous beliefs and cultural practices [9, 10], with many local nonphysician healers believing and preaching that the uvula is the main organ responsible for all throat and chest problems and should be removed as early as possible in childhood [11]. Despite being a common cultural practice, traditional uvulectomy has been associated with substantial number of harmful outcomes with significant morbidity and mortality largely from haemorrhage and sepsis [9, 11, 12].

In Tanzania, the practice of uvulectomy is a relatively common phenomenon [10, 13] carried out by traditional healers, most of who are not recognized by the ministry of health, despite the government stance on discouraging dangerous traditional practices. The prevalence of traditional uvulectomy in Tanzania has been estimated at 3.6% [14]. There are reports of traditional practitioners using the same instruments to perform the procedure in multiple patients without cleaning, disinfecting, or sterilizing, thus potentially exposing the children to life threatening communicable infections [15].

In this retrospective chart review study, we reviewed the records of all pediatric patients seen in the emergency department of a large national hospital during the year 2012 to describe the clinical presentations and outcomes of children presenting with complications from traditional uvulectomy.

## 2. Methods

*2.1. Study Setting.* The investigation was conducted at the Muhimbili National Hospital (MNH) Emergency Department (ED) in Dar es Salaam, Tanzania. Established in 2010, the MNH ED is the first full-capacity ED in Tanzania and is the clinical training site for the country's first emergency medicine residency program.

The department is staffed by interns (fresh graduates from medical school), registrars (registered medical practitioners each with 1–3 years of clinical experience following internship), and emergency medicine residents (all had already worked as registrars before joining the 3-year residency program). These doctors work under the clinical supervision of the locally trained emergency physician faculty with support and consultation from board-certified emergency physicians from the USA, Canada, and South Africa.

MNH is the largest tertiary care center in Tanzania and the ED serves a high acuity patient population from within Dar es Salaam as well as referral patients from throughout the country. Of the 36000 adult and pediatric patients seen each year, only 20% are discharged home from the ED. The top five categories of complaints seen in the department are trauma, infectious, mental health, neoplastic, and pregnancy-related issues [16].

*2.2. Study Design.* This was a prespecified subgroup analysis of a retrospective chart review of all children (less than 18 years old) seen in the MNH ED from 1 January 2012 to 31 December 2012. Trained physician abstractors reviewed the ED and inpatient records for all children presenting to the MNH ED during the study period. Data were recorded on a structured case report form, including basic demographics, reported initial complaints, final EMD diagnoses, and final hospital discharge diagnosis.

For this investigation, we examined all presentations associated with complications of traditional uvulectomy, including the clinical findings, treatment rendered, and patient outcomes.

*2.3. Statistical Analysis.* Data were imported into an Excel spreadsheet (Microsoft Corporation, Redmond, WA, USA), cleaned, and analyzed with StatsDirect (v 3.0.133, Cheshire, UK). We report descriptive statistics, including mean and standard deviations, medians and interquartile ranges, and counts and percentages as appropriate for the data type and distribution. Confidence intervals were calculated by the Clopper-Pearson (exact) method. Categorical values were compared between groups using the Chi Square test.

Table 1: Baseline characteristics of the patients.

| Variable | All ($N = 56$)* |
|---|---|
| Age | |
| Overall: median (interquartile range) | 1.3 years (7 months–2 years) |
| 1–6 months | 7 (13) |
| 6 months–<1 year | 18 (32) |
| 1 year–5 years | 30 (54) |
| >5 years | 1 (2) |
| Gender | |
| Male | 30 (54) |
| Female | 26 (46) |

*Except as specified, values are counts (percentages).

*2.4. Ethics.* The Senate research and publication committee of the Muhimbili University of Health and Allied Sciences reviewed the study protocol and granted ethical approval, including waiver of informed consent.

## 3. Results

According to the patient logs, a total of 5774 children presented to the MNH ED from 1 January 2012 to 31 December 2012. Of these, 5540 (96%) patient files were available for review and data abstraction. A total of 56 patients (1.0%, 95% CI: 0.7–1.3%) met our inclusion criteria of presentation due to complaint associated with recent traditional uvulectomy. Of those included, 30 (53.6%) of the study populations were male, with median age of 1.3 years (interquartile range: 7 months to 2 years), and 55 (98%) were below 5 years of age (Table 1).

The main presenting symptoms were cough in 46 (82%), report of fever prior to presentation in 26 (46%), and hematemesis in 21 (38%). The main physical examination findings documents in the ED charts were fever in 30 (54%), tachypnea in 17 (30%), tachycardia in 14 (25%), and hypoxia in 6 (11%) (Table 2).

The most common final ED diagnoses were pneumonia in 23 (41%), severe anemia, classified according to the World Health Organization definition as a hemoglobin measurement of less than 7 g/dL [17], in 20 (36%), and upper GI bleeding in 20 (36%). Bronchitis was the least common final ED Diagnosis (Table 3).

The most common final hospital discharge diagnoses were pneumonia in 23 patients (44%), upper GI bleeding in 24 patients (46%), Malaria in 22 patients (42%), HIV in 11 patients (21%), and severe anemia and malnutrition in 10 patients (19%). As was seen with the ED diagnoses, bronchitis was the least common hospital discharge diagnosis (Table 4).

Treatment included intravenous antibiotics for 35 patients (63%, 95% CI: 49–75%), blood transfusions for 11

TABLE 2: Clinical findings during EMD presentation.

| Presenting symptoms | $N = 56^*$ |
|---|---|
| Cough | 46 (82) |
| Report of fever prior to presentation | 26 (46) |
| Vomiting blood | 21 (38) |
| Difficulty in breathing | 12 (21) |
| Abdominal distension | 6 (11) |
| Chest pain | 5 (9) |
| Others** | 10 (18) |
| **Physical findings and vital signs** | $N = 56^*$ |
| Temperature > 37.5°C | 30 (54) |
| Tachypnea | 17 (30) |
| Tachycardia | 14 (25) |
| Oxygen saturation < 90% | 6 (11) |
| Bradycardia (<80 beats/min) | 5 (9) |

*Values are counts (percentages).
**Others include black stool, bleeding, convulsions, and oral ulcers.

TABLE 3: Final ED diagnoses.

| Diagnoses | $N = 56^*$ |
|---|---|
| Pneumonia | 23 (41) |
| Upper GI bleeding | 20 (36) |
| Severe anemia | 20 (36) |
| Malaria | 10 (18) |
| HIV | 8 (14) |
| Tuberculosis | 3 (5) |
| Bronchitis | 1 (2) |

*Values are counts (percentages). Some patients had more than one diagnosis listed.

TABLE 4: Final hospital diagnoses.

| Diagnoses | $N = 52^*$ |
|---|---|
| Upper GI bleeding | 24 (46%) |
| Pneumonia | 23 (44%) |
| Malaria | 22 (42%) |
| HIV | 11 (21%) |
| Severe anemia | 10 (19%) |
| Malnutrition | 10 (19%) |
| Septicemia | 3 (6%) |
| Tuberculosis | 3 (6%) |
| Bronchitis | 1 (2%) |

*Values are counts (percentages). 4 patients who died in the ED were excluded. Some patients had more than one diagnosis listed.

(20%, 95% CI: 10–32%), and surgical interventions for 3 (5%, 95% CI: 1–15%); these surgical interventions included suture ligation for hemostasis, packing, and electrical cauterization to achieve hemostasis. Four patients (7%, 95% CI: 2–17%) died in the ED and the rest were admitted to the hospital: 42 (75%) to the general pediatric ward, 7 (13%) to the pediatric intensive care unit, and 3 (5%) to the pediatric surgical service. Eight of the admitted patients died in the hospital for a total mortality of 12 (21%, 95% CI: 12–34%) among the study cohort (Table 5). By comparison, 498 (9%, 95% CI: 8–10%) of the 5484 children with complete data who presented to the ED for reasons not related to complications of uvulectomy died ($p = 0.003$).

TABLE 5: Disposition.

| Disposition | All $(N = 56)^*$ |
|---|---|
| General pediatric ward | 42 (75) |
| Intensive care unit | 7 (13) |
| Pediatric surgery | 3 (5) |
| Died at EMD | 4 (7) |
| **Clinical outcome** | All $(N = 56)^{**}$ |
| Survived to discharge | 44 (79; 66–88) |
| Died (both in the ward and EMD) | 12 (21; 12–34) |

*Values are counts (percentages).
**Values are counts (percentages; 95% confidence intervals).

## 4. Discussion

Our investigation found that 1% of children presenting to the MNH ED in the year 2012 had complaints related to a recent traditional uvulectomy and nearly all were under the age of 5 years. These findings are similar to those seen in other African countries [9, 12], where the procedure is predominantly performed in the early years of life due to the belief that the elongated uvula is responsible for myriad potential maladies, including sleep disturbances, respiratory infections, and even suffocation of children in their sleep [18].

The predominant symptoms at ED presentation in our cohort were cough, difficulty in breathing, fever, and hematemesis. All the children had at least one abnormal physical finding or vital sign at the time of presentation to the emergency medicine department, with more than half of the patients presenting with fever. Other observed abnormalities included tachypnea, tachycardia, and hypoxia. We were not able to establish with certainty that the presenting symptoms of our cohort were due to complications of the procedure or from preexisting medical conditions that prompted the procedure. Regardless, the observed mortality was more than twice that of all other children presenting to the ED during the study period. Previous studies from throughout Africa have shown that cough, throat pain, dysphagia, and loss of appetite are among the most common indications for traditional uvulectomy as stated by the traditional healers [19].

The top final ED diagnoses were pneumonia, upper GI bleeding, and severe anemia. The most common hospital discharge diagnoses were similar but also included malaria. Prior work in similar settings has demonstrated that respiratory infections and malaria remain among the top causes of hospital admission [20–22]. Acknowledging the previously mentioned clinical uncertainty, it is likely that these diagnoses were responsible for the initial presentation to the traditional healers that resulted in the uvulectomy. Though respiratory infections and malaria remain among the top causes of death [23] in children under the age of 5 years, these conditions are imminently treatable and curable with timely and appropriate clinical intervention. Not only is uvulectomy ineffective but also it carries the threat of significant morbidity and mortality while delaying treatment of any significant underlying medical condition.

None of the children in this group were discharged from the emergency department, 63% received intravenous antibiotics, 20% received a blood transfusion, and 5% required immediate surgical intervention for hemorrhage control. Prior studies have reported infections and bleeding as the major complications of uvulectomy, including one in which hemorrhage was present in over 50% of the patients, with the majority requiring surgical intervention to achieve hemostasis [13, 19].

The overall mortality rate of our cohort was high (21%) with one-third of those children dying in the ED and the rest succumbing during their hospital admission. This observed morality among those presenting following a recent uvulectomy was more than double that of all other children presenting to the ED during the study period (21% versus 9%, resp., $p = 0.003$). While our study design cannot prove causation, we believe that the significantly higher mortality rate is likely due, at least in part, to a harmful traditional practice that confers no known benefit to the patient. We believe that emergency care providers should advocate for legal and public health interventions to eliminate this dangerous and unnecessary practice.

## 5. Limitations

The limitations of this study include the retrospective design and the relative paucity of clinical data available from the patients' charts. Due to the nature of the study, we were unable to reliably identify the symptoms that prompted the uvulectomy. Hence, we cannot reliably differentiate between the initial symptoms and the subsequent complications of the procedure. Likewise, we were unable to demonstrate the exact cause of death for the 12 patients who died and are unable to definitively prove whether the uvulectomy contributed to their demise.

## 6. Conclusion

In our cohort of 56 patients, representing nearly 1% of all children presenting to the MNH ED in 2012, traditional uvulectomy was associated with significant morbidity as evidenced by the need for antibiotic therapy, blood transfusions, and surgical intervention. The observed mortality rate of 21% was more than twice that of all other children presenting to the ED during the study period. These findings are alarming given that the procedure confers no clinical benefit. Emergency care providers should advocate for legal and public health interventions to eliminate this dangerous practice.

## Abbreviations

ED: Emergency Department
GI: Gastrointestinal
HIV: Human immunodeficiency virus
MNH: Muhimbili National Hospital
MUHAS: Muhimbili University of Health and Allied Sciences
UK: United Kingdom
USA: United States of America.

## Conflict of Interests

The authors declare that there is no conflict of interests regarding the publication of this paper.

## References

[1] H. Nathan, I. Hershkovitz, B. Arensburg, Y. Kobyliansky, and M. Goldschmidt-Nathan, "Mutilation of the uvula among Bedouins of the South Sinai," *Israel Journal of Medical Sciences*, vol. 18, no. 7, pp. 774–778, 1982.

[2] G. T. A. Ijaduola, "Uvulectomy in Nigeria," *Journal of Laryngology and Otology*, vol. 95, no. 11, pp. 1127–1133, 1981.

[3] B. E. J. Hartley and J. Rowe-Jones, "Uvulectomy to prevent throat infections," *Journal of Laryngology and Otology*, vol. 108, no. 1, pp. 65–66, 1994.

[4] M. J. L. Ravesloot and N. de Vries, "'A good shepherd, but with obstructive sleep apnoea syndrome': traditional uvulectomy case series and literature review," *Journal of Laryngology and Otology*, vol. 125, no. 9, pp. 982–986, 2011.

[5] Y. V. Kamami, "Laser CO2 for snoring. Preliminary results," *Acta Oto-Rhino-Laryngologica Belgica*, vol. 44, no. 4, pp. 451–456, 1990.

[6] Y. P. Krespi, S. J. Pearlman, and A. Keidar, "Laser-assisted uvula-palatoplasty for snoring," *Journal of Otolaryngology*, vol. 23, no. 5, pp. 328–334, 1994.

[7] A. M. Lauretano, R. K. Khosla, G. Richardson et al., "Efficacy of laser-assisted uvulopalatoplasty," *Lasers in Surgery and Medicine*, vol. 21, no. 2, pp. 109–116, 1997.

[8] World Health Organization, *WHO Guidelines for Safe Surgery 2009: Safe Surgery Saves Lives*, World Health Organization, Geneva, Switzerland, 2009, http://www.ncbi.nlm.nih.gov/books/NBK143243/.

[9] E. M. Einterz, R. M. Einterz, and M. E. Bates, "Traditional uvulectomy in northern Cameroon," *The Lancet*, vol. 343, no. 8913, p. 1644, 1994.

[10] J. J. Manni, "Uvulectomy, a traditional surgical procedure in Tanzania," *Annals of Tropical Medicine and Parasitology*, vol. 78, no. 1, pp. 49–53, 1984.

[11] B. L. Ajibade, J. O. Okunlade, and O. A. Kolade, "Harmful cultural practices: parents perceived effects of traditional uvulectomy on the under-five-children in Jigawa State, Nigeria," *Journal of Dental and Medical Sciences*, vol. 9, no. 5, pp. 8–13, 2013.

[12] Save the Children Norway, *Baseline Survey on the Most Prevalent Harmful Traditional Practices (HTPs) and Sanitation Practices in Hamer, Dassenech and Nyangtom Woredas of South Omo Zone of SNNPR, Ethiopia*, North American Aerospace Defense Command (NORAD), 2011.

[13] K. Mboneko and F. Fabian, "Traditional uvulectomy and reported complications in under-five children in Mkuranga district Pwani region, Eastern Tanzania," *Tanzania Dental Journal*, vol. 12, no. 2, pp. 65–69, 2006.

[14] F. Taylor, "The practice of uvulectomy and related complications among children aged below 6 years in Ilemela district, Mwanza, Tanzania," *Tanzania Dental Journal*, vol. 15, no. 1, 2009.

[15] M. C. Gessler, D. E. Msuya, M. H. H. Nkunya, A. Schär, M. Heinrich, and M. Tanner, "Traditional healers in Tanzania:

sociocultural profile and three short portraits," *Journal of Ethnopharmacology*, vol. 48, no. 3, pp. 145–160, 1995.

[16] T. Reynolds, H. Sawe, N. Lobue, and V. Mwafongo, "107 most frequent adult and pediatric diagnoses among 60,000 patients seen in a new urban emergency department in Dar Es Salaam, Tanzania," *Annals of Emergency Medicine*, vol. 60, supplement, no. 4, p. S39, 2012.

[17] WHO, *Haemoglobin Concentrations for the Diagnosis of Anaemia and Assessment of Severity*, WHO, 2011, http://www.who.int/vmnis/indicators/haemoglobin/en/.

[18] A. Prual, Y. Gamatie, M. Djakounda, and D. Huguet, "Traditional uvulectomy in Niger: a public health problem?" *Social Science and Medicine*, vol. 39, no. 8, pp. 1077–1082, 1994.

[19] A. A. Adoga and T. L. Nimkur, "The traditionally amputated uvula amongst nigerians: still an ongoing practice," *ISRN Otolaryngology*, vol. 2011, Article ID 704924, 4 pages, 2011.

[20] J. D. Campbell, S. O. Sow, M. M. Levine, and K. L. Kotloff, "The causes of hospital admission and death among children in Bamako, Mali," *Journal of Tropical Pediatrics*, vol. 50, no. 3, pp. 158–163, 2004.

[21] I. Menge, F. Esamai, D. van Reken, and G. Anabwani, "Paediatric morbidity and mortality at the Eldoret District Hospital, Kenya," *East African Medical Journal*, vol. 72, no. 3, pp. 165–169, 1995.

[22] P. L. C. Petit and J. K. van Ginneken, "Analysis of hospital records in four African countries, 1975–1990, with emphasis on infectious diseases," *The Journal of Tropical Medicine and Hygiene*, vol. 98, no. 4, pp. 217–227, 1995.

[23] WHO, *The Global Burden Of Disease*, 2008.

# 2

# Basic Life Support: A Questionnaire Survey to Assess Proficiency of Radiologists and Radiology Residents in Managing Adult Life Support in Cardiopulmonary Arrest and Acute Anaphylactic Reaction

**Tariq Alam,[1] Yasir Jamil Khattak,[1] Muhammad Anwar,[1] and Asif Alam Khan[2]**

[1] *The Aga Khan University Hospital, Pakistan*
[2] *Khyber Medical College Peshawar, Pakistan*

Correspondence should be addressed to Muhammad Anwar; masaeed@excite.com

Academic Editor: Chee-Fah Chong

The aim of this paper is to assess proficiency of radiologists and radiology residents in managing adult life support in cardiopulmonary arrest and acute anaphylactic reaction.

## 1. Introduction

In the current modern era due to extensive advances in supportive care, radiology departments frequently receive critically ill patients for different procedures.

Despite supportive care for stabilization before radiologic procedures, such patients still have chances of cardiopulmonary arrests [1]. Cardiopulmonary resuscitation (CPR) in such patients is an important link in the Chain of Survival and can get life-saving time between early access to emergency care and early defibrillation.

Quick initiation of CPR, as well as high quality CPR, is crucial to survival.

Delay in commencing effective life support can result in a very poor outcome for the individual, with the highest chance of survival being, if CPR is commenced by well trained staff within 2 minutes of an arrest [2].

Though being a real important issue, there is still too less attention within the curriculum of training programs of both radiologists and radiology residents for teaching basic life support skills in an attractive way. Therefore they are not confident enough in such situations to initiate a CPR as they have not received enough satisfactory training relevant to applying CPR.

In order to assess this serious issue we conducted a questionnaire survey in Pakistan to assess ability of radiologists and radiology residents in managing adult life support in cardiopulmonary arrest and acute anaphylaxis reaction.

## 2. Material and Methods

This was a multicentre questionnaire survey used to assess knowledge of radiologists and radiology residents in managing adult cardiorespiratory arrest.

List of radiology residents was taken from the College of Physician and Surgeon, Pakistan.

124 radiologists and residents from 6 postgraduate teaching hospitals in 4 major cities of Pakistan participated and were included in the study.

A pilot study at our department was conducted to assess recent training and knowledge of adult basic life support. A questionnaire was designed for assessment of clarity and completeness in the participants. The final questionnaire was finalized without any change.

The questionnaires along with a covering letter explaining the purpose of study were sent to selected radiology residents by postal service in the respective.

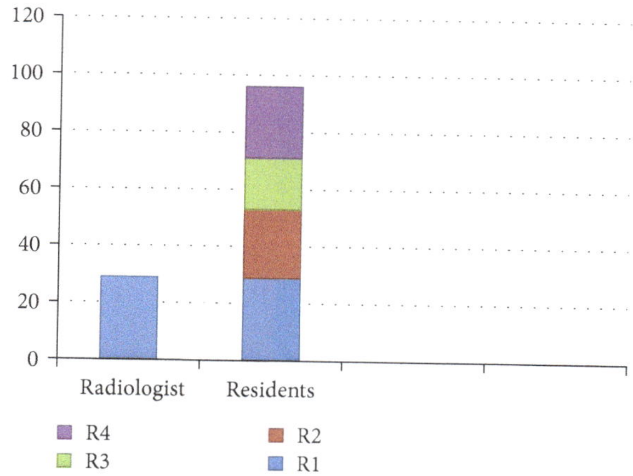


FIGURE 1

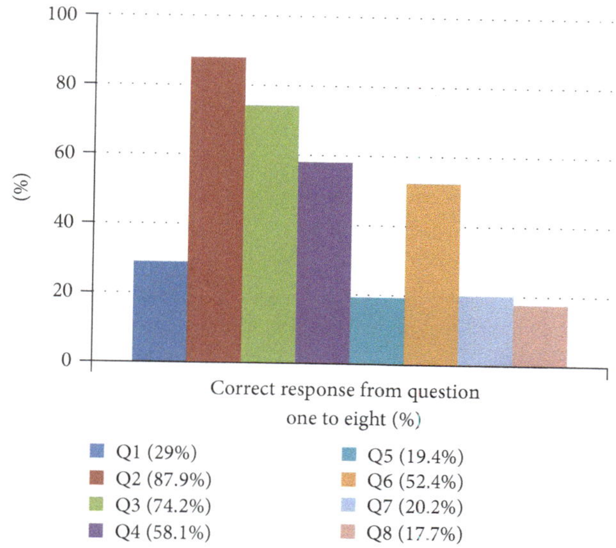


FIGURE 2

The questionnaire included demographic details and following questions are related to recent training and knowledge regarding adult basic life support:

(1) the most appropriate rate of CPR for an adult (chest compressions: breaths);

(2) check for pulse timing;

(3) maneuver that can be used to open the air way;

(4) the next appropriate step, if no pulse is present;

(5) the next appropriate step, if pulse is present;

(6) knowledge of signs/symptoms of an adverse reaction to contrast;

(7) confidence in initiating BLS;

(8) assistance by staff members (radiographers, assistants, etc.) in BLS.

The radiology residents were asked to fill the questionnaire from the residents at the same time during morning or evening sessions.

The questions regarding recent training and knowledge of adult basic life support have multiple responses. The participants were asked to encircle the appropriate response.

The respondents were given an explanation that their involvement was voluntary and confidentiality would be maintained.

## 3. Results

Of the 124 participants 29 were consultants and 95 were residents from year 1 to 4 (Figure 1). Nearly 44.85 percent of them answered correctly regarding basic life support. The correct responses for question one to eight were 29.0, 87.9, 74.2, 58.1, 19.4, 52.4, 20.2, and 17.7 percent, respectively. Only 29 percent of the respondents correctly told the most appropriate rate of CPR for an adult (chest compressions: breaths). Over 88 percent knew that pulse should be checked for no more than 10 seconds. About two-thirds (74 percent) told the correct maneuver that can be used to open the air way.

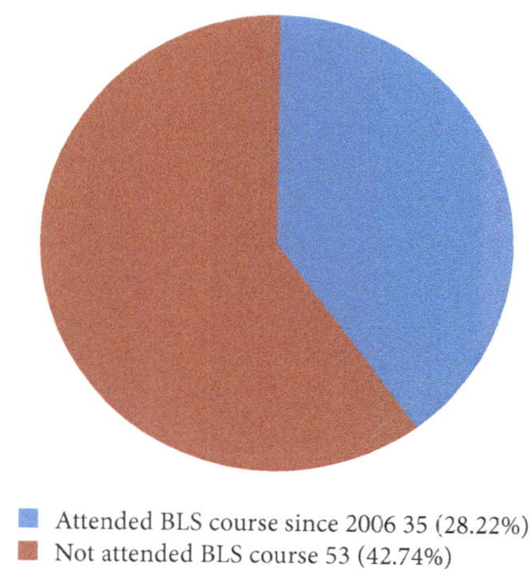


FIGURE 3

The majority (58 percent) knew the next appropriate step to be taken if no pulse is present.

The response for the next appropriate step if pulse is present was very poor (19.4 percent).

More than half knew the signs/symptoms of an adverse reaction to contrast.

The alarming point was that only 20.2 percent were confident to initiate BLS.

More astonishing was that only 17.7 percent felt that staff members around them (radiographers, assistants, etc.) would be able to assist in BLS (Figure 2).

Overall average score was calculated as 3.41 and 3.64 for consultants and residents, respectively.

Only 35 (28.22%) responders had attended life support course since 2006 whereas 53 (42.74%) responders did not attend the course at all (Figure 3). Of them 15.1% were radiologists and 84.9% residents. Those who attended life support course more recently were more likely to respond correctly.

## 4. Discussion

Despite the fact that CPR is an important link in the Chain of Survival and can buy life-saving time between early access to emergency care and early defibrillation, our study shows that most of the radiology residents and radiologists lack knowledge of the basics of adult basic life support.

Due to extensive advances, the radiology department receives critically ill patients for different procedures. The increase in number of patients cardiac arrest at radiology department is likely to increase. Therefore it needs of time to enhance capabilities of the radiology radiologists to perform effective CPR.

Our study showed that only 35 (28.2%) responders had attended basic life support course since 2006. While 53 (42.7%) responders have not attended course at all, of them 15.1% were radiologists and 84.9% residents. Health care professionals should take notice of this alarming factor.

The main reason for the inability and underconfidence is to initiate BLS by the radiology residents and radiologist is inadequate training. It is obvious that who has attended the BLS course performed well in comparison to those who did not attend the course.

Similarly, those who attended the BLS course recently performed well in comparison to those who attended the course quite some time back. In this regards our results are comparable to Tapping and Culverwell [3].

A great percentage of the respondents did not answer correctly to the question on the last guidelines of the American Heart Association Basic Life Support, 2010 that were relevant to the appropriate ratio of thoracic compressions to ventilations.

A significant factor which reinforces radiology residents and radiologists attitude to initiate CPR and perform correctly is the working experience and attitude. Most of the time they do not come across cardiopulmonary arrest situation which requires CPR; therefore, they feel less confident to initiate or perform it. As evident from the alarming results of our study there is still too less attention within the curriculum at medical universities for teaching life support skills in an attractive way.

A better way to change this attitude and increase the confidence of radiology residents and radiologist in initiating and performing CPR is systematic CPR training programs at regular intervals and incorporating them in curriculum.

Retention of knowledge and skills during and after training in CPR is difficult and requires a more systematic training as well as methods that will ensure better retention of skills and information [4].

In a study conducted by Oh and Han 47 professional nurses were tested on their skill of CPR 3 times at an interval of 4 months. From the results, it was confirmed that re-education clearly affects nurse's knowledge and skills by maintaining their knowledge and enhancing their skills [5].

Repeating training helps staff retain knowledge in CPR [6, 7].

## 5. Conclusion

Radiology consultants and residents in Pakistan do not meet objectives of basic life support and are unable to manage adult cardio respiratory arrest scenario. BLS training programs and refresher courses should be mandatory during residency in order to acquire required competency level for BLS.

## Appendix

### Basic Life Support: A Questionnaire Survey of Radiologists and Radiology Residents in Pakistan

*Questionnaire*

Please encircle one response.

Level: consultant [].

Resident: R1, R2, R3, R4.

Last basic life support course attended: 2001–2003, 2004–2006, 2007-2008, 2009–2011.

(1) The most appropriate rate of CPR for an adult (chest compressions : breaths):

(A) 5 : 2, (B) 10 : 2, (C) 15 : 2, (D) 30 : 2.

(2) Check for pulse for no more than

(A) 10 seconds, (B) 5 seconds, (C) 15 seconds.

(3) Which maneuver can be used to open the air way?

(A) sweep finger in mouth, (B) head tilt-chin lift, (C) chin tilt-head lift.

(4) If no pulse is present, the next appropriate step is to

(A) begin chest compressions, (B) ask for help, (C) administer 2 breaths.

(5) If pulse is present, the next appropriate step is to

(A) administer rescue breaths, (B) begin compressions, (C) no intervention required.

(6) Do you know the signs/symptoms of an adverse reaction to contrast?

(A) yes, (B) no.

(7) Would you feel confident initiating BLS?

(A) yes, (B) no, (C) do not know.

(8) Do you feel that staff members around you (radiographers, assistants, etc.) would be able to assist you in BLS?

(A) yes, (B) no, (C) do not know.

## Conflict of Interests

The authors declare that there is no conflict of interests regarding the publication of this paper.

## References

[1] W. W. Hope, K. Von Der Embse, G. Mostafa et al., "Cardiopulmonary arrest occurring in the radiology department: patient characteristics, incidence, and outcomes," *American Surgeon*, vol. 77, no. 3, pp. 273–276, 2011.

[2] Z.-J. Zheng, J. B. Croft, W. H. Giles, and G. A. Mensah, "Sudden cardiac death in the United States, 1989 to 1998," *Circulation*, vol. 104, no. 18, pp. 2158–2163, 2001.

[3] C. R. Tapping and A. D. Culverwell, "Are radiologists able to manage serious anaphylactic reactions and cardiopulmonary arrest?" *British Journal of Radiology*, vol. 82, no. 982, pp. 793–799, 2009.

[4] R. Hamilton, "Nurses' knowledge and skill retention following cardiopulmonary resuscitation training: a review of the literature," *Journal of Advanced Nursing*, vol. 51, no. 3, pp. 288–297, 2005.

[5] S.-I. Oh and S.-S. Han, "A study on the sustainable effects of reeducation on cardiopulmonary resuscitation on nurses' knowledge and skills," *Journal of Korean Academy of Nursing*, vol. 38, no. 3, pp. 383–392, 2008.

[6] H. J. J. M. Berden, F. F. Willems, J. M. A. Hendrick, N. H. J. Pijls, and J. T. A. Knape, "How frequently should basic cardiopulmonary resuscitation training be repeated to maintain adequate skills?" *British Medical Journal*, vol. 306, no. 6892, pp. 1576–1577, 1993.

[7] H. Kuhnigk, P. Sefrin, and T. Paulus, "Skills and self-assessment in cardio-pulmonary resuscitation of the hospital nursing staff," *European Journal of Emergency Medicine*, vol. 1, no. 4, pp. 193–198, 1994.

# 3

# Indications of Brain Computed Tomography Scan in Children Younger Than 3 Years of Age with Minor Head Trauma

**İsmail Gülşen,[1] Hakan Ak,[2] Sevdegül Karadaş,[3] İsmail Demır,[4] Mehmet Deniz Bulut,[5] and Soner Yaycioğlu[6]**

[1] *Yüzüncü Yıl University, School of Medicine, Department of Neurosurgery, Van, Turkey*
[2] *Bozok University, School of Medicine, Department of Neurosurgery, Yozgat, Turkey*
[3] *Yüzüncü Yıl University, School of Medicine, Department of Emergency Medicine, Van, Turkey*
[4] *Van Regional Training and Teaching Hospital, Clinic of Neurosurgery, Van, Turkey*
[5] *Yüzüncü Yıl University, School of Medicine, Department of Radiology, Van, Turkey*
[6] *Adnan Menderes University, School of Medicine, Department of Neurosurgery, Aydın, Turkey*

Correspondence should be addressed to Hakan Ak; nrsdrhakanak@yahoo.com

Academic Editor: Christian Wrede

*Objective*. To investigate the indications to receive brain computed tomography (CT) scan and to define the pathological findings in children younger than three years of age with minor head trauma in emergency departments. *Methods*. In this study, hospital case notes of 1350 children attending the emergency department of Bitlis State Hospital between January 2011 and June 2013 were retrospectively reviewed. 508 children under 3 years of age with minor head trauma were included in this study. We also asked 37 physicians about the indications for requiring CT in these children. *Results*. This study included 508 children, 233 (45,9%) of whom were female and 275 were male. In 476 (93,7%) children, the brain CT was completely normal. 89,2% of physicians asked in the emergency department during that time interval reported that they requested CT scan to protect themselves against malpractice litigation. *Conclusion*. In infants and children with minor head trauma, most CT scans were unnecessary and the fear of malpractice litigation of physicians was the most common reason for requesting a CT.

## 1. Introduction

Head trauma is the leading cause of mortality and morbidity in children [1]. Minor head trauma (MHT) constitutes a significant proportion of head injuries in children, about 90% [1, 2]. The prevalence, morbidity, and costs related to it make it an important health problem [2]. However, the incidence of intracranial pathology in MHT is about 3–5% [1]. As a general rule, in pediatric trauma patients with a Glasgow Coma Scale (GCS) less than 13, focal neurological deficits, and deteriorating consciousness should receive CT scan. However, for children with milder head injury, there is no clear consensus about requesting CT [3].

Most of the children with minor head trauma attend the emergency department nonsymptomatically or with minimal symptoms. Neurological examination is difficult in children, especially in newborns, infants (between one month and 12 months), and those under 3 years of age. Also, concern of the parents for their children and fear of malpractice litigation may force the physicians to request radiological imaging, especially the CT. The rate of requesting CT scans in children with MHT is between 5 and 50% [1]. The literature does not have sufficient data about the need for CT in this age group attending with MHT.

In this present study, we retrospectively evaluated CT findings in infants and in children under 3 years of age with MHT and the indications for their request.

## 2. Methods

In this study, hospital case notes of 1350 children attending the emergency department of Bitlis State Hospital between January 2011 and June 2013 were retrospectively reviewed. 508

Table 1: Physician groups and their reasons for requesting CT scan.

| Group | Malpractice litigation | Request of the family | Not knowing indications | Not wanting to follow up |
|---|---|---|---|---|
| G1 ($n = 2$) | – | – | – | – |
| G2 ($n = 2$) | – | – | – | – |
| G3 ($n = 9$) | + | + | – | + (6 of them) |
| G4 ($n = 12$) | + | – | + | + (4 of them) |
| G5 ($n = 12$) | + | + | + | + (4 of them) |

children younger than 3 years of age with MHT (Modified GCS 14 or GCS 15) were included in the study. Patients with insufficient data or those considered as child abuse were excluded. Information about age, gender, type of trauma, physical and neurological examination findings, CT result, and last status (discharge, hospitalization, or referral) was obtained from patients' hospital case notes.

37 physicians who worked during this time were asked about their reasons for requesting the CT scan. These roughly divided into four groups: protecting themselves against malpractice litigation, request of the family, not knowing indications for requesting the scan, and not wanting to follow up the patient in the emergency room.

## 3. Statistical Analysis

The statistical analyses were performed using software (SPSS 18.0). Parametric values were given as mean ± standard deviation, and nonparametric values were given as a percentage. To compare parametric continuous variables, student's $t$-test or analysis of variance was used; to compare nonparametric continuous variables, the Mann-Whitney $U$ test or the Kruskal-Wallis test was used. Categorical data were compared by Chi-square distribution. Two-tailed $P$ values of less than 0.05 were considered to indicate statistical significance.

## 4. Results

508 children younger than 3 years of age with minor head trauma were included in the study. 233 (45,9%) of them were female and 275 (54,1%) were male. 157 of them (30,9%) were younger than one year of age. 216 (42,5%) and 135 (26,6%) of them were between one and two years of age and two and three years of age, respectively. 89,5% of them were totally asymptomatic. In others presenting symptoms were vomiting in 38 (7,5%) and loss of consciousness for less than 5 seconds in 23 (4,5%) children. In 8 children, the presenting symptom was both vomiting and loss of consciousness.

Physical examination was totally normal except 40 (7,9%) cases. Brain CT scan revealed no pathological findings, cephalohematoma, linear fracture, cerebral contusion, epidural hematoma, and subdural hematoma in 476 (93,7%), 3 (0,6%), 18 (3,6%), 5 (1%), 2 (0,4%), and 4 (0,8%) of children, respectively. None of these children with pathological CT findings required operation. 476 (93,7%) of them had been discharged about 3 hours after trauma. The 18 children with linear fracture had been followed in the emergency service for about 24 hours. 14 children with cerebral contusion, epidural hematoma, and subdural hematomas were hospitalized for clinical followup for about 48 hours in the neurosurgery clinic.

There was a statistically significant relationship between vomiting and pathological physical examination findings ($P$ = 0,001; $R$ = 0,945). A similar relationship between loss of consciousness and pathological physical examination findings was detected ($P$ = 0,001; $R$ = 0,253).

There were significant correlations between vomiting and pathological CT findings ($P$ = 0,001; $R$ = 0,542), loss of consciousness and pathological CT findings ($P$ = 0,001; $R$ = 0,450), and pathological physical examination findings and pathological CT findings ($P$ = 0,001; $R$ = 0,556).

The physicians and reasons of requesting CT divided into groups. Physicians divided into five groups. These are neurosurgeons (group 1, $n$ = 2), specialists in emergency medicine (group 2, $n$ = 2), specialists in internal sciences (group 3, $n$ = 9), specialists in surgical sciences (group 4, $n$ = 12), and general practitioners (group 5, $n$ = 12). Answers were grouped as protecting themselves against malpractice litigation, request of the family, not knowing indications of requesting CT scan, and not wanting to follow up the patient in the emergency room. 33 (89,2%) physicians (groups 3, 4, and 5) stated that they requested CT to protect themselves against malpractice litigation. 21 (56,8%) (groups 3 and 5) physicians stated their indication as the request of the family. 24 (64,9%) (groups 4 and 5) physicians answered this question as not wanting to follow up the child in the emergency room. 14 (37,8%) physicians (6 physicians in group 3, 4 physicians in group 4, and 4 physicians in group 5) stated their answers as not being sure about indications of CT scanning in head trauma (Table 1).

Physicians in group 1 requested 20 CTs and there was a pathological CT finding on all of them. Physicians in group 2 requested 33 CTs and there was a pathological CT finding on 12 of them. Physicians requested 170, 100, and 185 CT scans in groups 3, 4, and 5, respectively.

## 5. Discussion

Head injury is common in pediatric population [1, 4]. In the presence of signs and symptoms of severe head injury like decreased GCS score, focal deficit/s, and deteriorating consciousness, the diagnosis of this pathology is relatively easy [1]. However, in MHT, which constitutes about 90% of childhood head trauma, the management of these patients is not so easy and there are some controversial points especially in appropriate diagnostic assessment [2, 3, 5]. Despite its very high prevalence, only 3–5% of children with MHT have traumatic brain injury and only less than 1% of them need emergent neurosurgical intervention [6]. Previous reports from different countries about pediatric minor head trauma indicated various results in clinical practice and examination of hospitalization rates [5].

Although in adult patients with MHT clinical decision rules for requesting CT have been well documented, performing a similar decision rule in children with MHT has two important difficulties [7, 8]. The first is difficulty in developing an appropriate data set, with adequate representation of all age groups and an adequate number of cases of traumatic brain injury. The second one is defining clinical variables that accurately predict traumatic brain injury in childhood [8].

Many of the previous studies about pediatric MHT in the literature have been retrospective from a single institution and have included a small number of patients. Also, these studies have included a limited number of infants and very young children [8]. Definite indications for CT scanning after a head trauma are a deteriorating clinical course, focal neurologic deficit, abnormal mental status, evidence of a skull fracture, and the presence of coagulopathy. Also, until additional evidence is available, loss of consciousness and persistent vomiting (more than 3) should be taken into consideration [9]. In a meta-analysis of 16 studies including 22420 children with MHT, Dunning et al. reported that the presence of skull fracture, focal neurologic signs, loss of consciousness, and GCS less than 15 was statistically associated with traumatic brain injury, whereas headache and vomiting were not. They also stated that the presence of seizures showed a trend toward an association with traumatic brain injury, but not a statistically significant association [10]. In a case control study, da Dalt et al. reported a similar conclusion that vomiting after an MHT was significantly related to personal or familial predisposition to vomit rather than to the presence of intracranial lesions [11]. However, in our study we observed strong relationship between vomiting and loss of consciousness and pathological CT findings.

There are two main problems concerning CT scans in children: most importantly the exposure to radiation and secondarily the cost. As we know, children, especially younger than 2 years of age, are considerably more sensitive to radiation than adults due to rapidly dividing cells associated with growth [12, 13]. Since children have longer life expectancies, they have more opportunity to express radiation damage, particularly cancer [12]. Additionally, we learned that a single head CT exposes children to 200–600 times as much radiation as typical posteroanterior and lateral chest radiographs [14].

According to the results of the present study, CT scans were requested unnecessarily in 93,7% of our patients. In fact, the aim of our study was to highlight this subject. For this purpose, we asked 37 physicians about the indications for requiring CT scans in these children to investigate the possible causes of high scanning rates. Our results clearly showed that the fear of malpractice litigation is the most important factor. Studdert et al. reported a similar conclusion in their study [15]. It was reported that, only in 2010, 9497 medical practice claims were filed in the United States and totally $3,177,305,000 were paid for these claims (average $334,559) [16]. Average payment constitutes about 5–10 times of the annual income of a physician in Turkey. The second most important factor is the request of the family. In our opinion, the request of the family should not have any effect in our daily practice; however, again the fear of malpractice litigation secondarily changes our practice. 14 physicians (37,8%) in our study stated that they were not sure about definite indications for brain CT in these children. Our results also indicate that neurosurgeons and specialists in emergency medicine had a high rate of detecting a pathological finding on CT. However, these physicians might miss some cases with pathological findings.

## 6. Conclusions

There is a need for further prospective, multicentered studies with a large number of patients to make decision rules especially for children in this age group.

The fear of malpractice litigation should be reduced by various measures which will protect physicians such as robust departmental guidelines.

In emergency departments, the number of specialists or qualified and certificated staff should be increased. Other physicians working in the emergency services should be trained intermittently in these issues.

*Limitations.* There are two main limitations in our study. These are the retrospective nature of the study and the fact that it is single centered.

## Disclosure

This paper has not been published anywhere before and is not under consideration by another journal. The final version of the paper was read by all of the authors.

## Conflict of Interests

The authors declare that there is no conflict of interests regarding the publication of this paper.

## References

[1] K. S. Quayle, D. M. Jaffe, N. Kuppermann et al., "Diagnostic testing for acute head injury in children: when are head computed tomography and skull radiographs indicated?" *Pediatrics*, vol. 99, no. 5, article e11, 1997.

[2] E. A. Savitsky and S. R. Votey, "Current controversies in the management of minor pediatric head injuries," *The American Journal of Emergency Medicine*, vol. 18, no. 1, pp. 96–101, 2000.

[3] B. Simon, P. Letourneau, E. Vitorino, and J. McCall, "Pediatric minor head trauma: indications for computed tomographic scanning revisited," *Journal of Trauma*, vol. 51, no. 2, pp. 231–238, 2001.

[4] S. A. Schutzman and D. S. Greenes, "Pediatric minor head trauma," *Annals of Emergency Medicine*, vol. 37, no. 1, pp. 65–74, 2001.

[5] C. J. Homer and L. Kleinman, “Technical report: minor head injury in children,” *Pediatrics*, vol. 104, no. 6, article e78, 1999.

[6] M. Özsaraç, Ö. Karçıoğlu, H. Topaçoğlu et al., “Clinical indicators of traumatic brain injury and skull fracture in pediatric head trauma patients,” *Turkish Journal of Emergency Medicine*, vol. 9, no. 4, pp. 153–158, 2009.

[7] M. J. Haydel, C. A. Preston, T. J. Mills, S. Luber, E. Blaudeau, and P. M. C. DeBlieux, “Indications for computed tomography in patients with minor head injury,” *The New England Journal of Medicine*, vol. 343, no. 2, pp. 100–105, 2000.

[8] D. S. Greenes, “Decision making in pediatric minor head trauma,” *Annals of Emergency Medicine*, vol. 42, no. 4, pp. 515–518, 2003.

[9] K. E. Gordon, “Pediatric minor traumatic brain injury,” *Seminars in Pediatric Neurology*, vol. 13, no. 4, pp. 243–255, 2006.

[10] J. Dunning, J. Batchelor, P. Stratford-Smith et al., “A meta-analysis of variables that predict significant intracranial injury in minor head trauma,” *Archives of Disease in Childhood*, vol. 89, no. 7, pp. 653–659, 2004.

[11] L. da Dalt, B. Andreola, P. Facchin, M. Gregolin, A. Vianello, and P. A. Battistella, “Characteristics of children with vomiting after minor head trauma: a case-control study,” *The Journal of Pediatrics*, vol. 150, no. 3, pp. 274–278, 2007.

[12] D. Schnadower, H. Vazquez, J. Lee, P. Dayan, and C. G. Roskind, “Controversies in the evaluation and management of minor blunt head trauma in children,” *Current Opinion in Pediatrics*, vol. 19, no. 3, pp. 258–264, 2007.

[13] N. Kuppermann, J. F. Holmes, P. S. Dayan et al., “Identification of children at very low risk of clinically-important brain injuries after head trauma: a prospective cohort study,” *The Lancet*, vol. 374, no. 9696, pp. 1160–1170, 2009.

[14] National Cancer Institute, *Radiation Risks and Pediatric Computed Tomography (CT): A Guide for Healthcare Providers*, National Cancer Institute, Bethesda, Md, USA, 2002.

[15] D. M. Studdert, M. M. Mello, W. M. Sage et al., “Defensive medicine among high-risk specialist physicians in a volatile malpractice environment,” *The Journal of the American Medical Association*, vol. 293, no. 21, pp. 2609–2617, 2005.

[16] D. A. Drukteinis, K. O’Keefe, T. Sanson, and D. Orban, “Preparing emergency physicians for malpractice litigation: a joint emergency medicine residency-law school mock trial competition,” *The Journal of Emergency Medicine*, vol. 46, no. 1, pp. 95–103, 2014.

# 4

# If Hunters End Up in the Emergency Room: A Retrospective Analysis of Hunting Injuries in a Swiss Emergency Department

**Valentina Bestetti, Emma E. Fisher, David S. Srivastava, Meret E. Ricklin, and Aristomenis K. Exadaktylos**

*Department of Emergency Medicine, University Hospital and University of Bern, Freiburgstrasse 16c, 3010 Bern, Switzerland*

Correspondence should be addressed to Meret E. Ricklin; meret.ricklin@insel.ch

Academic Editor: Robert W. Derlet

*Aim.* to characterize the mechanisms, patterns, and outcomes of nonfatal hunting-related injuries in patients presenting to Bern University Hospital, Switzerland, and compare these to reports of hunting injuries worldwide. *Methods.* patients presenting with hunting-related injuries to the Emergency Department at Bern University hospital from 2000 to 2014 were identified by retrospectively searching the department database using the keyword "hunt." Each case was analyzed in terms of the patient age and gender, the mechanism and pattern of injury, and management and patient follow-up. *Results.* 19 patients were identified. 16 were male with a mean age of 50 years (range: 16–74). Mechanisms of injury included firearm-related injuries, falls, and knife wounds. The most common patterns of injury were head injuries (7), followed by injuries to the upper (5) or lower limb (5) and trunk (2). Over half of the patients were admitted, and nine required emergency surgery. *Conclusion.* Nonfatal hunting accidents in Bern, Switzerland, are largely caused by firearms and falls and tend to occur in male hunters with a mean age of 50 years. The most common patterns of injury are orthopedic and head injuries, often requiring surgery. These findings are consistent with international studies of nonfatal hunting accidents.

## 1. Introduction

Hunting is a popular hobby in Switzerland, involving about 30,000 people each year [1]. Hunting injuries, especially those that have fatal consequences, attract a great deal of media attention. However, the literature on hunting injuries, particularly those that are nonfatal, is disappointingly scarce. This is most likely due to underreporting of nonfatal hunting accidents and a lack of national databases for recording these incidents in regions where hunting is popular, including Switzerland, Scandinavia, and Germany. In Switzerland, it is only compulsory to report fatal hunting accidents to the Advisory Centre for Accident Prevention. In contrast, the National Electronic Injury Surveillance System (NEISS) and the International Hunter Education Association (IHEA) in the USA collect data about both fatal and nonfatal hunting accidents across the country. The USA has therefore provided much of the existing data on the causes, mechanisms, and outcomes of nonfatal hunting accidents as well as the characteristics of the hunters involved.

Hunting is an even more popular recreational activity in the USA than in Switzerland; in 2014 over 16 million Americans obtained a hunter's license, which equates to about 5% of the total population [2]. According to the NEISS, which collects data from one hundred emergency departments across the USA, over 7,000 Americans were involved in hunting accidents due to firearms or tree-stand falls in 2013 [3]. Most of these accidents were nonfatal. However, the IHEA, who also have a key role in gathering data about hunting-related incidents, estimates that 10% of the 1000 hunting-related firearm injuries recorded annually in USA are fatal [4].

In terms of hunter demographics, studies of hunting-related accidents from Denmark, Germany, and the USA have discovered that those involved tend to be males with hunting experience and with a mean age of 40–50 years old [5–8]. Younger hunters appear to be involved in fewer accidents, despite evidence that they engage in more risky hunting behaviors, such as use of camouflage [5, 9]. There is also evidence from studies of Danish and Swedish hunters that people involved in accidents tend to be those that hunt most frequently [5, 9].

Regarding hunting accidents themselves, most occur during the hunt rather than at home or in the car before or after the hunt [6, 9]. The majority are caused by firearms or falls from hides [10]. Much of the literature to date has focused on hunting accidents caused by the former. The firearm injury surveillance study found that there were 1.8 million presentations of firearm-related injuries across emergency departments in the USA from 1993 to 2008 and just under 2% of these were caused by hunting accidents [11]. Reasons for firearm-related hunting accidents include not seeing the victim, not using the weapon appropriately, swinging the weapon whilst shooting, and, less commonly, mistaking the victim for game [5, 6].

Research has shown that the pattern of injury depends on the mechanism of the hunting accident. A study of deer hunting-related injuries in Wisconsin found that injuries from firearms were evenly split between orthopedics and general surgery, whilst 90% of tree-stand related injuries were orthopedic in nature [7]. Common orthopedic injuries due to falls from tree stands include spinal, pelvis, and extremity fractures [10]. Tree-stand falls also carry a substantial risk of high impact head injury and neurological deficit [12].

With respect to the prevention of hunting accidents, a study of the behavior and attitudes of Swedish hunters found that most believe safer weapon handling and better hunt planning can prevent hunting accidents [9]. In accordance with these findings, efforts to minimize hunting-related accidents in most countries have focused on increasing the visibility of hunters by encouraging them to don "hunters' orange" and educating hunters in gun safety [10]. However, hunting injuries appear to be on the increase in the USA despite these measures, and recently attention has turned to the safety issues surrounding the use of tree stands for large game hunting [10, 12].

The aim of this study is to analyze the causes, patterns, and management and outcomes of nonfatal hunting-related injuries in a series of patients presenting to Bern University hospital, Switzerland, and to compare these to reports of hunting injuries worldwide. To our knowledge, this is the first time that data on nonfatal hunting accidents in Switzerland has been analyzed in this way.

## 2. Materials and Methods

The Emergency Department of Bern University Hospital provides emergency care for a population of 1.8 million inhabitants and treats more than 35,000 adults each year.

Our study covers an observational period of 14 years, from November 2000 to November 2014, and includes adult patients treated in the Emergency Department of Bern University Hospital for hunting-related injuries.

Table 1: Mechanisms of injury.

| Mechanism of injury | Number | Percentage |
|---|---|---|
| Firearm projectile | 4 | 21 |
| Firearm backfiring | 3 | 16 |
| Knife | 4 | 21 |
| Fall | 6 | 32 |
| Other | 2 | 10 |

The emergency department database, starting in 2000, of health-related patient data allows authorized healthcare professionals to access clinical reports, radiographs, laboratory results, and other relevant medical documents. During the observational period, two database systems were implemented: Qualicare (Qualidoc AG, Trimbach, Switzerland) was used from November 2000 to July 2012 and E.Care (E.care bvba, Turnhout, Belgium) from July 2012 to November 2014.

The database search was performed by the emergency department's database manager using the keyword "hunt." The search also included possible misspellings of this word to optimise the search results.

The data were then reviewed by the first author to check the relevance of the search results to the study. Cases that were judged relevant by the first author were classified by gender, age, mechanism and pattern of injury, management, and the need for follow-up at one month and one year.

## 3. Results

*3.1. Hunter Demographics.* From 2000 to 2014, 19 patients presented to Bern University Emergency Department with hunting-related injuries. 16 of these patients were male and the mean age was 50 years (range: 16–74 years).

*3.2. Mechanisms of Injury.* Most injuries ($n = 18$; 95%) were self-inflicted; only one person in this study was shot by a third party. Four patients were admitted with injuries from firearm projectiles and three with injuries from firearms backfiring. Four patients sustained penetrating knife wounds and six patients were admitted with injuries related to falls whilst hunting, be this from an elevated hunting stand or walking in the wilderness. One patient was admitted with sciatica and another with footwear-related pressure sores. See Table 1.

*3.3. Patterns of Injury.* The patterns of hunting-related injuries were also analysed. Seven patients suffered head injuries, five sustained injuries to the upper limb, and another five patients injured the lower limb. Two patients sustained injuries to the trunk. See Table 2.

*3.4. Management of Hunting-Related Injuries.* Over half of the patients ($n = 11$) with hunting-related injuries were admitted and the remaining eight were treated in the emergency department and discharged without any further complications. Eight of the eleven inpatients required emergency surgery: four required emergency orthopaedic surgeries for

Table 2: Patterns of injury.

| Location | Number | Percentage |
|---|---|---|
| Head | 7 | 37 |
| Upper extremity | 5 | 26 |
| Lower extremity | 5 | 26 |
| Trunk | 2 | 11 |

soft tissue injuries or in one case, subluxation of the hip; three required urgent hand surgery for soft tissue injuries and one patient underwent neurosurgery for a subdural haematoma. The three remaining patients that were admitted did not require surgery and were managed conservatively by various specialties (cardiology, rheumatology, and ENT).

*3.5. Follow-Up.* Five of the patients that were admitted were discharged with no further follow-up and did not return to hospital within the first year following their accident. Three of the inpatients were discharged with outpatient follow-up scheduled within 30 days of discharge. One patient required a plaster cast for two months and was then successfully discharged from outpatient care. Another patient required a longer follow-up period of three months, during which he had five outpatient appointments. He was then discharged from outpatient care without further complications. The patient that underwent neurosurgery was readmitted 20 days after discharge due to relapse of the subdural hematoma. No further information was available on the emergency department database about his follow-up since his second admission.

## 4. Discussion

Hunting continues to be a popular pastime for many people in Switzerland. Hunting accidents are inevitable and those that are fatal must be reported to the Swiss Advisory Centre for Accident Prevention. However there is no national registry of nonfatal hunting accidents in Switzerland in contrast to the USA where two organizations systematically document fatal and nonfatal hunting accidents nationwide. Until now, the mechanisms, patterns of injury, and outcomes of nonfatal hunting accidents in Switzerland have not been investigated. To our knowledge, this is the first Swiss study to examine hunting-related injuries, with respect to patient characteristics, mechanisms and patterns of injury, management, and patient outcomes.

The results of this study are largely consistent with the limited existing international data on nonfatal hunting accidents. We found that most nonfatal hunting accidents involved men with a mean age of 50 years, which is similar to the results of studies from Denmark, Germany, and the USA [5–8].

In addition, the most commonly involved weapon was a shotgun, followed by knives. This finding supports the results of Therbo and Van der Osten who found that 88% of hunting accidents in a group of Danish hunters were caused by shotguns and only 6% by knives [5]. Another finding from this study was that most injuries were self-inflicted rather than caused by another person: this supports the finding that over half of hunting-related accidents in central Ohio are self-inflicted [8]. In contrast, studies of German and Danish hunters have found that the majority of fire-arm-related hunting injuries involve a third party [5, 6]. One possible explanation for these mixed results could be differences in the teaching and content of firearm training and hunting examinations in different countries.

Our results support recent evidence from the USA that falls, as opposed to direct injury from firearm projectiles, are the principal cause of nonfatal hunting-related injuries [10, 12]. In this study, over almost a third of hunting-related injuries were associated with falls but not all from elevated tree stands; some injuries were sustained from falls whilst hunting in difficult terrain. In the USA, falls from tree stands may account for up to two-thirds of all hunting-related injuries and 8% result in permanent neurological injury or death [7, 8]. Common causes for falls from tree stands include poor tree stand construction, loss of balance, and falling asleep in the hide [12].

The results of this study also reveal that the most common patterns of injury from nonfatal hunting accidents are injuries to the head and extremities; however, in this study, no fractures were recorded. This finding supports other studies that have shown a high incidence of head injuries in hunters that fall from tree stands. About 60% of the patients in this study required operative intervention, which is 20% less than what Crockett et al. found in their study of hunting-related injuries in Ohio [8]. The most frequently involved specialty in the management of our series of hunting-related accidents was orthopedics, which is consistent with findings of Halanski and Corden [7].

Analysis of patient follow-up demonstrates that most patients that are admitted after hunting-related accidents can be discharged after initial management of their injuries with no further or very minimal follow-up as outpatients. Similarly, in a study of neurological injuries from hunting-related tree stand falls in New York, 72% of patients were discharged without follow-up and a further 11% with outpatient follow-up [12]. Two patients in our study required an extended period of follow-up before being discharged successfully, and only one patient in this case series required readmission.

Whilst our study may offer a unique insight into nonfatal hunting injuries in Switzerland, it is not without its limitations. Firstly, this study only evaluated nonfatal hunting injuries that were deemed severe enough by hunters to present to our emergency department. It is entirely conceivable that there were other nonfatal hunting injuries in the region during the period of study that never presented to our emergency department. Secondly, we only had access to cases of hunting injuries that were clearly labelled as such in the emergency department database. As mentioned previously, there is no national database of hunting accidents in Switzerland and therefore extrapolating our results to the rest of the country may not be entirely accurate. Finally, we cannot completely exclude the possibility that some cases of hunting-related injuries in the emergency department database were missed by the search criteria due to unstandardized data entry.

## 5. Conclusion

Nonfatal hunting accidents in Bern, Switzerland, are largely caused by firearms and falls and tend to occur in male hunters with a mean age of 50 years. The most common patterns of injury are orthopedic and head injuries, often requiring surgery. These findings are consistent with international studies of nonfatal hunting accidents but highlight a need for a national database documenting all hunting accidents in Switzerland.

## Conflict of Interests

The authors declare that there is no conflict of interests regarding the publication of this paper.

## References

[1] BAFU, Helvetic statistics of hunting activities.

[2] National Shooting Sports Foundation, *Industry Intelligence Reports*, National Shooting Sports Foundation, 2014.

[3] Consumer Products Safety Commission (CPSC) National Electronic Injury Surveillance System (NEISS) estimates, 2013.

[4] International Hunter Education Association Incident report, 2014.

[5] M. Therbo and C. Von Der Osten, "Firearm-related hunting accidents in Denmark," *Journal of Trauma—Injury, Infection and Critical Care*, vol. 67, no. 6, pp. 1265–1268, 2009.

[6] B. Karger, F. Wissmann, D. Gerlach, and B. Brinkmann, "Firearm fatalities and injuries from hunting accidents in Germany," *International Journal of Legal Medicine*, vol. 108, no. 5, pp. 252–255, 1996.

[7] M. A. Halanski and T. E. Corden, "Wisconsin firearm deer hunting season: injuries at a level I trauma center, 1999–2004," *Wisconsin Medical Journal*, vol. 107, no. 1, pp. 20–24, 2008.

[8] A. Crockett, S. P. Stawicki, Y. M. Thomas et al., "Tree stands, not guns, are the midwestern hunter's most dangerous weapon," *American Surgeon*, vol. 76, no. 9, pp. 1006–1010, 2010.

[9] M. Junuzovic, P. Midlöv, S. L. Lönn, and A. Eriksson, "Swedish hunters' safety behavior and experience of firearm incidents," *Accident Analysis and Prevention*, vol. 60, pp. 64–70, 2013.

[10] G. F. Lebus, C. A. Krueger, D. J. Stinner, and H. R. Mir, "Hunting stand-related injuries in orthopedics," *Southern Medical Journal*, vol. 107, no. 9, pp. 574–577, 2014.

[11] R. T. Loder, "Temporal variation in United States firearm injuries 1993–2008: results from an international database," *Journal of Injury and Violence Research*, vol. 6, no. 1, pp. 1–15, 2014.

[12] C. A. Pierre, B. A. Plog, V. Srinivasan, K. Srinivasan, A. L. Petraglia, and J. H. Huang, "Tree stand falls: a persistent cause of neurological injury in hunting," *World Journal of Clinical Cases*, vol. 2, no. 8, pp. 345–350, 2014.

# 5

# Nonconcordance between Clinical and Head CT Findings: The Specter of Overdiagnosis

**Kelli N. O'Laughlin,[1,2] Jerome R. Hoffman,[3] Steven Go,[4] Gelareh Z. Gabayan,[5,6,7] Erum Iqbal,[8] Guy Merchant,[9] Roberto A. Lopez-Freeman,[10] Michael I. Zucker,[3] and William R. Mower[3,6,11]**

[1] *Department of Emergency Medicine, Brigham & Women's Hospital, 75 Francis Street, Boston, MA 02115, USA*
[2] *Harvard Medical School, 25 Shattuck Street, Boston, MA 02115, USA*
[3] *University of California, Los Angeles (UCLA) David Geffen School of Medicine, 10833 Le Conte Avenue No. 12138, Los Angeles, CA 90095, USA*
[4] *Department of Emergency Medicine, University of Missouri-Kansas City (UMKC) School of Medicine, 2411 Holmes Street, Kansas City, MO 64108, USA*
[5] *Greater Los Angeles Veterans Affairs Healthcare System, 11301 Wilshire Blvd, Los Angeles, CA 90073, USA*
[6] *Ronald Reagan UCLA, Emergency Medicine Center, 757 Westwood Plaza, Los Angeles, CA 90095, USA*
[7] *Department of Medicine, University of California, Los Angeles (UCLA), 757 Westwood Plaza, Los Angeles, CA 90095, Irvine, USA*
[8] *School of Medicine, University of California, Irvine, 1001 Health Sciences Road, 252 Irvine Hall, Irvine, CA 92697-3950, USA*
[9] *UCLA Medical Center, 757 Westwood Plaza, Los Angeles, CA 90095, USA*
[10] *Department of Emergency Medicine, University of Cincinnati, 234 Goodman Street, Cincinnati, OH 45219, USA*
[11] *Emergency Medicine Center, University of California, Los Angeles (UCLA), 924 Westwood Blvd., Suite 300, Los Angeles, CA 90095, USA*

Correspondence should be addressed to Kelli N. O'Laughlin; kolaughlin@post.harvard.edu

Academic Editor: Tobias Lindner

*Background.* It is unclear whether history and physical examination findings can predict abnormalities on head computed tomography (CT) believed to indicate increased risk of lumbar-puncture- (LP-) induced brain herniation. The objectives of this study were to (1) identify head CT findings felt to be associated with increased risk of brain herniation and (2) to assess the ability of history and physical examination to predict those findings. *Methods.* Using a modified Delphi survey technique, an expert panel defined CT abnormalities felt to predict increased risk of LP-induced brain herniation. Presence of such findings on CT was compared with history and physical examination (H&P) variables in 47 patients. *Results.* No H&P variable predicted "high-risk" CT; combining H&P variables to improve sensitivity led to extremely low specificity and still failed to identify *all* patients with high-risk CT. *Conclusions.* "High-risk" CT is not uncommon in patients with clinical characteristics known to predict an absence of actual risk from LP, and thus it may not be *clinically relevant*. "Overdiagnosis" will be increasingly problematic as technological advances identify increasingly subtle deviations from "normal."

## 1. Introduction

There is substantial evidence in the medical literature that lumbar puncture (LP) is extremely safe [1–3], particularly in the setting of patients who are immunologically normal and who do not manifest abnormal mental status, papilledema, or focal neurological deficit [3–5]. Nevertheless, many clinicians are concerned that LP could lead to tonsillar herniation [6–11] in patients with increased intracranial pressure (ICP), by decreasing cerebrospinal fluid pressure in the subarachnoid space, and thus creating a pressure gradient that could displace cerebral and brainstem structures [7, 12].

There are only a small number of reports, however, suggesting catastrophic deterioration related to LP [9, 13, 14], and even the validity of these observations has been questioned [15–17]. Nevertheless, despite the substantial evidence that few, if any patients, are at risk from LP, many clinicians worry about potential harm, and it has been suggested that head computed tomography (CT) be obtained prior to LP, in the hope that it might be able to identify the few patients in whom the procedure would purportedly be dangerous [5, 18]. There are no studies, however, which define what if any findings on head CT actually do predict increased risk of tonsillar herniation following LP [3, 4, 19].

We designed this study to assess the prevalence of "high-risk" CT findings in patients who undergo head CT for any reason and in particular whether and how often such findings occur in patients whose clinical presentations make it extremely unlikely that they would be harmed by LP. Because of the absence of any gold standard for "high-risk" CT findings, we convened an expert panel and asked its member to define what CT findings indicate increased risk of tonsillar herniation following LP; we then used clinical data that had been prospectively recorded on a large cohort of patients for whom CT had been ordered to assess the relationship between selected history and physical examination (H&P) findings and the presence of those CT characteristics defined by the expert panel as conferring increased risk.

## 2. Methods

*2.1. Ethics Statement.* This study was approved by the University of California, Los Angeles (UCLA) Institutional Review Committee. Informed consent was not required as the clinical data collected was deidentified and did not impact clinical care.

*2.2. Study Design.* We designed this study in two parts. First, given the absence of any prior criterion standard regarding which if any head CT findings predict increased hazard from performance of LP, we convened an expert panel to determine if it was possible for them to agree on any set of head CT characteristics that could be defined as predicting "high risk" of LP-induced brain hemiation (Part I). Second, we used prospectively collected data from the large NEXUS 2 cohort of emergency department patients for whom head CT had been ordered, for whatever reason, to evaluate how closely clinical findings correlate with the presence or absence of any of these "high-risk" CT findings (Part II). We did not make any assumptions regarding what would have happened to any of the *individual* patients in our study had an LP been performed on them. (We did assume, on the other hand, based on substantial evidence from the literature, that at most a very few patients in this cohort might have been harmed by LP, particularly among that subset of patients who had been prospectively found not to have papilledema, altered mentation, or focal neurological findings.)

*Part I: The Modified Delphi Technique to Define Predictive Head CT Abnormalities.* We employed a modified Delphi survey technique [20–23] to allow a group of content experts, who perform LP and/or interpret head CT regularly, to generate a list of head CT abnormalities that they believed to predict high risk of herniation with LP and thus contraindicate this procedure. Of the 16 physicians asked to participate, 13 agreed. The panel included academic physicians in emergency medicine (2), internal medicine (1), infectious disease (1), neurology (4), neurosurgery (2), and radiology (3) including one general radiologist, one neuroradiologist, and one emergency radiologist), from four academic medical centers in the Midwest and the West Coast of the United States.

A structured e-mail survey regarding potential LP contraindications was sent to the panelists, each of whom then indicated his or her level of agreement (0 = "strongly disagree," and 5 = "strongly agree") with the following statement: "This CT finding should contraindicate performance of an LP," for a series of possible CT findings (see Appendix information at "Information and Survey Sent to the Delphi Panel"). Narrative explanations of the experts' responses were solicited, and panelists were asked to suggest any additional CT findings they felt should contraindicate LP. For subsequent rounds, survey participants were asked to read the anonymous narrative explanations submitted by all of the panelists and then to rerate each CT finding. While three survey rounds are generally considered adequate to achieve a valid consensus opinion [24], when an additional potential LP contraindication was first suggested in the third round, one final survey round was added. Panelists were blinded to the identities of other panel members, but they were allowed to use outside references and to discuss the survey with colleagues. In order to maximize sensitivity, we included in the final list of "contraindications" any finding assigned a level of 4 or 5 by one-third of the panelists.

*Part II: Study Subjects.* We included all of the 1737 patients for whom a head CT scan had been ordered at an academic, urban, level I emergency department (ED) between April 2006 and February 2007, as part of a prior study in which the treating clinician prospectively recorded the presence or absence of specific H&P findings at the time the CT was ordered and before it was actually done [25]. The only exclusion criterion was a history of a prior neurosurgical intervention. A neuroradiologist interpreted all CT images. Two physician reviewers, blinded to H&P findings, then independently classified the written head CT radiology reports as reflecting that the patient either was at increased risk (if *any* of the expert panel's increased-risk findings were present (Table 1)) or was not at increased risk (if *none* of these findings were present). When both reviewers independently agreed that the written report was definitive regarding presence or absence of the increased-risk findings, they were classified as such. In any case where *either* of the physicians was uncertain on how to classify this, based solely on the written report, the actual CT images were reviewed by an expert radiologist, who then prospectively characterized each study with regard to the presence or absence of increased-risk findings. If the emergency radiologist was uncertain, a senior emergency physician conducted an additional review of the CT images. To be as conservative as possible in these few remaining, this physician labeled the CT scan as showing "increased risk" only if any one of the following additional findings was present: dilation, enlargement or compression of the 4th ventricle or the brainstem, hydrocephalus, effaced cerebral sulci, local mass effect, or evidence of edema.

*2.3. Primary Data Analysis.* We calculated the sensitivity, specificity, and positive and negative predictive values for each of the individual H&P findings in predicting the presence of increased risk of herniation with LP on head CT (as defined by the expert panel). We also analyzed the test characteristics of the complete neurologic examination and all aspects of the H&P, assuming that the presence of any single abnormal finding predicts increased risk as determined by CT.

## 3. Results

*3.1. Part I: The Modified Delphi Results.* The expert panel ultimately agreed on five findings on head CT that were felt to increase risk of LP sufficiently so as to contraindicate performance of this procedure (Table 1). There was complete agreement on inclusion of subtentorial or tonsillar herniation, strong agreement on obliteration of the fourth ventricle, and majority agreement on lateral shift of midline structures and loss of basilar cisterns; a sufficient minority (at least one-third of the panel) felt that the obliteration of the superior cerebellar cistern and the quadrigeminal plate cistern should be included. Three other findings (isolated dilation of the temporal horns of the lateral ventricles, intracranial abscess in an immunocompromised patient, and Chiari I malformation with a tethered cord) had at least one vote for inclusion, but they were ultimately excluded because they were not endorsed by an adequate number of panelists.

*3.2. Part II: Study Subjects Results.* Of the 1737 patients initially included, 445 had abnormal head CTs. Of these, 122 were excluded because of a previous neurosurgical intervention, leaving 323 patients for the final analysis. The average age of study subjects was 57.8 years (range, 1–99 years), and 58% were male. Other demographic characteristics are listed in Table 2.

In categorizing the CT scan reports, both of the physician reviewers independently agreed that the written radiology report definitively indicated the presence, or absence, of the high-risk findings, in 68% of the cases. The emergency radiologist who then reviewed the actual CT images in the remaining 32% of cases was able to categorize findings as clearly present or absent in all but 2%; these few cases were then categorized by a senior emergency physician, using the conservative criteria described above (with cases classified as high risk only if they showed definitive dilation, enlargement or compression of the 4th ventricle or the brainstem, hydrocephalus, effaced cerebral sulci, local mass effect, or evidence of edema). Overall, 47 (14.6%) of the CT scans had at least one of the high-risk findings defined by the expert panel (Figure 1).

None of the individual elements of H&P were sensitive in identifying patients with increased risk based on head CT findings (Table 3). The highest sensitivity for any single clinical characteristic was 68.9% (CI 53.4, 81.8), for presence of a focal neurological deficit on examination; this finding had a specificity of 73.5% (CI 67.8, 78.7). When the neurological examination was considered as a whole, with the presence of any single abnormality on examination compared with presence or absence of high-risk CT, sensitivity was still only 87.0% (CI 73.7, 95.1), and specificity was 39.3% (CI 33.5, 45.3). If the presence of any single abnormality on either history or physical examination was considered positive, sensitivity was increased to 95.7% (CI 85.5, 99.5), but specificity was further decreased to only 17.8% (CI 13.5, 22.9); this approach still failed to identify 2 of 47 patients with "high-risk" CT findings.

Table 1: Head CT abnormalities identified as contraindications to LP by the Delphi panel.

| Head CT abnormalities | Percentage of the Delphi panel who rated the abnormality as 4 or 5 (out of 5) |
|---|---|
| Lateral shift of midline structures | 73 |
| Loss of basilar cisterns | 73 |
| Obliteration of the fourth ventricle | 91 |
| Subtentorial herniation or tonsillar herniation | 100 |
| Obliteration of the superior cerebellar cistern and the quadrigeminal plate cistern with sparing of the ambient cisterns | 36 |

Table 2: Demographic and clinical characteristics of study subjects, $N = 323$.

| | |
|---|---|
| Sex | |
| Male | 188 (58.2) |
| Age | |
| Range | 1 to 99 |
| Mean | 57.8 |
| Median | 62 |
| Interquartile range (IQR) | 47–87 |
| Pediatric ages | |
| ≤3 | 8 |
| 3 to 6 | 3 |
| 6 to 18 | 11 |
| Race | |
| White | 189 |
| Black | 17 |
| Hispanic | 57 |
| Asian | 22 |
| Middle Eastern | 17 |
| Others/unknown | 21 |

Table 3: Test characteristics of history and physical examination findings in relation to clinically abnormal head CTs.

| | *N* | Sensitivity | CI | Specificity | CI | NPV | CI | PPV | CI |
|---|---|---|---|---|---|---|---|---|---|
| Blunt head injury | 139/307 | 47.7 | (32.5, 63.3) | 55.1 | (48.9, 61.3) | 86.3 | (80.2, 91.1) | 15.1 | (9.6, 22.5) |
| Dangerous mechanism | 105/285 | 33.3 | (19.6, 49.6) | 62.6 | (56.1, 68.7) | 84.4 | (78.3, 89.4) | 13.3 | (7.5, 21.4) |
| Vomiting | 23/318 | 8.9 | (2.5, 21.2) | 93 | (89.4, 95.8) | 86.1 | (81.6, 89.3) | 17.4 | (5.0, 38.7) |
| Coagulopathy | 36/280 | 8.3 | (1.8, 22.5) | 86.5 | (81.5, 90.5) | 86.5 | (81.5, 90.5) | 8.3 | (1.8, 22.5) |
| Skull fracture | 21/319 | 11.6 | (3.8, 24.6) | 94.2 | (90.7, 96.64) | 86.9 | (82.6, 90.5) | 23.8 | (8.2, 47.2) |
| Scalp hematoma | 81/319 | 26 | (14.2, 41.1) | 74.7 | (69.1, 79.8) | 85.7 | (80.6, 89.9) | 14.8 | (7.9, 24.5) |
| Neuro deficit | 102/313 | 68.9 | (53.4, 81.8) | 73.5 | (67.8, 78.7) | 93.4 | (89.1, 96.3) | 30.4 | (21.7, 40.3) |
| ALOC | 134/316 | 67.4 | (52.0, 80.5) | 61.9 | (55.8, 67.7) | 91.8 | (86.8, 95.3) | 23.1 | (16.3, 31.2) |
| Abnormal behavior | 100/314 | 53.3 | (37.9, 68.3) | 71.8 | (66.0, 77.1) | 90.2 | (85.4, 93.8) | 24 | (16.0, 33.6) |
| No spontaneous eye opening | 61/316 | 34.1 | (20.5, 49.9) | 83.1 | (78.1, 87.3) | 88.6 | (88.1, 92.3) | 24.6 | (14.5, 37.3) |
| Not oriented | 189/305 | 65.1 | (49.1, 79.0) | 66.4 | (60.3, 72.1) | 92.1 | (87.3, 95.5) | 24.1 | (16.7, 33.0) |
| Not following commands | 76/310 | 43.2 | (28.34, 59.0) | 78.6 | (73.2, 83.4) | 89.3 | (84.6, 93.0) | 25 | (15.8, 36.3) |
| Amnestic | 28/224 | 18.5 | (6.3, 38.1) | 88.3 | (83.0, 92.5) | 88.8 | (83.5, 92.8) | 17.9 | (6.1, 36.9) |
| Combined criteria | 271/322 | 95.7 | (85.5, 99.5) | 17.8 | (13.5, 22.9) | 96.1 | (86.5, 99.5) | 16.6 | (12.4, 21.6) |
| Abnormal neuro exam | 207/321 | 87 | (73.7, 95.1) | 39.3 | (33.5, 45.3) | 94.7 | (88.9, 98.0) | 19.3 | (14.2, 25.4) |
| Abnl neuro exam or vomiting | 217/321 | 87 | (73.7, 95.1) | 36 | (30.3, 42.0) | 94.3 | (88.0, 97.9) | 18.5 | (13.6, 24.4) |

*N*: number, CI: confidence interval, PPV: positive predictive value, NPV: negative predictive value, Abnl: abnormal, and Neuro: neurological.

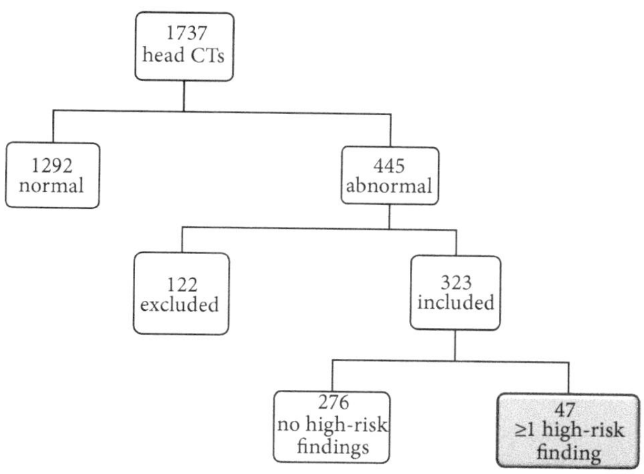


Figure 1: Study subject selection.

## 4. Discussion

There is substantial evidence in the medical literature that brain herniation secondary to lumbar puncture is extremely uncommon; this is particularly true among patients who do not have high-risk clinical findings, such as altered mentation or focal neurological deficits. Because of concerns about this catastrophic possibility, however, several authors have suggested that head CT scanning be performed prior to LP, to help identify patients at increased risk.

Because of the absence of any prior criterion standard regarding "high-risk" CT findings, we performed Part I of our study to define a group of such findings about which experts would agree that they represent an increased risk of LP-induced brain herniation on head CT findings. Using standard accepted methodology of a modified Delphi technique, our expert panel was able to reach consensus, and at least one of their "high-risk" findings was present in about one of every seven patients in our cohort; a majority of these patients at "high risk" as indicated by their CT findings had clinical findings (as *prospectively* recorded) that suggested very little or no actual likelihood of danger from LP. The method used to characterize high-risk findings on CT scans (to rely on written radiology reports *only* when they were definitive and to have images prospectively reviewed when such written reports were not absolutely clear) was intentionally conservative and intended to bias against our hypothesis that CTs lead to overdiagnosis by showing "high-risk findings." While we of course cannot know with any certainty what would or would not have happened to any individual in our cohort had he or she been subjected to LP, it is clear that this number is far larger than the rate of deterioration that should be expected amongst this group.

There are two very different possible explanations for this discordance between clinical findings in individual patients and "high-risk" elements on CT. One explanation is based on the *assumption* that when a technologically advanced test like CT identifies some problem not identified by clinical exam, the former always provides more accurate evidence of the patient's true condition; this type of reasoning is extremely widespread in modern medical practice. In the clinical scenario addressed by our study, that would mean that clinical findings are insufficient to identify patients in whom LP would be dangerous—and that CT should be performed routinely prior to LP—to identify a substantial group of patients with a clinically occult risk from this procedure. However, it is also possible that CT findings (as defined by this expert panel and as reflected in opinion papers in the medical literature [14]) are overly sensitive and identify a fairly large group of patients the large majority of whom are *not* in fact at any risk. It is not possible to say with certainty which of these interpretations is correct, based on this or any other currently available study.

We believe that this disjunction between sophisticated technology and traditional diagnostic evaluation is not unique to head CT scanning and the risk of herniation and that the importance of our findings extends far beyond the narrow question of whether routine imaging (which also carries well-described medical and economic costs [3, 26, 27]), prior to LP, would on balance be beneficial or harmful. Modern technological approach to pulmonary embolism (PE), for example, has led to a vast increase in the number of patients given this diagnosis, but a concomitant vast decrease in the case-fatality rate associated with it [28], which appears to be largely independent of any benefit from advances in treatment. In addition, a recent decision analysis suggests that while an effort to identify PE in a cohort of reasonably low-risk patients using CT angiography may benefit a few patients, it will harm many more, increasing not only morbidity but also mortality [28]. Our observations about the use of CT to predict risk of brain herniation should thus be viewed in terms of this much larger question about technology in general and suggest that this question needs urgent attention from both the research community and the practicing physicians, since simply *assuming* that the former must be a better "gold standard" may in fact lead to major harm to patients [28, 29].

Although it is tempting to assume that technology is both more reliable and more accurate than clinical examination, there are several reasons to question this belief. First, there are numerous examples where some finding identified by some type of advanced technology is given the same name as a previously well-known clinical event, but it actually implies a far less dangerous clinical entity. As in the case of PE, described above, a hyphema diagnosed by slit-lamp examination is less worrisome (and should be approached differently) than a hyphema visible to the naked eye; similarly, CT-defined pneumothorax is clinically different than pneumothorax seen on a chest X-ray, acute myocardial infarction (MI) defined on the basis of troponin leak is not the same as the clinically apparent MI, and asymptomatic microscopic prostate "cancer" diagnosed by biopsy, after screening, implies a very different prognosis (and should be approached differently) than does cancer searched for and found because of clinical symptoms.

With regard to the specific clinical issue raised in our study, a recent publication reported head CT "evidence of herniation" in many patients who were clinically entirely stable [30]. The meaning of such "herniation" is obviously different than is tonsillar herniation associated with catastrophic clinical deterioration. Because clinicians have long used clinical findings to decide who can safely undergo LP without a head CT and because with this approach tonsillar herniation rarely if ever occurs (especially in patients with normal mental status and no focal deficit), we believe that the CT criteria defined by our experts are likely to be overly sensitive and identify "risk" in many patients who could undergo LP with almost no chance of clinical deterioration.

Since clinical brain herniation almost inevitably results in death, it is appropriate that CT criteria for safe performance of LP should err on the side of high sensitivity. On the other hand, failure to recognize that "findings" on head CT may not have the meaning traditionally attributed to the same "abnormalities" ("lesions" and "diseases") identified on the basis of clinical condition could lead to dramatic overdiagnosis [29], which could in turn result in substantial harm to patients. In our scenario, this could lead to an insistence on routine CT scanning prior to LP, despite the long history of safe performance of LP without CT; furthermore, findings on those CT scans would almost certainly then lead to avoidance of LP in many patients in whom this test would not only be enormously safe but could also provide important diagnostic information.

In a broader sense, our study raises generic concerns about the danger of *assuming* that as technology advances, it will always provide a better and better diagnostic gold standard. We can easily envision, for example, a time when the *N*th generation CT scanners, using electron microscope-type resolution, might identify a "thyroid nodule" in just about everyone—which might be proved on biopsy to be "cancer" in many—even though the vast majority would never know about this "cancer" had the "advanced imaging" not been performed. The same could be true for "renal cysts", or lesions on supermammography, or even "pulmonary emboli" in many if not all normal pulmonary arteries leading to obvious and profound conundrums about both the meaning of such findings and the appropriate way to separate disease, which might benefit from treatment, from overdiagnosis of normal (or at least clinically unimportant) variation. Surveillance bias has been described as "the more you look, the more you find," [31]. The type of overdiagnosis we believe we have identified appears to be a closely related variant, where "the closer you look (with more and more powerful tools), the more you find."

The head CT criteria defined by our panel as representing "increased risk" of herniation are based on expert opinion, rather than experimental evidence, which does not exist. Although many specialties were represented in the expert panel, not all regularly perform LP, which may have resulted in an overly conservative list of "contraindications." Our expert panel also suffered a degree of expert attrition, with one neurosurgeon, one neurologist, and one neuroradiologist failing to complete the entire sequence of surveys. Peer pressure can influence expert panels [32], so this could conceivably have biased our results.

Nevertheless, our study provides strong evidence that no H&P findings, alone or in combination, are adequately sensitive to detect head CT abnormalities believed by a panel of experts to predict enhanced potential for brain herniation during LP. Since clinical brain herniation is extremely rare following LP and these CT findings are far more common, it is likely that these criteria are overly sensitive and that their application to patients needs to be reconsidered. Furthermore, our study suggests that there is an urgent need to question the assumption that "advanced" technology defines the criterion standard when there is a clear disjunction between abnormalities defined clinically and "abnormalities" given the same name, despite an absence of clinical correlates, when identified by such technology.

## Appendix

### Information and Survey Sent to the Delphi Panel

Dear Colleague:

Thank you for agreeing to be part of an expert panel to help determine CT contraindications to LP. This is round 1 of 3 questionnaires regarding the topic.

For the following 3 items:

(1) *Please indicate your level of agreement that the CT finding listed is a contraindication for performing an lumbar puncture* using a 5 point scale (0 indicates strong disagreement and 5 strong agreement).

(2) Please *explain the reasons for your choice* in the space provided.

(3) Please *add any additional CT findings* that are contraindications to LP you feel should be on the list.

*Please return this questionnaire by email or fax.*

Your Name: ________________________

(1) The CT finding of a *lateral shift of the midline structures* is a contraindication to performing an LP.

Strongly disagree 0 1 2 3 4 5 Strongly agree

Your level of agreement with statement #1: ________

*Please explain* the reason(s) for your answer:

(2) The CT finding of a *loss of the basilar cisterns* is a contraindication to performing an LP.

Strongly disagree 0 1 2 3 4 5 Strongly agree

Your level of agreement with statement #2: ________

*Please explain* the reason(s) for your answer:

(3) The CT finding of an *obliteration of the fourth ventricle* is a contraindication to performing an LP.

Strongly disagree 0 1 2 3 4 5 Strongly agree

Your level of agreement with statement #3: ________

*Please explain* the reason(s) for your answer:

(4) The CT finding of an *obliteration of the superior cerebellar cistern and the quadrigeminal plate cistern with sparing of the ambient cisterns* is a contraindication to performing an LP.

Strongly disagree 0 1 2 3 4 5 Strongly agree

Your level of agreement with statement #4: ________

*Please explain* the reason(s) for your answer:

(5) Please suggest any additional CT findings that are contraindications to LP that you feel should be included in this list, and briefly explain why.

## Disclosure

No direct funding was received for this study. The authors were personally salaried by their institutions during the period of writing (although no specific salary was set aside or given for the writing of this paper).

## Conflict of Interests

The authors declare that they have no conflict of interests.

## Authors' Contribution

William R. Mower, Steven Go, and Kelli N. O'Laughlin conceived and designed the study. Steven Go supervised the expert panel process and data collection. William R. Mower and Guy Merchant supervised the collection and management of data related to head CTs and radiology reports. Kelli N. O'Laughlin, Gelareh Z. Gabayan, Erum Iqbal, and Roberto A. Lopez-Freeman assisted with data collection. Kelli N. O'Laughlin and Gelareh Z. Gabayan categorized radiology reports, and Michael Zucker and Jerome R. Hoffman served as arbitrators. Kelli N. O'Laughlin analyzed the data and William R. Mower served as senior advisor providing guidance on data analysis. Kelli N. O'Laughlin drafted the paper except for the sections related to the expert panel, which were drafted by Steven Go. Jerome R. Hoffman revised the paper (including particularly the Discussion), Gelareh Z. Gabayan participated in paper revision, and Kelli N. O'Laughlin, Jerome R. Hoffman, and William R. Mower took responsibility for the final paper revisions. Kelli N. O'Laughlin, Jerome R. Hoffman, and William R. Mower took responsibility for the paper as a whole.

## References

[1] G. Linker, N. Mirza, G. Manetti, M. Meyer, K. T. Putnam, and T. Sunderland, "Fine-needle, negative-pressure lumbar puncture: a safe technique for collecting CSF," *Neurology*, vol. 59, no. 12, pp. 2008–2009, 2002.

[2] M. K. Patel and M. A. Clarke, "Lumbar puncture and subarachnoid haemorrhage," *Postgraduate Medical Journal*, vol. 62, no. 733, pp. 1021–1024, 1986.

[3] R. Hasbun, J. Abrahams, J. Jekel, and V. J. Quagliarello, "Computed tomography of the head before lumbar puncture in adults with suspected meningitis," *The New England Journal of Medicine*, vol. 345, no. 24, pp. 1727–1733, 2001.

[4] A. K. Gopal, J. D. Whitehouse, D. L. Simel, and G. R. Corey, "Cranial computed tomography before lumbar puncture: a prospective clinical evaluation," *Archives of Internal Medicine*, vol. 159, no. 22, pp. 2681–2685, 1999.

[5] P. R. Greig and D. Goroszeniuk, "Role of computed tomography before lumbar puncture: a survey of clinical practice," *Postgraduate Medical Journal*, vol. 82, no. 965, pp. 162–165, 2006.

[6] F. Simonetti, P. Pergami, M. Ceroni, A. H. Ropper, and R. Viviani, "About the original description of cerebellar tonsil herniation by Pierre Marie," *Journal of Neurology Neurosurgery and Psychiatry*, vol. 63, no. 3, p. 412, 1997.

[7] N. H. Steigbigel, "Computed tomography of the head before a lumbar puncture in suspected meningitis—is it helpful?" *The New England Journal of Medicine*, vol. 345, no. 24, pp. 1768–1770, 2001.

[8] W. Waldman and R. Laureno, "Precautions for lumbar puncture: a survey of neurologic educators," *Neurology*, vol. 52, no. 6, p. 1296, 1999.

[9] G. P. Duffy, "Lumbar puncture in the presence of raised intracranial pressure," *British Medical Journal*, vol. 1, no. 641, pp. 407–409, 1969.

[10] P. R. Dodge and M. N. Swartz, "Bacterial meningitis—a review of selected aspects. ii. special neurologic problems, postmeningitic complacations and clinicopathological correlations," *The New England Journal of Medicine*, vol. 272, pp. 954–960, 1965.

[11] S. Kastenbauer, F. Winkler, H.-W. Pfister et al., "Cranial CT before lumbar puncture in suspected meningitis (multiple letters)," *The New England Journal of Medicine*, vol. 346, no. 16, pp. 1248–1251, 2002.

[12] H. van Crevel, A. Hijdra, and J. De Gans, "Lumbar puncture and the risk of herniation: when should we first perform CT," *Journal of Neurology*, vol. 249, no. 2, pp. 129–137, 2002.

[13] G. P. Duffy, "Lumbar puncture in spontaneous subarachnoid haemorrhage," *British Medical Journal*, vol. 285, no. 6349, pp. 1163–1164, 1982.

[14] D. J. Gower, A. Baker, W. Bell, and M. R. Ball, "Contraindications to lumbar puncture as defined by computed cranial tomography," *Journal of Neurology Neurosurgery and Psychiatry*, vol. 50, no. 8, pp. 1071–1074, 1987.

[15] B. D. Archer, "Computed tomography before lumbar puncture in acute meningitis: a review of the risks and benefits," *Canadian Medical Association Journal*, vol. 148, no. 6, pp. 961–965, 1993.

[16] W. J. Oliver, T. C. Shope, and L. R. Kuhns, "Fatal lumbar puncture: fact versus fiction—an approach to a clinical dilemma," *Pediatrics*, vol. 112, no. 3, pp. e174–e176, 2003.

[17] J. Zisfein and A. J. Tuchman, "Risks of lumbar puncture in the presence of intracranial mass lesions," *Mount Sinai Journal of Medicine*, vol. 55, no. 4, pp. 283–287, 1988.

[18] J. J. Perry, I. G. Stiell, G. A. Wells et al., "Attitudes and judgment of emergency physicians in the management of patients with acute headache," *Academic Emergency Medicine*, vol. 12, no. 1, pp. 33–37, 2005.

[19] N. D. Baker, H. Kharazi, L. Laurent et al., "The efficacy of routine head computed tomography (CT scan) prior to lumbar puncture in the emergency department," *Journal of Emergency Medicine*, vol. 12, no. 5, pp. 597–601, 1994.

[20] H. A. Linstone and M. Turoff, *The Delphi Method: Techniques and Applications*, Addison-Wesley, Reading, Mass, USA, 1975.

[21] N. Dalkey and O. Helmer, "An experimental application of the delphi method to the use of experts," *Management Science*, vol. 9, pp. 458–467, 1963.

[22] R. L. Custer SJ and B. R. Stewart, "The modified delphi technique—a rotational modification," *Journal of Vocational and Technical Education*, vol. 15, 1999.

[23] A. Ali, "Using the delphi technique to search for empirical measures of local planning agency power," *The Qualitative Report*, vol. 10, pp. 718–744, 2005.

[24] K. W. Brooks, "Delphi technique: expanding applications," *North Central Association Quarterly*, vol. 54, pp. 377–385, 1979.

[25] W. R. Mower, J. R. Hoffman, M. Herbert, A. B. Wolfson, C. V. Pollack Jr., and M. I. Zucker, "Developing a clinical decision instrument to rule out intracranial injuries in patients with minor head trauma: methodology of the NEXUS II investigation," *Annals of Emergency Medicine*, vol. 40, no. 5, pp. 505–514, 2002.

[26] A. Sodickson, P. F. Baeyens, K. P. Andriole et al., "Recurrent CT, cumulative radiation exposure, and associated radiation-induced cancer risks from CT of adults," *Radiology*, vol. 251, no. 1, pp. 175–184, 2009.

[27] R. T. Griffey and A. Sodickson, "Cumulative radiation exposure and cancer risk estimates in emergency department patients undergoing repeat or multiple CT," *American Journal of Roentgenology*, vol. 192, no. 4, pp. 887–892, 2009.

[28] D. H. Newman and D. L. Schriger, "Rethinking testing for pulmonary embolism: less is more," *Annals of Emergency Medicine*, vol. 57, no. 6, pp. 622–627, 2011.

[29] G. Welch, L. Schwartz, and S. Woloshin, *Over-Diagnosed: Making People Sick in the Pursuit of Health*, Beacon Press, Boston, Mass, USA, 2011.

[30] L. J. Baraff, R. L. Byyny, M. A. Probst, N. Salamon, M. Linetsky, and W. R. Mower, "Prevalence of herniation and intracranial shift on cranial tomography in patients with subarachnoid hemorrhage and a normal neurologic examination," *Academic Emergency Medicine*, vol. 17, no. 4, pp. 423–428, 2010.

[31] E. R. Haut and P. J. Pronovost, "Surveillance bias in outcomes reporting," *Journal of the American Medical Association*, vol. 305, no. 23, pp. 2462–2463, 2011.

[32] F. Woudenberg, "An evaluation of delphi," *Technological Forecasting and Social Change*, vol. 40, no. 2, pp. 131–150, 1991.

# 6

# Assessment of a New E-Learning System on Thorax, Trachea, and Lung Ultrasound

**Colleen Cuca,[1] Patrick Scheiermann,[2] Dorothea Hempel,[3] Gabriele Via,[4] Armin Seibel,[1,5] Magnus Barth,[1] Tim O. Hirche,[6] Felix Walcher,[1,7] and Raoul Breitkreutz[1,8]**

[1] *Ultrasound Regional Network SonoABCD and Frankfurter Institut für Notfallmedizin und Simulationstraining, Fachbereich Medizin der Johann Wolfgang Goethe-Universität, Klinikum der Johann Wolfgang Goethe-Universität, 60528 Frankfurt am Main, Germany*

[2] *Klinik für Anaesthesiologie, Klinikum der Universität München, Campus Grosshadern, 81377 München, Germany*

[3] *II. Medizinische Klinik und Poliklinik, Universitätsmedizin Mainz, 55131 Mainz, Germany*

[4] *Anestesia e Rianimazione I, Fondazione IRCCS, Policlinico San Matteo, 27100 Pavia, Italy*

[5] *Klinik für Anästhesiologie, Intensiv- und Notfallmedizin, Diakonie Klinikum Jung Stilling, 57074 Siegen, Germany*

[6] *Fachbereich Pneumologie, Deutsche Klinik für Diagnostik GmbH, 65191 Wiesbaden, Germany*

[7] *Klinik für Unfall-, Hand- und Wiederherstellungschirurgie, Klinikum der Johann Wolfgang Goethe-Universität, 60590 Frankfurt am Main, Germany*

[8] *Zentrale Notaufnahme, Klinikum Frankfurt Höchst, 65929 Frankfurt am Main, Germany*

Correspondence should be addressed to Raoul Breitkreutz; raoul.breitkreutz@gmail.com

Academic Editor: Aristomenis K. Exadaktylos

*Background.* Lung ultrasound has become an emerging tool in acute and critical care medicine. Combined theoretical and hands-on training has been required to teach ultrasound diagnostics. Current computer technology allows for display, explanation, and animation of information in a remote-learning environment. *Objective.* Development and assessment of an e-learning program for lung ultrasound. *Methods.* An interactive online tutorial was created. A prospective learning success study was conducted with medical students using a multiple-choice test (Trial A). This e-learning program was used as preparation for a certified course followed by an evaluation of trained doctors (Trial B) by linear analogue scales. Pretests were compared with postcourse tests and sustainability tests as well as a posttest of a one-day custom classroom training. *Results.* In Trial A, during the learning success study ($n = 29$), the increase of correct answers was 11.7 to 17/20 in the post-test and to 16.6/20 in the sustainability test (relative change 45.1%, $P < 0.0001$). E-learning almost equalled scores of classroom-based training regarding gain and retention of factual knowledge. In Trial B, nineteen participating doctors found a 79.5% increase of knowledge (median, 95% CI: 69%; 88%). *Conclusion.* The basics of lung ultrasound can be taught in a highly effective manner using e-learning.

## 1. Introduction

The increasing demand for ultrasound applications in critical care medicine requires a discerning analysis of current and emerging training methods. In particular, ultrasound diagnostics of thorax, trachea, and lungs remain underutilized, although it has been shown to deliver more specific and sensitive results than chest X-ray, for example in cases of pulmonary edema regarding B-line differential diagnostics [1], pneumothorax [2–4], or pulmonary consolidation [5–8]. The safety and accuracy of ultrasound-guided interventions have similarly been demonstrated in critical care scenarios such as thoracocentesis [9, 10]. Pulmonary ultrasound is considered of utmost importance in critical care ultrasound curricula [11, 12] and encompasses the impartment of cognitive and psychomotor skills for accurate interpretation and acquisition of sonographic images.

Lecture- and seminar-based events, the current standards for ultrasound training, are often inaccessible due to time or financial constraints, posing a substantial hurdle to interested parties from medical students to board-certified doctors. While practical ultrasound skills may be quickly acquired in brief training courses [13, 14], the advancement of computer- and online-based training calls into question the necessity of a training seminar to convey pure theoretical knowledge of basic ultrasound concepts [15].

An online e-learning program can reduce the time, staff, and financial commitments of lecture-based training and promote active user involvement with the course material. The broad scope of e-learning and its accessibility enables knowledge to be conveyed quickly and effectively, ensuring its place in current and future learning applications [16]. Previous studies examining the effectiveness of e-learning programs in ultrasound training [17, 18] have primarily concentrated on using Internet media to present classical frontal lectures or enable a platform for tutoring, thereby removing the spatial drawback of attendance-based courses but retaining the typical teacher-student configuration. "Activation" of a learner is considered to be much more effective than passive listening to classical lectures [19].

We developed an interactive online training program as part of a critical care ultrasound training and aimed to analyze the success of independent theoretical skill development through an individual e-learning course as compared to a day-long training seminar with personal attendance provided by http://www.SonoABCD.de. http://www.SonoABCD.de is a network of multiple participating hospitals and institutions providing ultrasound education in Germany [13, 14, 20].

Our study was designed to determine the effectiveness and sustainability of content conveyed through the e-learning training program, as assessed by medical doctors and medical students. Further we compared factual knowledge gain with a generic attendance training.

## 2. Methods

*2.1. Contents of the E-Learning System.* The tutorial explains the basics of sonography and the most important physiological and pathological sonographic patterns of lung and pleura as defined by the International Consensus Conference on Lung Ultrasound [8]. Target groups were medical doctors and medical students. The module content is structured in 5 chapters: basics and pleural effusion, pneumothorax, pulmonary edema and consolidations, trachea, and workflow of a protocol-based lung ultrasound exam with exercises. Those 5 chapters contain a total of 21 units, which represent one screen each (Table 1).

*2.2. Didactic Concept and Script.* The theoretical approach was based on constructivism, which emphasizes a setting in which the learner arrives at his/her own conclusions and the "teacher" plays a more passive role in comparison to a classic frontal-lecture environment [21]. The script consists of 21 screens: one screen for each unit of the online tutorial. An important part in the learning process is interaction, whereupon the newly acquired knowledge is actively applied [22]. The units consist of ultrasound, X-ray and anatomical pictures, learning texts with key facts, and corresponding exercises: drag and drop, multiple choice, radio button, and fill-in-the-blank. An overview of the video clips and still images, including their respective sources, is provided (Table 1).

*2.3. Production of the Online Tutorial.* The anatomical sketches were drawn in coloured pencil and converted to Joint Photographic Experts Group (JPEG) standard format. All ultrasound videos were converted from their various formats to a flash-specific format using the Adobe Flash CS3 Video Encoder (Adobe Systems Inc., San Jose, CA, USA). The videos were cut in width and height as well as in duration to anonymize content as necessary and run in endless loops to facilitate uninterrupted viewing. Adobe Flash CS3 Version 9.0 was used as the main development tool, as its player plug-in allows presentation of videos and animations over the Internet in over 99% of browser programs installed in North America and Europe [23]. Each unit was saved as a source file (.fla), allowing later changes to be made, as well as an object file (.swf) for online display. Several learning units contain animations in terms of moving lines and arrows to denote specific structures in the sonographic videos. These animations were constructed by adding a layer for each object on the timeline on top of the videos, which creates the appearance of being inside or reaching into the videos.

The Web Kit Freiburg [24] was used as a template for the flash files. The Web Kit Freiburg itself was created in Flash (Adobe Systems Inc., San Jose, CA, USA) and delivered the framework and empty exercises originally created from the WEBGEO [25], in which a large number of the geography college courses were implemented as online tutorials. The user of the online tutorial loads an HTML file, which subsequently refers to all flash files containing the units. The online tutorial was first created in German language and later translated into English. The project's development, testing, and file sharing platform were hosted by the Basic Support for Cooperative Work (BSCW) Internet server of the Goethe-University of Frankfurt am Main, Germany [26].

*2.4. Learning Success Study with Medical Students (Trial A).* A learning success study was conducted only with medical students. The entire study was done over the Internet, enabling every student to work through the online tutorial and take the tests at his own pace without any custom or hands-on training during the trial period. The online tutorial leveraged the WebCT platform [27] which offers the possibility of online testing and to which all students of Frankfurt University have access. The learning success study was composed of 20 multiple-choice questions with 4 answers each, out of which exactly one was correct. This test was copied from a former learning success study about a one-day course program with a combination of lecture and hands-on training entitled "Thorax and Lung Ultrasound in Emergencies/THOLUUSE [13, 14]." The participants of the THOLUUSE study were used as a reference group for comparison. Students took the test three times as pre-test, posttest, and sustainability test, with varied question and answer sequences. The pretest was available for one week, after which the online tutorial became

TABLE 1: Source index of sonographic films and still images used in the online e-learning program modules.

| No. | Image (Name) | Description | Source |
|---|---|---|---|
| 1 | Pleura anatomical sketch | Drawing of pleura, lung, recess, diaphragm, liver | M. Barth |
| 1 | Orientation film | Sonographic film of pleura, lung, recess, diaphragm, liver | T. Hirche |
| 2 | Artifact film | Sonographic film of physiological lung | R. Breitkreutz |
| 3 | Thorax photography | Photography with marked position of the probe | M. Barth |
| 3 | Curtain film | Sonographic film of the curtain phenomenon of the liver | R. Breitkreutz |
| 4 | Dorsal extinction film | Sonographic film of a rip over the lung | T. Hirche |
| 4 | Dorsal gain film | Sonographic film of blood vessels | T. Hirche |
| 5 | Pleural effusion film | Sonographic film of pleural effusion with atelectasis | T. Hirche |
| 5 | Pleural effusion in x-ray | X-ray of pleural effusion, right | T. Hirche |
| 6 | Reverberation film | Sonographic film of Reverberations | R. Breitkreutz |
| 7 | Seashore-Sign film | Sonographic film of a physiological lung in M-Mode | R. Breitkreutz |
| 7 | Bar-code-Sign film | Sonographic film of a pneumothorax in M-Mode | R. Breitkreutz |
| 8 | Pneumothorax | Sonographic film of a pneumothorax in B-Mode | R. Breitkreutz |
| 8 | Pneumothorax x-ray | X-ray of Pneumothorax, left | [28] |
| 9 | Lung point in B-mode | Sonographic film of lung point in B-mode | [29] |
| 9 | Lung point in M-mode | Sonographic image of lung point in M-mode | [30] |
| 9 | Lung point schematic sketch | Schematic explanation of the lung point | [30] |
| 10 | Lung pulse in M-mode | Sonographic film of lung pulse in M-mode | R. Breitkreutz |
| 10 | Lung pulse in B-mode | Sonographic film of lung pulse in B-mode with Doppler | T. Hirche |
| 11 | Trachea anatomical sketch | Drawing of the trachea in transversal sectional image | M. Barth |
| 11 | Trachea longitudinal sonogram | Sonographic longitudinal image of the trachea | R. Breitkreutz |
| 12 | Neck anatomical sketch transversal | Drawing of transversal sectional image of the neck | M. Barth |
| 12 | Trachea transversal sonogram | Sonographic transversal image of the trachea | R. Breitkreutz |
| 13 | Pneumothorax split screen | Sonographic image of a pneumothorax in split screen B-mode and M-mode | [30] |
| 13 | Lung point split screen | Sonographic image of the lung point in split screen B-mode and M-mode | [30] |
| 14 | Lung split screen | Sonographic film of physiological lung in split screen B-mode and M-mode | R. Breitkreutz |
| 15 | Thorax with probe | Thorax with ultrasound probe and 6 sectors for examination | R. Breitkreutz |
| 15 | Lung 6 split screens | 6 images in split screen B-mode and M-mode of different sectors of the thorax, one of which with pneumothorax | R. Breitkreutz |

Table 1: Continued.

| No. | Image (Name) | Description | Source |
|---|---|---|---|
| 16 | Trachea longitudinal for practice | Sonographic longitudinal image of the trachea | R. Breitkreutz |
| 16 | Trachea transversal for practice | Sonographic transversal image of trachea | R. Breitkreutz |
| 17 | Pleural effusion film | Sonographic film of pleural effusion with atelectasis (as on screen No. 5) | T. Hirche |
| 18 | Alveolointerstitial syndrome | Sonographic film lung contusion, multiple B-lines | [29] |
| 18 | Lung consolidation | Sonographic film of consolidated lung parenchyma | R. Breitkreutz |
| 18 | peripheral parenchymal lesions | Sonographic image with multiple peripheral parenchymal lesions | [29] |
| 18 | peripheral parenchymal lesion | Sonographic image with multiple peripheral parenchymal lesion and B-line | [29] |
| 19 | Air bronchogram | Sonographic image of lunge with air bronchogram | [31] |
| 20 | Lung infarction | Sonographic image of lung infarction after pulmonary embolism | [31] |
| 20 | Triangular lung infarction | Sonographic image of triangular lung infarction after pulmonary embolism | [32] |
| 20 | Rounded lung infarction | Sonographic image of rounded lung infarction after pulmonary embolism | [32] |
| 21 | Pulmonary edema with 5 B-lines | Sonographic film of a pulmonary edema with 5 B-lines | [33] |
| 21 | Pulmonary edema with confluent B-lines | Sonographic film of a pulmonary edema with confluent B-lines | [34] |

M. Barth, T. Hirche and R. Breitkreutz provided pictures from their private archives.

available for two weeks. Following the tutorial, the posttest was administered within the 4th week, after which the online tutorial was no longer available for knowledge refreshment. After a two-week waiting period without access to the e-learning program, participants were allowed for one week at the seventh week of the study to take the sustainability test. At no time during the trial were the participants given access to the answer key. To augment participation compliance, ten monetary prizes between 20 and 50 Euros were distributed to the top scorers. According to the study design, only those students who participated in all three tests were incorporated into the final statistical consideration (Figure 1).

*2.5. Evaluation of the Online Tutorial by Medical Students.* The participants of the learning success study were subsequently asked to evaluate the online tutorial. This evaluation was carried out using the Internet tool survey monkey [35] and the questions were scaled discretely from 0 to 10 (Table 2). The participants were additionally asked about the time (in minutes) they spent working through the online tutorial.

*2.6. Evaluation of the Online Tutorial by Medical Doctors (Trial B).* Four weeks prior to the one-day training courses on thorax, trachea, and lung sonography, the online tutorial was provided to medical doctors as a preparation for the course [13]. The participants received logins and passwords for the BSCW server. After their training course, they were asked to evaluate the online tutorial using a 13-question linear analogue self-assessment (LASA) survey. Each question was displayed individually on an A4 landscape-format page accompanied by a single, horizontal, 20 cm line without numbers. Participants could mark the line in between two extremes (example question as warm up "How was the coffee today?" ranging from "very bad" to "very good"). The marks were measured to an accuracy of 1 mm and those measurements converted into percent values (Table 3). The participating medical doctors were also given the opportunity to make additional comments on the second page of the survey.

*2.7. Statistical Methods.* Data analysis and sample size planning were performed using BIAS 9.04 (BIAS, epsilon Verlag, Frankfurt, Germany). Wilcoxon matched pairs test was used for analysis of pre- and postintervention test results. A $P$ value of less than 0.05 was considered to be significant, thus indicating group differences. Distributions of variables are indicated as mean, median, and 25th/75th percentiles and shown as box plots. We aimed for descriptive explorative data analysis only. Case number calculation by a biostatistician control centre (Dr. H. Ackermann, Institute for Biostatistics and Mathematical Modeling, Hospital of the University of Frankfurt, Frankfurt am Main, Germany)

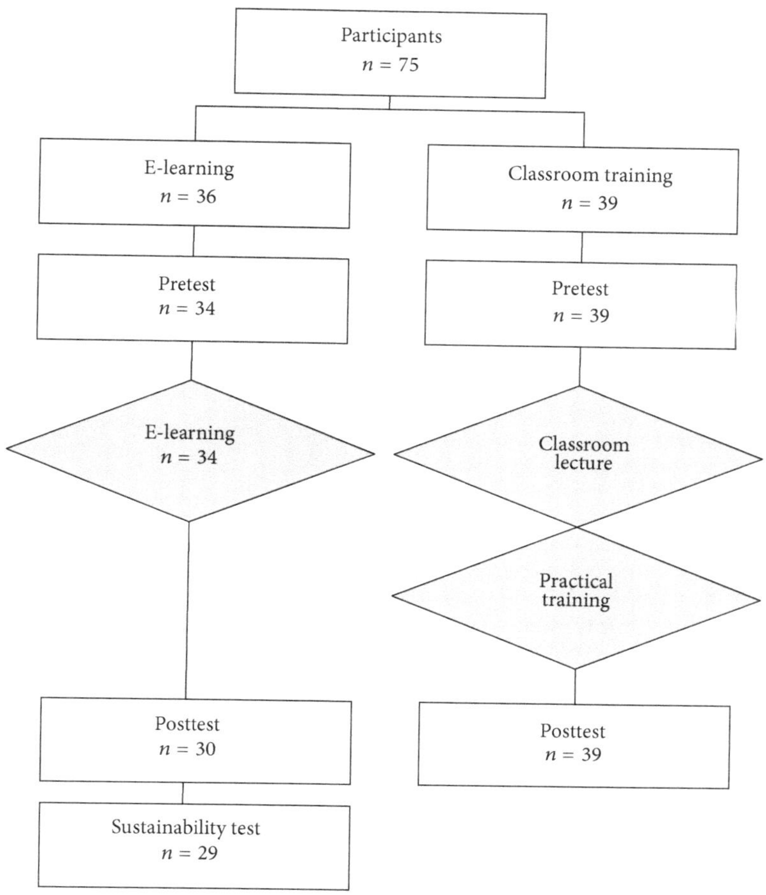


FIGURE 1: Flow diagram of all study participants. The classroom training cohort was part of the THOLUUSE study (with permission [14]).

revealed a minimum number of students completing all study parts of fifteen.

## 3. Results

*3.1. Expert Evaluation.* Before the e-learning was used by our test group, an English version was evaluated by nine experts of the International Lung Ultrasound Consensus Conference [8]. This assured the quality of the tutorial prior to the start of testing and the conformity to consensus terminology. Thus, limitations in completeness and precision were improved, although not all of the 73 consensus statements were included as we did not want to integrate highly specialized lessons (e.g., ARDS) in the tutorial (Table 1). Remarkably, both main questions related to prelearning and use in their own training programmes were answered with a score of more than 90% (Figure 2).

### *3.2. Quantitative and Qualitative Evaluation by Students (Trial A)*

*3.2.1. Quantitative Evaluation.* Of the 36 registered participants, 29 completed all three tests (81%), thus exceeding the required number ($n = 15$) determined by the study design.

TABLE 2: Questions of qualitative evaluation survey of the e-learning program using the internet tool Survey Monkey. Questions were scaled discretely from 0 to 10.

| |
|---|
| The 6 questions regarding study and program setup and organization, personal initiative and learning success read as follows:" |
| (1) How well was the study organized? |
| (2) How good was your prior knowledge of sonography? |
| (3) How suitable was WebCT as a framework for the e-learning program? |
| (4) How high was your motivation for the e-learning program? |
| (5) How good was your overall impression of the e-learning program? |
| (6) How great was your learning success? |

The participating students scored significantly higher in the posttest and sustainability test than they did in the pretest (Figure 3).

*3.2.2. Pretest versus Posttest.* The mean score on the pretest was 11.7 (median 12, 25%; 75% percentile 9.5; 13.5,) while the mean of the posttest was 17.0 (median 17, 25%; 75%

Table 3: Questions of qualitative evaluation survey of the e-learning program using linear analogue self-assessment by medical doctors.

| |
|---|
| (1) How do you evaluate the subject matter? |
| (2) How well were the modules defined? |
| (3) Were enough details presented? |
| (4) Could you recognize the structures on the ultrasound clips? |
| (5) Was a central theme apparent throughout the modules? |
| (6) How significant was your knowledge gain? |
| (7) Was the time requirement acceptable? |
| (8) How well prepared do you feel for the practical course? |
| (9) How much time were you able to invest in the e-learning course? |
| (10) How many units did you complete? |
| (11) How well were you able to operate the e-learning program? |
| (12) How solvable were the tasks in the e-Learning program? |
| (13) How high was your motivation level for e-Learning? |

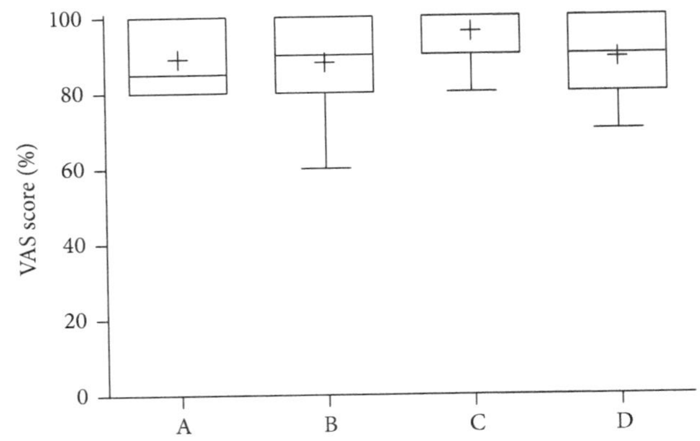


Figure 2: Evaluation of the online tutorials by lung ultrasound experts ($n = 9$, members of Volpicelli et al. [8]). Experts revised as peer group the e-learning by grading the content within a data sheet blinded to each other. Questions aimed to assess key questions: A: completeness? B: precision? C: sufficient as prelearning? D: would you use it at your own training programme?

percentile 16; 19), equalling a relative improvement of 45.1% ($P < 0.0001$ in Wilcoxon's matched pairs test). Individually, 26 of 29 students displayed an improvement in score, two had a decline (which were also the worst scores in the posttest overall), and one had no change in score. Nearly half (14/29) of all participants achieved a score of 18/20 or higher (90%), suggesting a very positive learning effect (Figure 3).

*3.2.3. Pretest versus Sustainability Test.* Similarly to that of the posttest, the sustainability test mean of 16.6 (median 17, 25%; 75% percentile 15; 18) was significantly higher than that of the pretest mean of 11.7 (median 12, 25%; 75% percentile 9.5; 13.5), displaying a relative improvement of 41.8% ($P < 0.0001$ in Wilcoxon's matched pairs test). Only one of the 29 participants had a lower score in the sustainability test as compared to the pretest (Figure 3).

*3.2.4. Posttest versus Sustainability Test.* In comparison to the pre-test, both the posttest and sustainability test showed significant improvement. The results of the posttest 17 (median 17, 25%; 75% percentile 16; 19) and sustainability test 16.6 mean (median 17, 25%; 75% percentile 15; 18) did not differ significantly from each other ($P = 0.237$), suggesting a positive long-term learning effect amongst the participants of the e-learning lung ultrasound program (Figure 3).

*3.2.5. Comparison of E-Learning with THOLUUSE.* Although the theoretical knowledge and learning success test were identical to that of the parent study, THOLUUSE [13] in which both theoretical and practical knowledge were conveyed in a day-long, attendance-based thorax and lung ultrasound course, it is important to acknowledge that the e-learning program is not able to incorporate the practical knowledge transfer that imparts the critical psychomotor skills required for ultrasound application. In addition to the identical multiple-choice test used, the results were also very similar in both studies. In both courses, the mean and median values of the pretest (e-learning mean: 11.7, median: 12, 25%;

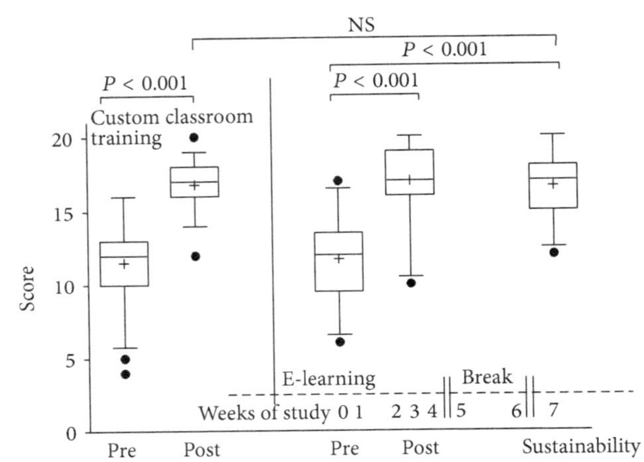


Figure 3: Comparison of two learning strategies: e-Learning versus custom classroom training. Absolute score indicates results of a pre- and posttest multiple choice questionnaire including 20 knowledge or image questions. Left of vertical line: results of learning success of a one-day presence only training on lung ultrasound "THOLUUSE" including 50% hands-on of ($n = 54$) medical doctors without E-Learning (taken from Breitkreutz et al. [14]). Right of dashed line: learning with e-learning but without custom classroom or hands-on training. E-Learning access was available within a learning phase of 4 weeks followed by a break without access of 2 weeks and completion with a sustainability test within the 7th week, results of $n = 29$ medical students. E-Learning was as effective as presence training regarding knowledge gain. (Boxslots contain median; line, box with 25/75 percentile, whiskers 5/95%, outliers, plus sign: mean), NS: not significant.

75% percentile: 9.5; 13.5, THOLUUSE mean: 11.5, median: 12, 25%; 75% percentile: 10; 13) as well as the posttest (e-learning mean: 17, median: 17, 25%; 75% percentile: 16; 19, THOLUUSE mean: 16.8, median: 17, 25%; 75% percentile 16; 18) and sustainability test (e-learning median 17, 25%; 75% percentile 15; 18) were identical. The average relative

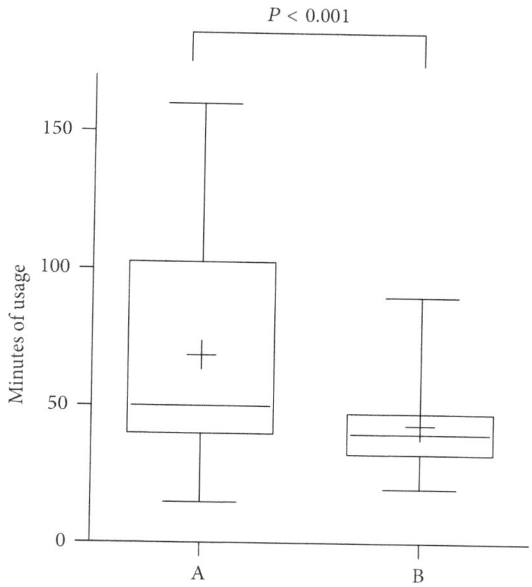


FIGURE 4: Self-evaluation of time spent with the online tutorial. A: $n = 14$; medical students after learning success study using survey monkey. B: $n = 13$; postgraduate medical doctors as part of the VAS questionnaires using paper-based questionnaires.

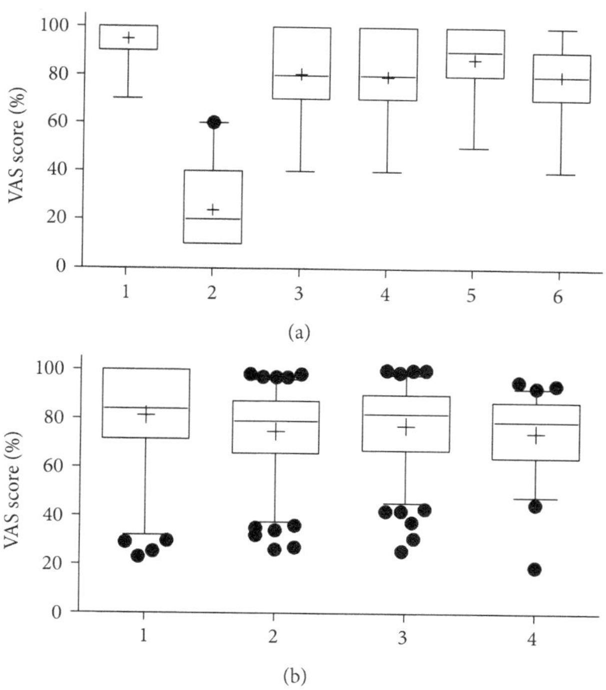


FIGURE 5: Self-evaluation at a discrete scale (0–10) of the online tutorial after completion, (a): of the learning success study by $n = 19$ medical students using Survey Monkey. 1: organization of the E-Learning, 2: own prior knowledge in lung ultrasound, 3: web-CT platform comfort, 4: own motivation, 5: general impression, 6: own learning success, (b): of $n = 34$ medical doctors after completion of preparation of the THOLUUSE training prelearning. Results of questions were grouped into areas of interest.1: personal effort, 2: scientific contents, 3: technical feasibility, 4: own learning success.

improvement in both tests was also very similar (45.1% and 41.81% e-learning, 45.71% THOLUUSE) (Figure 3).

*3.2.6. Qualitative Evaluation of Medical Students.* Of the 34 students who were asked to do so, 19 returned both a completed evaluation of the program and all tests they had participated in. In addition to 6 questions assessing the effectiveness of the program (Table 2), the students were also asked to estimate the time they took to complete the units. This question was answered by 14 of the 19 students and indicated that most ($n = 8$) users completed the program within a 40 to 60 minute time frame, corresponding to approximately 2-3 minutes per unit. Two students completed all units within 15–20 minutes, averaging less than 1 minute per unit, and three students took between 6 and 8 minutes per unit (Figure 4).

With the clear exception of question 2, the responses were overwhelmingly positive (Figure 4). The study organization was rated highest amongst the students (mean 90, median 100, 25%; 75% percentile 90; 100). The lowest rating, prior knowledge (mean: 20, median: 20, 25%; 75% percentile 10; 40), indicates that the majority of participants in the student-based study had no previous exposure to sonography. The rather high ratings of question 3 (mean: 80, median: 80, 25%; 75% percentile 70; 100) likely reflect the fact that many medical students in Frankfurt are familiar with the WebCT program and therefore had few or no problems operating it. The students rated their individual motivation predominantly positively (mean: 70, median: 80, 25%; 75% percentile 70; 100), corresponding to the positive self-assessment of motivation in the qualitative post-training survey of medical doctors. The e-learning program itself was rated second highest (mean: 80, median: 90, 25%; 75% percentile 80; 100), which likely indicates that many students have been exposed to similar pathways of online study and could use these for comparison. Personal assessment of individual learning success was also rated positively (mean: 80, median: 80, 25%; 75% percentile 70; 90), similar to the feedback of the identical question posed to the medical doctors (Figure 5).

*3.3. Qualitative Evaluation by Medical Doctors (Trial B).* 13 of the 34 completed surveys answered the question, "how long did the e-learning program take you in minutes?" Nine participants required between 30 and 50 minutes to complete the e-learning modules, two took more than 50 minutes, and two fewer than 30. Eleven doctors indicated that they had completed all answers in this reported time (Figure 5).

A total of 34 of 50 distributed surveys were returned with completed evaluations of the 13 questions using LASA.

The medians of each of the 13 questions surpassed 70. The response to question 10, "how significant was your knowledge gain?" (mean: 91, median: 100, 25%; 75% percentile 95; 100) was particularly positive (Figure 5).

The 13 individual questions were grouped into four categories: individual effort (Questions 9, 10, and 13), content evaluation (1, 3, 5, 12), practical application (2, 4, 7, 11), and success (6, 8) (Figure 5).

The category for individual effort received the highest ratings (mean: 79, median: 84, 25%; 75% percentile 72; 100), reflecting the fact that most of the doctors completed the entire program. Ratings were similarly high in the objective evaluations of program content (mean: 75, median: 79, 25%; 75% percentile 66; 87) and user-friendliness (mean: 77, median: 82, 25%; 75% percentile 67; 90) as well as in the subjective assessment of personal learning success (mean: 74, median: 79, 25%; 75% percentile 64; 87) (Figure 5).

The participating medical doctors were given the opportunity to make additional comments on the second page of the survey. Four doctors wrote that they were unable to complete the survey due to time constraints; another reported an unspecified error message, which prevented him from completing the program. Three participants in the first course commented that a user guide for the e-learning program would have been helpful; this was then assembled and distributed in the second course. Several positive comments were received from the participants regarding course and program organisation.

## 4. Discussion

Ultrasound is regarded to be a crucial diagnostic tool in many clinical questions of critical care medicine [36]. It is therefore imperative that ultrasound training is concisely and effectively conveyed to course participants. Appropriate application of ultrasound requires the ability to cognitively recognize and interpret pathological images as well as acquire the images using an ultrasonic device and psychomotor skills, the latter of which must be taught through practical hands-on training. Image recognition and theoretical basics, however, were demonstrated by our study to be effectively conveyed by an online e-learning program which requires neither the financial nor the time commitment that an attendance-based training demands.

The knowledge gain in image recognition and basic sonographic theory is nearly identical to that of its parent study THOLUUSE [13, 14] which was able to demonstrate the effectiveness of a one-day classroom-based training (for thorax, trachea, and lung ultrasound). This strongly suggests that the theoretical portion of such a course could be completed at the participant's convenience previous to the practical, hands-on teaching.

In the evaluations received from the medical doctors, the median values of each of the 13 questions surpassed the score of 70%, enabling the conclusion that most participants were generally satisfied with the organization and content of the e-learning program.

The often-proven advantage of interactive learning in comparison to a lecture-based setting [37–39] is an additional argument for the application of e-learning programs to convey theoretical knowledge. Many previous e-learning studies have confined themselves to classical frontal lecture or student-teacher compositions [17, 18], thereby wasting the opportunity to exploit the advantage of an interactive learning system. The single study utilizing interactive e-learning in ultrasound [40] concerns procedural skills as opposed to the sonoanatomical knowledge the current study conveys. As critical as the psychomotor component of image acquisition is, it is mandatory to acquire the cognitive ability to recognize normal and pathological findings within the images [41]. The necessary interaction required by our e-learning program yielded the positive results that prove that the learned theoretical material is stored beyond the short-term memory of the participant, providing a solid base on which the practical skills of ultrasound diagnostics can be built.

Critics of e-learning question the effectiveness of such a program, which depends heavily not only on the competence of the learner, but also on his or her motivation to set learning goals and realize the steps to achieve them [42]. While motivation did not seem to be a hindrance within the boundaries of our study, further studies need to be carried out to compare actual (as opposed to self-estimated) performance on the practical portion of the training. A possible way to achieve this would be to merge the current study with the THOLUUSE study as a blended learning concept: offering the theoretical portion as e-learning and comparing the results of the subsequent practical training with that of THOLUUSE and as a future expanded concept adding further trainee-centred tools such as work books, quizzes, training in scenarios, and postcourse trainer/trainee interaction.

## 5. Limitations

Study limitations include the inability to randomize the study and the fact that participants were aware in advance of the intention and basic content of the e-learning program. Furthermore, participants were volunteers, which may have skewed motivation-related results in a more positive direction than if the modules had been completed by all students of a particular semester, for example. Several students seemed to speed through the e-learning program at an average rate of 1 minute per module, thus suggesting an overly rash preoccupation with their contents. The high mean scores of the posttest and sustainability test dispute this: despite the relatively quick processing of new knowledge, these inexperienced sonographers were able to apply their skills appropriately and effectively. Another limiting factor is that no sustainability test was performed by the medical doctors. A subsequent study would have to analyze both e-learning and classroom-based learning in a randomized fashion with both pretests and sustainability tests.

## 6. Conclusions

E-learning has great potential to provide a substantial theoretical basis of sonographic principles and image recognition, the results of which are comparable to attendance-based courses. We recommend the use of e-learning to provide this knowledge to the widest audience possible, ensuring long-term retention of learned tenets and provoking interest in further practical training. E-learning is set to become a vital part of theoretical training in lung ultrasound and may induce future trainee-centred blended learning programs.

## Acknowledgment

The authors want to thank Dr. H. Ackermann (Institute for Biostatistics and Mathematical Modeling, Hospital of the University of Frankfurt, Frankfurt am Main, Germany) for his help with the power calculation.

## References

[1] L. Gargani, F. Frassi, G. Soldati, P. Tesorio, M. Gheorghiade, and E. Picano, "Ultrasound lung comets for the differential diagnosis of acute cardiogenic dyspnoea: a comparison with natriuretic peptides," *European Journal of Heart Failure*, vol. 10, no. 1, pp. 70–77, 2008.

[2] R. G. Wilkerson and M. B. Stone, "Sensitivity of bedside ultrasound and supine anteroposterior chest radiographs for the identification of pneumothorax after blunt trauma," *Academic Emergency Medicine*, vol. 17, no. 1, pp. 11–17, 2010.

[3] C. G. Ball, A. W. Kirkpatrick, and D. V. Feliciano, "The occult pneumothorax: what have we learned?" *Canadian Journal of Surgery*, vol. 52, no. 5, pp. E173–E179, 2009.

[4] A. W. Kirkpatrick, R. Brown, S. Crickmer et al., "Hand-held portable sonography for the on-mountain exclusion of a pneumothorax," *Wilderness and Environmental Medicine*, vol. 12, no. 4, pp. 270–272, 2001.

[5] G. Bedetti, L. Gargani, A. Corbisiero, F. Frassi, E. Poggianti, and G. Mottola, "Evaluation of ultrasound lung comets by hand-held echocardiography," *Cardiovascular Ultrasound*, vol. 4, article 34, 2006.

[6] G. Soldati and S. Sher, "Bedside lung ultrasound in critical care practice," *Minerva Anestesiologica*, vol. 75, no. 9, pp. 509–517, 2009.

[7] N. Xirouchaki, E. Magkanas, K. Vaporidi et al., "Lung ultrasound in critically ill patients: comparison with bedside chest radiography," *Intensive Care Medicine*, vol. 37, no. 9, pp. 1488–1493, 2011.

[8] G. Volpicelli, M. Elbarbary, and M. Blaivas, "International evidence-based recommendations for point-of-care lung ultrasound," *Intensive Care Medicine*, vol. 38, no. 4, 2012.

[9] D. Lichtenstein, J.-S. Hulot, A. Rabiller, I. Tostivint, and G. Mezière, "Feasibility and safety of ultrasound-aided thoracentesis in mechanically ventilated patients," *Intensive Care Medicine*, vol. 25, no. 9, pp. 955–958, 1999.

[10] P. H. Mayo, H. R. Goltz, M. Tafreshi, and P. Doelken, "Safety of ultrasound-guided thoracentesis in patients receiving mechanical ventilation," *Chest*, vol. 125, no. 3, pp. 1059–1062, 2004.

[11] S. Röhrig, A. Seibel, P. M. Zechner et al., "Thoracoabdominal sonography (E-FAST plus)—AI training module 5 in anaesthesiologist: performed focussed sonography," *Anästhesiologie, Intensivmedizin, Notfallmedizin, Schmerztherapie*, vol. 46, no. 11-12, pp. 772–781, 2011.

[12] P. H. Mayo, Y. Beaulieu, P. Doelken et al., "American college of chest physicians/la societédé réanimation de langue française statement on competence in critical care ultrasonography," *Chest*, vol. 135, no. 4, pp. 1050–1060, 2009.

[13] M. Steigerwald, *THOLUUSE (Thorax-, Trachea- und Lungensonographie in der Intensiv- und Notfallmedizin): Entwicklung und Überprüfung eines neuen Kurskonzeptes, Fachbereich Medizin [Med Dissertation]*, Johann Wolfgang Goethe Universität, Frankfurt , Germany, 2009.

[14] R. Breitkreutz, M. Steigerwald, P. Scheiermann et al., "Thorax, trachea and lung ultrasonography in emergency and critical care medicine (THOLUUSE): assessment of an objective structured training concept," *Emergency Medicine International*. In press.

[15] E. Platz, A. Liteplo, S. Hurwitz, and J. Hwang, "Are live instructors replaceable? Computer vs. classroom lectures for EFAST training," *Journal of Emergency Medicine*, vol. 40, no. 5, pp. 534–538, 2011.

[16] J. Sandars and M. Langlois, "E-learning and the educator in primary care: responding to the challenge," *Education for Primary Care*, vol. 16, no. 2, pp. 129–133, 2005.

[17] E. Filippucci, G. Meenagh, A. Ciapetti, A. Iagnocco, A. Taggart, and W. Grassi, "E-learning in ultrasonography: a web-based approach," *Annals of the Rheumatic Diseases*, vol. 66, no. 7, pp. 962–965, 2007.

[18] E. Platz, K. Goldflam, M. Mennicke, E. Parisini, M. Christ, and C. Hohenstein, "Comparison of web-versus classroom-based basic ultrasonographic and efast training in 2 European hospitals," *Annals of Emergency Medicine*, vol. 56, no. 6, pp. 660.e1–667.e1, 2010.

[19] P. Haidet, R. O. Morgan, K. O'Malley, B. J. Moran, and B. F. Richards, "A controlled trial of active versus passive learning strategies in a large group setting," *Advances in Health Sciences Education*, vol. 9, no. 1, pp. 15–27, 2004.

[20] http://www.SonoABCD.org.

[21] Schulmeister, *Grundlagen Hypermedialer Lernsysteme, Theorie-Didaktik-Design*, Oldenbourg Wissenschaftsverlag, 2007.

[22] R. Gagne, *The Conditions of Learning*, Holt Rinehart & Winston, New York, NY, USA, 4th edition, 1985.

[23] Adobe Flash Player, Adobe Systems, San Jose, Calif, USA, 2010, http://www.adobe.com/products/flashruntimes/statistics.html.

[24] Web-Kit-Freiburg, Eine Entwicklungsumgebung für Online-Lernmodule mit Macromedia Flash Dokumentation 2.0.0, 2007, http://www.rz.uni-freiburg.de/services/elearning/ewerkzeuge/autorentools/webkitfr.

[25] WEBGEO, June 2013, http://www.webgeo.de.

[26] BSCW: Basic Support for Cooperative Work, 2010, http://bscw.de.

[27] Blackboard, 2007, http://www.blackboard.com.

[28] Wikipedia, http://en.wikipedia.org/wiki/File:Pneumothorax_CXR.jpg.

[29] G. Soldati, A. Testa, F. R. Silva, L. Carbone, G. Portale, and N. G. Silveri, "Chest ultrasonography in lung contusion," *Chest*, vol. 130, no. 2, pp. 533–538, 2006.

[30] D. A. Lichtenstein, G. Mezière, N. Lascols et al., " Ultrasound diagnosis of occult pneumothorax," *Critical Care Medicine*, vol. 33, no. 6, pp. 1231–1238, 2005.

[31] G. Mathis, "Thoraxsonographie—teil 2: subpleurale lungenläsionen," *PRAXIS*, vol. 93, no. 17, pp. 719–724, 2004.

[32] G. Mathis, W. Blank, A. Reissig et al., "Thoracic ultrasound for diagnosing pulmonary embolism: a prospective multicenter study of 352 patients," *Chest*, vol. 128, no. 3, pp. 1531–1538, 2005.

[33] B. Bouhemad, M. Zhang, Q. Lu, and J.-J. Rouby, "Clinical review: bedside lung ultrasound in critical care practice," *Critical Care*, vol. 11, article 205, 2007, http://www.ncbi.nlm.nih.gov/pmc/articles/PMC2151891/bin/cc5668-S2.avi.

[34] B. Bouhemad, M. Zhang, Q. Lu, and J.-J. Rouby, "Clinical review: bedside lung ultrasound in critical care practice," *Critical Care2007*, vol. 11, article 205, http://www.ncbi.nlm.nih.gov/pmc/articles/PMC2151891/bin/cc5668-S3.avi.

[35] Survey Monkey, http://www.surveymonkey.com/.

[36] L. Neri, E. Storti, and D. Lichtenstein, "Toward an ultrasound curriculum for critical care medicine," *Critical Care Medicine*, vol. 35, no. 5, pp. S290–S304, 2007.

[37] B. S. Bryner, D. Saddawi-Konefka, and T. R. Gest, "The impact of interactive, computerized educational modules on preclinical medical education," *Anatomical Sciences Education*, vol. 1, no. 6, pp. 247–251, 2008.

[38] P. J. O'Byrne, A. Patry, and J. A. Carnegie, "The development of interactive online learning tools for the study of Anatomy," *Medical Teacher*, vol. 30, no. 8, pp. e260–e271, 2008.

[39] J. Sweller, "Cognitive load theory, learning difficulty, and instructional design," *Learning and Instruction*, vol. 4, no. 4, pp. 295–312, 1994.

[40] J. Chenkin, S. Lee, T. Huynh, and G. Bandiera, "Procedures can be learned on the web: a randomized study of ultrasound-guided vascular access training," *Academic Emergency Medicine*, vol. 15, no. 10, pp. 949–954, 2008.

[41] N. Flindt, "E-learning. Theoriekonzepte und Praxiswirklichkeit," Saarbrücken, Germany: VDM Dr. Müller, 397s, 2007.

[42] S. Price, H. Ilper, S. Uddin et al., "Peri-resuscitation echocardiography: training the novice practitioner," *Resuscitation*, vol. 81, no. 11, pp. 1534–1539, 2010.

# 7

# The Impact on Emergency Department Utilization and Patient Flows after Integrating with a General Practitioner Cooperative

**W. A. M. H. Thijssen,[1,2,3] M. Wijnen-van Houts,[1] J. Koetsenruijter,[2] P. Giesen,[2] and M. Wensing[2]**

[1] *Catharina Hospital, Michelangelolaan 2, P.O. Box 1350, 5602ZA NB Eindhoven, The Netherlands*
[2] *IQ Scientific Institute for Quality of Healthcare (IQ Healthcare), Radboud University Nijmegen Medical Centre, IQ P.O. Box 9101, Healthcare 114, 6500HBGLO Nijmegen, The Netherlands*
[3] *Emergency Department, Catharina Hospital, Eindhoven P.O. Box 1350, 5602ZA NB Eindhoven, The Netherlands*

Correspondence should be addressed to W. A. M. H. Thijssen; wendy.thijssen@cze.nl

Academic Editor: Chak W. Kam

*Introduction*. A new model, an emergency care access point (ECAP) for after-hours emergency care, is emerging in The Netherlands. This study assessed the effect on emergency department (ED) utilization and patient flows. *Methods*. Routinely recorded clinical ED patient data, covering a six-year period, was collected. Segmented regression analysis was used to analyze after-hours changes over time. *Results*. 59.182 patients attended the ED before the start of the ECAP and 51.513 patients after, a decrease of 13%. Self-referred ED patients decreased 99.5% (OR 0.003; 95% CI 0.002–0.004). Referred patients increased by 213.4% and ED hospital admissions increased by 20.2%. A planned outpatient follow-up increased by 5.8% (OR 1.968 95% CI 1.870–2.071). The latter changed from fewer contacts to more contacts (OR 1.015 95% CI 1.013–1.017). Consultations at the regional genereral practitioner cooperative (GPC) increased by 26.0% (183.782 versus 232.246). *Conclusion*. ECAP implementation resulted in a decrease in ED utilization, a near absence of self-referring patients, and a higher probability of hospital admission and clinical follow-up. This suggests either an increase of ED patients with a higher acuity or a lower threshold of admitting referred patients compared to self-referred patients. Overall, increased collaboration with after-hours primary care and emergency care seemed to optimize ED utilization.

## 1. Introduction

Organizing after-hours care is an important challenge in many countries. After-hours care is provided between 5 p.m. and 8 a.m., on weekends and national holidays. In most western countries emergency departments (EDs) are confronted with overcrowding, while general practitioners (GPs) are not all easily accessible, especially after hours. Differences in national healthcare systems have a noticeable effect on redirecting patients to primary care services. In the United States, studies show an increase of 23–27% in ED visits between 1997 and 2008 [1, 2]. Simultaneously, delivering primary care access after hours decreased from 40% of the GPs in 2006 to 29% in 2009 and different models exist [3–5]. In western Europe, the GP plays a significant role in providing after-hours care, with 77% of the GPs in Italy, 89% in the UK, and 97% in The Netherlands providing after-hours arrangements [3]. Across Europe, different models of after-hours primary care exist, varying from local rotation groups to large General Practitioner Cooperatives (GPCs) [6, 7]. Despite good primary care access, high and rising ED visits are also an issue in Europe [8].

In the Dutch healthcare system, precise numbers are lacking, but an estimated average of 1.9–2.1 million patients visited the ED per year between 2004 and 2008, with 135 treatments per 1000 inhabitants per year [9]. The GP is the coordinator of access to the hospital specialist for the majority of emergency care. Primary care is provided

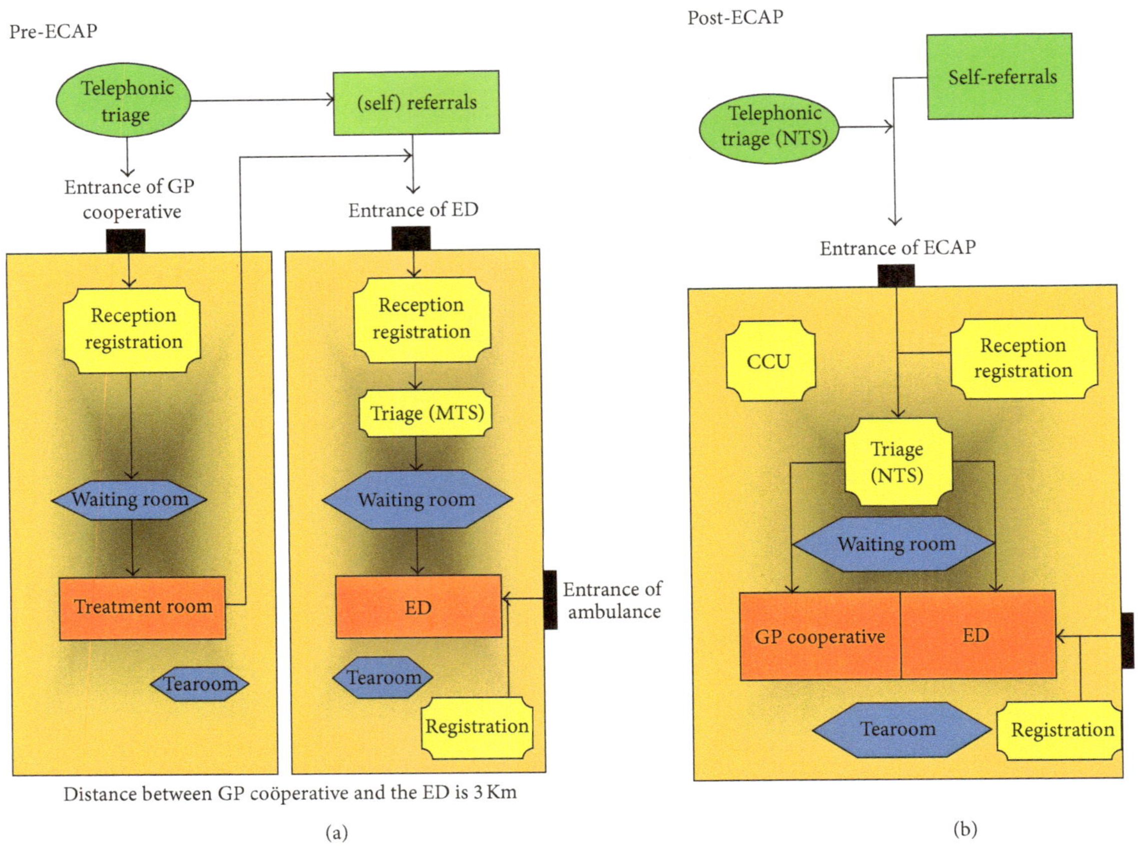


FIGURE 1: The GP can order blood tests during ECAP hours and order X-rays until 10 p.m., without referring the patient to the ED. This is similar to office hours.

24 hours a day, 7 days a week. It is always free at the point of entry, while patient copayments are required for visits to the ED. During office hours, GPs provide patient care in their office-based practices, including emergency care. Patients can contact their GP through the practice phone number for a telephone advice, a consultation or a home visit. Self-referred patients, who present to the ED during office hours and who are eligible for a GP consultation, are given the option to contact their own GP for an appointment. If they insist on receiving medical care in the ED, they are registered for treatment in the ED. The organization of after-hours primary care has changed in recent years from rota groups to GPCs, mainly to reduce GPs' workload and also to improve the quality of after-hours care. Since 2000, large-scale GPCs have emerged in the Netherlands, with around 130 GPCs serving the Dutch population of nearly 17 million inhabitants [6, 9, 10]. Nonetheless, there is a rise in self-referrals to the ED, because patients can still choose to visit the ED directly and bypass the GPC. To enhance efficiency, decrease overcrowding and costs of after-hours care by redirecting the patient that does not need hospital care to the GP, an organizational model has been proposed that integrates the GPC and the ED into a colocation with one emergency care access point (ECAP), Figure 1.

At this integrated emergency care access point (ECAP), triage will determine whether patients will be seen by a GP or by a physician in the ED. Only a few integrated models exist at this point. Influenced by local successes, several GPCs and EDs are planning to integrate in the near future. Despite the growing interest, little is known of the ECAP effect on flow of ED patients and their planned follow-up. Several small studies over a short period show different results varying from no flow change to a shift of 15–53% of patients from the ED to the GPC [11–20].

In our study, we took advantage of a natural organizational change, which occurred in the south east region of The Netherlands. The local GPC integrated with the ED of an inner city hospital during after-hours care, creating a colocation with one emergency care access point.

The objective of this study was to examine the effect of an ECAP on ED utilization and planned patient follow-up. We expected that a large part of the self-referrals could be redirected to the GPC, leading to a decrease in ED utilization. Furthermore we expected an increase of hospital admissions and out-patient clinical follow-up, since the GP is more likely to refer patients to the colocated ED then to another hospital.

## 2. Materials and Methods

We conducted a longitudinal observational study in an integrated after-hours care model between an urban emergency department (ED) and a general practitioner cooperative

(i) One entrance with one desk for both GP and ED patients
(ii) Preferred access via a single regional telephone number
(iii) Access daily from 5 p.m. till 8 a.m. and on weekends and national holidays
(iv) Trained chauffeurs in recognizable fully equipped GP cars for home visits
(v) ICT support including electronic patient files and electronic feedback to the patient's own GP
(vi) Triage nurses (GP or ED nurses) in contact by telephone and on side
(vii) GP shifts of 6–8 hours
(ix) Ambulance patients are directly seen in the ED

Box 1: Features of an integrated GPC and ED (ECAP).

(GPC) in the southeast region of The Netherlands, serving a population of around 325.000 people. In this model, the ED and the GPC, who formerly worked separately, now integrated forming a colocation with one emergency care access point (ECAP), (Figure 1). To determine the ECAP effect on the trend of ED patient flows, we compared routinely collected ED data three years before and three years after the implementation of the ECAP. Since there is no colocation during office hours, meaning that patients can bypass the GP, we also collected ED data during non-ECAP hours to see overall changes in trends. We hypothesized an increase in GPC patients and, therefore, also collected GPC data to analyze changes before and after the ECAP implementation. The medical ethical committee of the hospital granted institutional review board exemption.

*2.1. Organizational Changes.* Before the study, the ED and the GPC were located in different areas in the city, 3 kilometres apart. Although patients were encouraged to contact the GPC first, they could choose to visit the ED at their own initiative. The collaboration of the ED and the GPC to form an ECAP with one triage system in December 2008 changed this. It meant a difference in the routing of the patient after-hours because the patient could no longer willingly bypass the GP (Box 1). The ECAP is open from 5 p.m. till 8 a.m. during weekdays, the weekend, and national holidays. As before the change, patients are encouraged to phone the GPC first via a regional telephone number, when they seek medical help during ECAP hours. The after-hours change into an ECAP and the ways to contact the GP were promoted by flyers in the ED, GPC, and in waiting rooms of both the hospital and all regional GPs and by advertisements in local newspapers, prior to the implementation. A call center for the regional telephone number is colocated with the ECAP and is manned by telephone operators who are trained in using The Netherlands triage system (NTS) to determine patient urgency. NTS is a triage system that is developed and validated in The Netherlands to work for the ambulance services, GPCs, and EDs [21]. It determines the urgency, type of medical advice (consult, home visit, or telephone advice) and type of healthcare provider (ambulance, GP, or ED). A GP at the call center supervises all phone calls. Depending on the complaint and telephone triage outcome, patients will either receive a telephone advice, an appointment with a GP at the ECAP, a GP home visit or they will be directly referred to the ED. If necessary, the ECAP can send out an ambulance as well. Independently of the ECAP, there is also the national emergency phone number, 112, that patients can phone 24/7, to request an ambulance. Self-referred patients who do not phone and turn up at the ECAP are registered and triaged with NTS by a trained triage nurse. Depending on their triage outcome, patients either receive a scheduled appointment at the GPC or are directly referred to the ED. The GP supervises the triage nurse; therefore, all patients that are directly referred to the ED after triage are registered as GP referrals. Patients who have been treated by a hospital physician either in the outpatient clinic or through a hospital admission, within three months prior to presenting at the ECAP, were automatically referred to the ED and registered as a return visit. This was a local agreement between GPs and hospital physicians prior to the start of the ECAP. The GP can request simple blood tests 24/7 and X-rays until 10 p.m., without having to refer the patient to the ED, similar to office hours.

*2.2. Study Setting.* The studied ED is the only ED in the city and is situated just outside the city centre, serving the major part of the city and the northern region outside the city. There used to be another hospital with a small ED that closed down in August 2008, during the time frame of our study, three months before the study intervention.

The GPC is a large cooperation that has three locations in the region, serving 510.000 people. Two locations are outside the city. The studied GPC in the city was initially located three kilometers from the ED before integrating.

*2.3. Measures.* For the ED, we gathered data from the CS-EZIS system, Chipsoft BV, which is a computerized system routinely used for real time management of patients. Every patient that presents to the ED is registered in this system. We collected clinical data of the ED, covering a six-year period from 2006 to 2012, three years before and three years after the start of the emergency care access point (ECAP). Because the ECAP started on 1 December 2008, we considered this a transition month and did not include this month in our data. For comparison reasons, we therefore also excluded data from December 2011, making the pre ECAP period and the post ECAP period equal, namely 35 months.

For the ECAP hours, we collected patient characteristics as gender and age. For patient origin, the EZIS system has 7 categories: self-referral, GP referral, ambulance referral, return visit, outpatient clinical referral, radiology referral

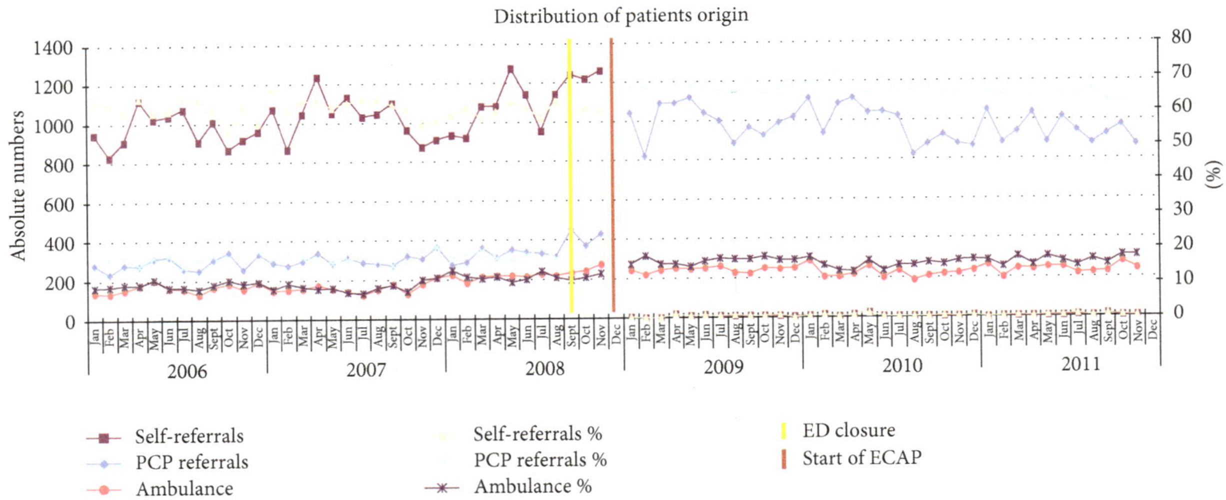


FIGURE 2: Distribution of patients origin. For visual reasons the percentage of revisits, referrals from outpatient clinics or other hospitals is not shown in this figure.

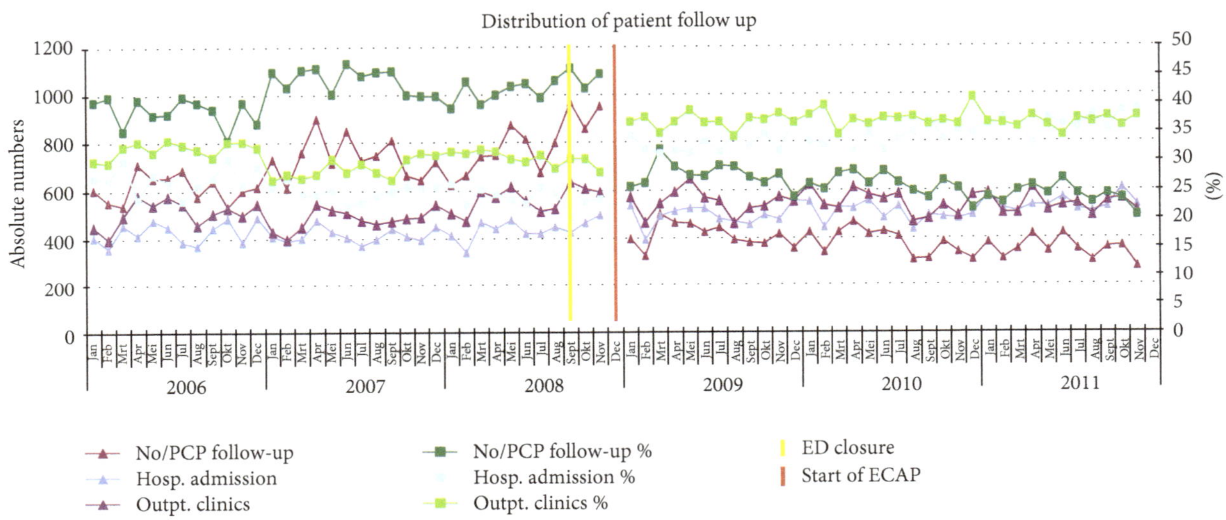


FIGURE 3: Distribution of patient follow-up. For visual reasons the percentage of deceased in the ED and transfer to another hospital is not shown in this figure. These percentages are very low and remained unchanged.

(e.g., a proven fracture), and referrals from another hospital. We also collected data about the next clinical step after the ED visit, where the EZIS system also has 7 categories: no follow-up, GP follow-up, outpatient clinical follow-up, hospital admission, transfer to another hospital, left without being seen, and either died in the ED or brought in dead.

We also collected absolute ED patient numbers from non-ECAP hours to look at the overall trend of ED visits. Finally we collected regional GPC data on the number of ECAP visits, telephone advice, and home visits before and after the start of the ECAP.

*2.4. Data Analysis.* For the comparison of descriptive characteristics of patients before and after the start of the ECAP, we used the chi-square test. We calculated numbers and percentages. A logistic segmented regression analysis was performed to test the changes after implementation of the ECAP as shown in Figures 2 and 3. This method estimates separately the change over time before the intervention, the direct effect of the intervention itself, and the change over time after the intervention. $P < 0.05$ was considered significant. Outcome variables were self-referrals versus non-self-referrals and an outpatient clinical follow-up contact versus no clinical follow-up contact (the combined categories of no follow-up contact and a GP follow-up contact). The regression model controlled for the effect of age and gender. We used SPSS 19.0 for our statistical analysis.

The following categories were used: hospital admission, outpatient clinical follow-up and no outpatient clinical follow-up (GP follow-up or no follow-up combined). Two periods were distinguished: before the start of the ECAP (1 January 2006 till 1 December 2008) and after the start of

Table 1: After-hours ED patient characteristics; numbers and percentages of patients, total of 3 years before and 3 years after the start of the ECAP.

| | Before 2006–2008* | | After[II] 2009–2011* | |
|---|---|---|---|---|
| | N | % | N | % |
| Total non-ECAP hours | | | | |
| 94.778 | 44.190 | — | 50.588 | — |
| Total ECAP hours | | | | |
| 110.696 | 59.182 | 100 | 51.513 | 100 |
| Gender | | | | |
| Male | 32.283 | 54.5 | 26.843 | 52.1 |
| Age in years | | | | |
| 1–17 | 13.873 | 23.4 | 10.264 | 19.9 |
| 18–29 | 10.701 | 18.1 | 7.591 | 14.7 |
| 30–49 | 13.698 | 23.1 | 10.674 | 20.7 |
| 50–64 | 8.604 | 14.5 | 8.679 | 16.8 |
| 65–84 | 10.698 | 18.1 | 11.980 | 23.3 |
| ≥85 | 1.608 | 2.7 | 2.325 | 4.5 |
| Time of visit | | | | |
| 8 a.m.–5 p.m.[†] | 16.285 | 27.5 | 14.304 | 27.8 |
| 5 p.m.–11 p.m.[‡] | 30.575 | 51.7 | 25.571 | 49.6 |
| 11 p.m.–8 a.m.[$] | 12.322 | 20.8 | 11.638 | 22.5 |

*Excluding December 2008 and December 2011; [†]weekend days and national holidays; [‡]7 days a week; [$]7 days a week; [II]all changes are significant after the ECAP using chi-square testing.

the ECAP (1 January 2009 till 1 December 2011), 35 months in each period.

## 3. Results

In the non-ECAP hours, a total of 94.778 patients attended the ED, 44.190 in the period before the start of the ECAP and 50.588 after the start, an increase of 14%. During ECAP hours over the same period, a total of 110.696 patients attended the ED, 59.182 ED patients before the start of the ECAP and 51.513 patients after the start, an overall decrease of 13%. During ECAP hours, the majority in both groups, pre- and post-ECAP, were males, 54.5% and 52.1%, respectively. The mean patient age shifted from 39 to 44 years old. The percentage of total ED patients in younger age groups (0–49 years) decreased and older age groups (50 and older) increased with 9.3%. The group of 65 and older increased by 16.2%. The majority of patients presented to the ED in the evening between 5 p.m. and 11 p.m. (51.7% and 49.6%). All changes were significant (Table 1).

Figure 2 shows that in the post-ECAP period, the number of ED self-referrals decreased by 99.5% (36.139 versus 181), GP referrals increased by 213.4% (10.876 versus 34.089) and the number of patients brought in by ambulance increased by 3.2% (6.244 versus 8.222). The logistic segmented regression analysis showed a slight decrease in self-referrals before the introduction of the ECAP (OR 0.997; 95% CI 0.995–0.999). After the intervention, there was an instant, considerable decrease in self-referrals (OR 0.003; 95% CI 0.002–0.004).

After the start of the ECAP, both hospital admissions, 14.854 versus 17.827, as well as outpatient clinical follow-up, 18.003 versus 19.047, increased with 20.2% and 5.8%, respectively. There was a decrease of 46.4% in ED patients referred back to their GP for follow-up or who did not need follow-up at all, 24.896 versus 13.342 (Figure 3). The regression analysis showed that the number of outpatient clinical follow-up contacts and hospital admissions decreased before the introduction of the ECAP (OR 0.993; 95% CI 0.991–0.995). Directly after the introduction of the ECAP, the number of follow-up contacts increased (OR 1.968; 95% CI 1.870–2.071) and the trend changed from less contact to more contacts (OR 1.015; 95% CI 1.013–1.017). All changes were significant.

Table 2 shows the effect of the closing of the other city's ED 3 months prior to starting the ECAP. There is an average increase of 430 ED patient visits per month (31.9%). There was no noticeable change in percentage of self-referrals (59.2% and 60.1%) or GP referrals (18.4 and 20.2%). The increasing trend of no/GP follow-up (5.2% and 1.8%) and decreasing trend of hospital admission (2.6% and 2.0%) remained unchanged after the closing.

Table 3 shows that after implementing the ECAP, the total number of patients having contact with the GPC increased by 30% (330.162 versus 412.545). Patients receiving a consult at the regional GPC increased by 26.0% (183.782 versus 232.246) and patient home visits decreased by 14.3% (33.618 versus 28.818).

## 4. Limitations

With the implementation of the ECAP, the triage system changed from the Manchester triage system (MTS) to The Netherlands triage standard (NTS), and both systems are not comparable. We therefore had to look at hospital admissions and outpatient clinical follow-up for comparison of patients acuity.

Three months before the organizational change, the only other emergency department in the city closed. This led to a shift in patients spreading out over other hospitals in the region, including the studied ED, and this might have affected total patient numbers but should not have had an effect on trends.

The observational design implies that factors outside the ECAP may have contributed to the results. The study used data that were retrospectively analyzed. This study took advantage of a naturally occurring change in a large geographical area, but its relevance for other settings has to be considered.

## 5. Discussion

The implementation of an ECAP led to a decreased ED utilization, with almost no self-referring patients and an increase in ED patients with a hospital admission or planned

TABLE 2: Effect of the closure of another city's ED on patient numbers and percentage on the researched ED.

| * | ECAP | Patient N | Origin Self-referral %[†] | GP referral | Ambulance | Follow-up No/GP follow-up %[†] | Hosp. admissions | Outpatient clinic |
|---|---|---|---|---|---|---|---|---|
| 2006 | Before | 4697 | 59.2 | 19.2 | 10.6 | 37.7 | 27.9 | 32.5 |
| 2007 | Before | 4902 | 59.8 | 18.4 | 9.8 | 42.9 | 25.3 | 29.5 |
| 2008 | Before | 6193 | 60.1 | 20.2 | 12.0 | 44.7 | 22.3 | 29.5 |
| 2009 | After | 4307 | 0.5 | 67.0 | 17.0 | 27.1 | 33.1 | 37.7 |
| 2010 | After | 4110 | 0.2 | 65.3 | 15.8 | 25.1 | 35.6 | 36.6 |
| 2011 | After | 4399 | 0.4 | 62.9 | 16.9 | 22.7 | 37.9 | 37.1 |

*Each year contains a three-month period covering September, October, and November. In the before period, the ECAP had not been implemented, and the ED closure in 2008 is the only regional change in the emergency healthcare setting. In the after period, the ECAP is implemented as well. [†]Mean percentage.

TABLE 3: Patient numbers at the regional GPC before and after the ECAP (after hours).

| Total | Pre-ECAP | | | | Post-ECAP | | | | Total |
|---|---|---|---|---|---|---|---|---|---|
| Year | 2006 | 2007 | 2008 | Subtotal | 2009 | 2010 | 2011 | Subtotal | |
| Telephone advice | 33.866 | 37.485 | 41.411 | **112.762** | 52.541 | 48.481 | 50,459 | **151.481** | **264.243** |
| GPC consultation | 58.062 | 62.345 | 63.375 | **183782** | 77.875 | 77.812 | 76,559 | **232.246** | **416.028** |
| Home visit | 10.773 | 11.385 | 11.460 | **33.618** | 10.741 | 9.156 | 8,921 | **28.818** | **72.436** |
| Total | **102.701** | **111.215** | **116.246** | **330.162** | **141.157** | **135.449** | **135.939** | **412.545** | **752.707** |

The regional GPC consists of three GPCs including the studied GPC. Separate GPC data is not available since it is not registered as such.

outpatient follow-up. These findings suggest that fewer but more patients with a higher acuity attended the ED after the start of the ECAP.

This is one of the first long-term studies to observe the changes in attending ED patients after implementing an ECAP, so it is difficult to compare it with available literature. We found a patient reduction of 13% after the start of the ECAP. It is plausible to assume that patient numbers would have followed the same trend after hours as during office hours (14% increase), had the ECAP not been implemented. The total effect of the ECAP would thus be a decrease of 27% of patients attending the ED. Earlier pilot studies, with short follow-up periods, found a shift of low acuity patients, mostly self-referrals, from the ED to the GPC varying from 15% to 53% [13–21]. Although we could not compare triage outcome, our data supports these findings, since the overall ED patient decrease in our study is mostly due to the shift of the younger, male patients, which is typically the low acuity self-referral. In referred patients the increase of 213% we found is much higher compared to other studies [15–21]. Several factors might have contributed to that increase difference, for instance the closing of the other ED, although overall patient numbers do not seem to imply that. It is more likely that, in contrast to most other studies, the patients in our study cannot bypass the GP and visit the ED directly. Furthermore, the protocol to refer every patient, who has been admitted or seen in the outpatient clinic for similar presenting complaints within the previous three months, is likely to lead to higher referral numbers. Decreasing this arbitrary 3-month period could further decrease the number of patients being referred. With respect to patients follow-up, we found an increase of 20.2% in hospital admissions. This differs from the decrease found in a smaller Dutch study and the 0.2% decrease found by Andersson in a study that was also confronted with closing EDs in the region [17, 18]. An explanation could be that starting an integrated ECAP is likely to increase the adherence with more GP referrals to this specific hospital. It is also likely that the GP has a lower threshold to refer patients to the ED next door rather than transporting to another ED. Similarly, the ED physician is likely to have a lower threshold to admit patients being referred by a GP compared to the self-referral. Apart from the increasing aging patient with comorbidities, this trend of increasing hospital admissions could be due to the ongoing development of rapid diagnostic technologies, early treatment availability, and public education campaigns in recognizing heart attacks and strokes [22].

Similar to a previous study in The Netherlands, we found an increase in number of patients staying within one setting for follow-up [23]. These previous studies show an increase as well as a decrease of outpatient clinical follow-up after an ED referral [17, 23].

Across the world, policy makers are looking for the optimal organization of emergency care [5, 8, 24, 25]. This study suggests that high involvement of primary care providers in emergency care can optimize the efficiency of ED utilization. Patients with serious conditions benefit from the facilities and skills at the ED, while patients with less serious conditions are treated in a primary care setting, reducing ED crowding. The high number of patients receiving planned clinical follow-up might indicate potential for further efficiency gains. Further research is also needed to examine health outcomes in patients attending the ECAP and receiving either primary care or treatment at the ED.

## 6. Conclusion

In summary, the introduction of a regional integrated ECAP in one region in The Netherlands was associated with substantial changes in the flow of patients, including an overall decrease in ED utilization, an almost disappearance of self-referring ED patients, and a higher probability of hospital admission and clinical follow-up at the ED. The latter suggests that either the proportion of patients presenting to the ED with a higher acuity increased or the threshold of admitting referred patient is lower than that of the self-referred patients. The integrated model for emergency care, in which the GP is the first point of contact for patients, works well for The Netherlands. Differences across healthcare systems and after-hours primary care models make it somewhat difficult to predict whether this also applies to other settings, but we suggest that it works well in countries with a well-developed primary care sector.

## Conflict of Interests

The first author of the paper works as an emergency physician in the researched ED. The second author has worked as an emergency medicine trainee in the researched hospital during the process of this research and writing the paper, but is currently working as an emergency physician in another hospital.

## References

[1] N. Tang, J. Stein, R. Y. Hsia, J. H. Maselli, and R. Gonzales, "Trends and characteristics of US emergency department visits, 1997–2007," *Journal of the American Medical Association*, vol. 304, no. 6, pp. 664–670, 2010.

[2] S. R. Pitts, J. M. Pines, M. T. Handrigan, and A. L. Kellermann, "National trends in Emergency Department Occupancy, 2001–2008: effect of inpatient admissions versus Emergency Department Practise intensity," *Annals of Emergency Medicine*, vol. 60, no. 6, pp. 679.e3–686.e3, 2012.

[3] C. Schoen, R. Osborn, P. T. Huynh, M. Doty, J. Peugh, and K. Zapert, "On the front lines of care: primary care doctors' office systems, experiences, and views in seven countries," *Health Affairs*, vol. 25, no. 6, pp. w555–w571, 2006.

[4] C. Schoen, R. Osborn, M. M. Doty, D. Squires, J. Peugh, and S. Applebaum, "A survey of primary care physicians in eleven countries, 2009: perspectives on care, costs, and experiences," *Health Affairs*, vol. 28, no. 6, pp. 1171–1183, 2009.

[5] S. A. O'Malley, D. Samuel, A. Bond, and E. Carrier, "After-hours care and its coordination with primary care in the US," *Journal of General Internal Medicine*, vol. 27, no. 11, pp. 1406–1415, 2012.

[6] L. Huibers, P. Giesen, M. Wensing, and R. Grol, "Out-of-hours care in western countries: assessment of different organizational models," *BMC Health Services Research*, vol. 9, article 105, 2009.

[7] R. Grol, P. Giesen, and C. van Uden, "After-hours care in the United Kingdom, Denmark, and the Netherlands: new models," *Health Affairs*, vol. 25, no. 6, pp. 1733–1737, 2006.

[8] A. Majeed, "Redesigning after-hours primary care," *Annals of Internal Medicine*, vol. 156, no. 1, part 1, pp. 67–68, 2012.

[9] P. C. E. Steenwijk, E. G. S. van der Sterren, C. J. van Vugt, and Samenwerking huisartsenposten en spoedeisende hulp (SEH), "Collaboration between GP cooperatives and Emergency Departments," Report from IQ healthcare in collaboration with The Netherlands GP cooperative Association, 2010.

[10] W. A. M. H. Thijssen, P. H. J. Giesen, and M. Wensing, "Emergency departments in the Netherlands," *Emergency Medicine Journal*, vol. 29, no. 1, pp. 6–9, 2012.

[11] P. Giesen, M. Smits, L. Huibers, R. Grol, and M. Wensing, "Quality of after-hours primary care in the Netherlands: a narrative review," *Annals of Internal Medicine*, vol. 155, no. 2, pp. 108–113, 2011.

[12] E. P. Moll van Charante, G. ter Riet, and P. Bindels, "Self-referrals to the A&E department during out-of-hours: patients' motives and characteristics," *Patient Education and Counseling*, vol. 70, no. 2, pp. 256–265, 2008.

[13] P. Giesen, E. Franssen, H. Mokkink, W. van den Bosch, A. van Vugt, and R. Grol, "Patient either contacting a general practice cooperative or accident and emergency department out of hours: a comparison," *Emergency Medicine Journal*, vol. 23, no. 9, pp. 731–734, 2006.

[14] R. B. Kool, D. J. Homberg, and H. C. M. Kamphuis, "Towards integration of general practitioner posts and accident and emergency departments: a case study of two integrated emergency posts in the Netherlands," *BMC Health Services Research*, vol. 8, article 225, 2008.

[15] C. J. T. van Uden, R. A. G. Winkens, G. Wesseling, H. F. B. M. Fiolet, O. C. P. van Schayck, and H. F. J. M. Crebolder, "The impact of a primary care physician cooperative on the caseload of an emergency department: the Maastricht integrated out-of-hours service," *Journal of General Internal Medicine*, vol. 20, no. 7, pp. 612–617, 2005.

[16] D. M. Pickin, A. O'Cathain, M. Fall, A. B. Morgan, A. Howe, and J. P. Nicholl, "The impact of a general practice co-operative on accident and emergency services, patient satisfaction and GP satisfaction," *Family Practice*, vol. 21, no. 2, pp. 180–182, 2004.

[17] G. Andersson and I. Karlberg, "Lack of integration, and seasonal variations in demand explained performance problems and waiting times for patients at emergency departments: a 3 years evaluation of the shift of responsibility between primary and secondary care by closure of two acute hospitals," *Health Policy*, vol. 55, no. 3, pp. 187–207, 2001.

[18] C. J. T. van Uden, R. A. G. Winkens, G. J. Wesseling, H. F. J. M. Crebolder, and C. P. van Schayck, "Use of out of hours services: a comparison between two organisations," *Emergency Medicine Journal*, vol. 20, no. 2, pp. 184–187, 2003.

[19] H. Philips, R. Remmen, P. van Royen et al., "What's the effect of the implementation of general practitioner cooperatives on caseload? Prospective intervention study on primary and secondary care," *BMC Health Services Research*, vol. 10, article 222, 2010.

[20] F. D. O'Kelly, C. Teljeur, I. Carter, and P. K. Plunkett, "Impact of a GP cooperative on lower acuity emergency department attendances," *Emergency Medicine Journal*, vol. 27, no. 10, pp. 770–773, 2010.

[21] C. J. T. van Uden and H. F. J. M. Crebolder, "Does setting up out of hours primary care cooperatives outside a hospital reduce demand for emergency care?" *Emergency Medicine Journal*, vol. 21, no. 6, pp. 722–723, 2004.

[22] J. D. Schuur and A. K. Venkatesh, "The growing role of Emergency Departments in hospital admissions," *The New England Journal of Medicine*, vol. 367, pp. 391–393, 2012.

[23] L. Huibers, W. Thijssen, J. Koetsenruijter, P. Giesen, R. Grol, and M. Wensing, "GP cooperative and emergency department:

an exploration of patient flows," *Journal of Evaluation in Clinical Practice*, vol. 19, no. 2, pp. 243–249, 2013.

[24] D. Margolius and T. Bodenheimer, "Redesigning after-hours primary care," *Annals of Internal Medicine*, vol. 155, no. 2, pp. 131–132, 2011.

[25] M. I. Gaakeer, C. L. van den Brand, and P. Patka, "Emergency medicine in the Netherlands: a short history provides a solid basis for future challenges," *European Journal of Emergency Medicine*, vol. 19, no. 3, pp. 131–135, 2012.

# 8

# Physiological-Social Scores in Predicting Outcomes of Prehospital Internal Patients

**Abbasali Ebrahimian,[1,2] Hesam Seyedin,[2] Roohangiz Jamshidi-Orak,[3] and Gholamreza Masoumi[4]**

[1] *School of Nursing and Allied Medical Sciences, Semnan University of Medical Sciences, Semnan, Iran*
[2] *Department of Health Services Management, School of Health Management and Information Sciences, Iran University of Medical Sciences, Tehran, Iran*
[3] *School of Health Management and Information Sciences, Iran University of Medical Sciences, No. 6, Rashid Yasemi Street, Vali-e-asr Avenue, Tehran 1995614111, Iran*
[4] *Emergency Department, 7th Tir Hospital, Iran University of Medical Sciences, Tehran, Iran*

Correspondence should be addressed to Roohangiz Jamshidi-Orak; jam_orak@yahoo.co.in

Academic Editor: Harold K. Simon

The physiological-social modified early warning score system is a newly developed instrument for the identification of patients at risk. The aim of this study was to investigate the feasibility of using the physiological-social modified early warning score system for the identification of patients that needed prehospital emergency care. This prospective cohort study was conducted with 2157 patients. This instrument was used as a measure to detect critical illness in patients hospitalised in internal wards. Judgment by an emergency medicine specialist was used as a measure of standard. Data were analyzed by using receiver operating characteristics curves and the area under the curve with 95% confidence interval. The mean score of the physiological-social modified early warning score system was $2.71 \pm 3.55$. Moreover, 97.6% patients with the score $\geq 4$ needed prehospital emergency services. The area under receiver operating characteristic curve was 0.738 (95% CI = 0.708–0.767). Emergency medical staffs can use PMEWS $\geq 4$ to identify those patients hospitalised in the internal ward as at risk patients. The physiological-social modified early warning score system is suggested to be used for decision-making of emergency staff about internal patients' wards in EMS situations.

## 1. Introduction

Emergency medical services (EMS) are at the front line of meeting patients' needs out of hospital environments. Emergency medical staffs are main persons who impact the decision for patients' transference to inpatient healthcare settings. Judgments by emergency medical staffs in prehospital situations are rarely evidence-based and are mainly rooted in subjective data and staffs' level of education and past experiences [1–3]. Sometimes, their decisions may result in inappropriate transfer of patients to hospitals by ambulance or leaving patients on their own, while they must be transferred to the hospital [4].

Unnecessary transfer and improper or excessive use of prehospital emergency services are unresolved issues in the EMS [5]. There are some reports about avoidable use of prehospital care in several countries, including the USA, UK, and Iran [6–8]. Improper use of prehospital EMS leads to wasting limited resources, idling real emergency patients to receive appropriate care, increasing morbidity and mortality rate of patients with conditions that require emergency services, low-quality performance, and job dissatisfaction in prehospital emergency staffs [5]. Therefore, establishing a control mechanism can reduce unnecessary patient transfer and inappropriate use of EMS [9].

There are some well-known methods to determine the severity of illness in various conditions of hospital environments such as the early warning scoring (EWS) systems [10–12]. The EWS systems commonly use vital sign criteria to warn medical staffs of patients' condition [13, 14]. The aim

Table 1: PMEWS admission algorithm.

Date:
Time:
Patient ID label:

| | Physiological data (MEWS) | | | | | | |
|---|---|---|---|---|---|---|---|
| Score | 3 | 2 | 1 | 0 | 1 | 2 | 3 |
| Resp. rates | ≤8 | | | 9–18 | 19–25 | 26–29 | ≥30 |
| O2 Stats. | <89 | 90–93 | 94–96 | >96 | | | |
| Heart rate | ≤40 | 41–50 | | 51–100 | 101–110 | 111–129 | ≥130 |
| Systolic BP | ≤70 | 71–90 | 91–100 | >100 | | | |
| Temp. | | ≤35 | 35.1–36 | 36.1–37.9 | 38–38.9 | ≥39 | |
| Neuro. | | | | Alert | Confused/agitated | Voice | Pain unconscious |

| | | |
|---|---|---|
| **Patient data:** Score 1 for each factor | | |
| Age > 65 | | |
| Social isolation (lives alone, no fixed abode) | | |
| Chronic disease (respiratory, cardiac, renal, immunosuppressed, and DM) | | |
| **Performance status** | **Score** | |
| Normal activity without restriction | 0 | **MEWS:** |
| Strenuous activity limited, can do light | 1 | **Patient data score:** |
| Limited activity but capable of self-care | 2 | **Total PMEWS:** |
| Limited activity, limited self-care | 3 | Name of assessor: |
| Confined to bed/chair, no self-care | 4 | Grade: |

of such systems is fast recognition of critical patients to trigger appropriate responses [15–17]. In the last decade, a few studies have been carried out related to prehospital patient harm events [18]. Moreover, in the prehospital environment, there are no suitable scoring systems for EMS to support decision-making regarding patients' transfer to hospital [19]. Thus, the development of a valid and reliable early warning score system is important to recognise at risk patients in the prehospital environment [20]. The modified early warning score (MEWS) is one of the simple scoring systems that can be used in emergency situations [21, 22].

In the previous study [8], the MEWS was applied to identify patients with medical (nontraumatic) conditions in prehospital emergency environments. It was shown that the MEWS was efficient in the identification of critically ill patients and its sensitivity was in an acceptable level. However, its sensitivity was mentioned to be low and was not efficient enough to determine doubtful patients who need prehospital emergency care [8]. A few studies have investigated the applicability of physiological-social modified scoring system (PMEWS) for patients hospitalised in the internal ward in prehospital care [4, 23]. Therefore, in this study, the authors used the PMEWS to identify the patients with medical (nontraumatic) conditions in prehospital emergency situations. The PMEWS also contain some social norms and is able to examine various variables in comparison to the MEWS. The aim of this study was to investigate the feasibility of using the PMEWS for the identification of patients that needed prehospital emergency care.

## 2. Method

This is a prospective, cohort study. All patients from 23 July to 22 September 2012 following a complaint of an internal pathology problem transferred to a hospital by the EMS in Tehran city were invited to participate in this study. We included only those patients complaining from internal diseases. Trauma patients, patient's less than 12 years of age, and pregnant and mentally ill patients were excluded from this study.

To access the participants, two sites out of four regions of emergency prehospital activities in Tehran were randomly selected. The data collection tool was a form composed of two parts. The first part consisted of the physiological parameters including systolic blood pressure, heart rate, respiratory rate, oxygen saturation percent, temperature, and status of consciousness (APVU; alert, verbal response, and no response to painful stimuli). The second part consisted of the data on social isolation as living alone or having no fixed abode, chronic diseases, age, and performance status.

Table 2: Patient's characteristics.

| Character | $N$ | % |
|---|---|---|
| Age > 65 | 694 | 32.2 |
| Male | 1192 | 55.3 |
| Female | 964 | 44.7 |
| Social isolation | 308 | 14.3 |
| Chronic disease | 1132 | 52.5 |
| Need of the EMS response | 682 | 68.4 |
| Did not require the EMS response | 1474 | 31.6 |
| | Mean | SD |
| Age | 50.58 | 22.15 |
| Physiological score | 1.97 | 2.86 |
| Social score | 0.75 | 1.16 |
| PMEWS | 2.71 | 3.55 |

These factors were combined to produce a physiological-social modified early warning score (Table 1) derived from previous studies [19, 23].

Prehospital emergency technicians filled in the patient's transference routine form and at the same time completed the PMEWS standards form. Then they classified the patients into two groups:

(1) patients who really required transfer to hospital,

(2) patients who did not require the EMS response.

This was done based on the emergency medicine specialist judgment as a gold standard in this study. The ROC curve was used to demonstrate the sensitivity and specificity of PMEWS form.

## 3. Results

A total of 2305 participants entered the study, and 2157 forms were properly completed (response rate 93.6%). The average and standard deviation of the patients' age were 50.58 ± 22.15. Also, 44.7% of the participants were men and 55.3% of them were women. Mean and standard deviation of physiological scores of transferred patients, social scores, and the PMEWS were reported to be 1.97 ± 2.86, 0.75 ± 1.16, and 2.71 ± 3.55, respectively (Table 2).

According to emergency medicine specialists' judgements, 68.4% of the patients who were transported to the hospital required emergency medical services and 31.6% of them did not require any emergency treatments (Table 2).

The results showed that with the increase in PMEWS scores the need for patients to be transferred is increased. 97.6% of patients with the score of 4 or more and all of the patients with the score of 10 needed emergency transport (Figure 1). The area under receiver operating characteristic curve (AUROC) using the PMEWS score as a discriminator for requiring emergency transportation was 0.738 (95% CI = 0.708–0.767) and for physiological score was 0.692 (95% CI = 0.660–0.724) and for social score was 0.667 (95% CI = 0.635–0.699) (Figure 2).

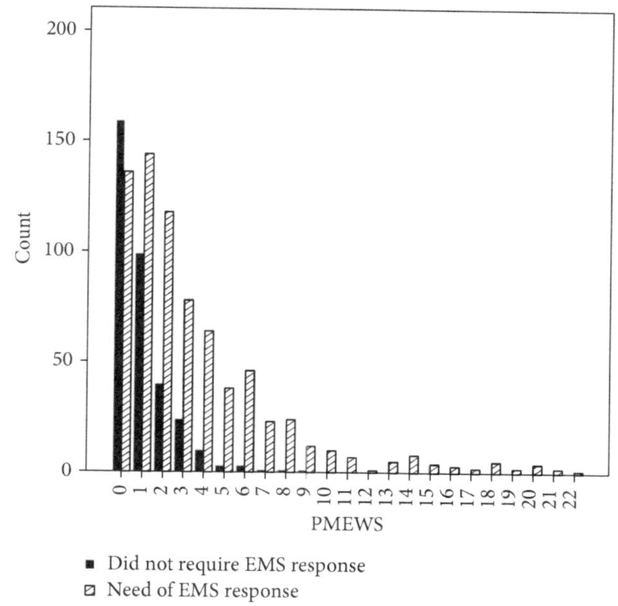


Figure 1: Distribution of the PMEWS in relation to final disposal.

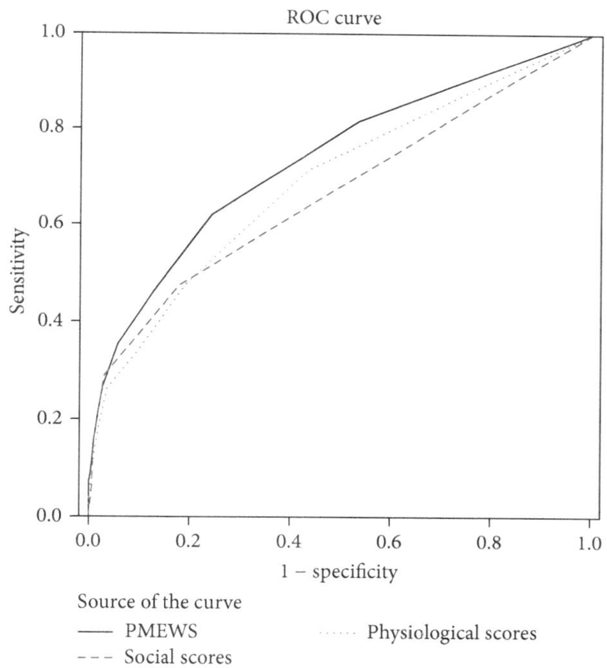


Figure 2: ROC curve for physiological, social, and PMEWS scores as predictors of need of the EMS response.

## 4. Discussion

Designing a system to identify patients in need of receiving prehospital emergency care has been emphasized in previous studies [8, 11, 19, 24]. Our findings revealed that when the PMEWS score is equal to or lower than 4, the PMEWS can predict the seriousness of critically-ill patients' need for receiving the EMS.

The sensitivity of this tool was mentioned to be 97.65, using 4 as a cutoff point. This cutoff point in the Fullerton et al. study was three [24] and two in Challen and Walter study [19]. The differences in cutoff points in these studies are due to a variety of research communities. The skills of prehospital emergency medical technicians may vary in different studies. Another reason could be the variation of the quality in hospital services and physicians' judgment in these hospitals. It is suggested that every society should use the PMEWS with an appropriate cutoff point based on its demographic and cultural components. Discovery of this cutoff point requires scientific research with a sufficient sample size.

The area under AUROC curve using the score as a discriminator for admission was 0.767. This finding is close to the area under AUROC curve in the studies by Challen and Walter (0.710), Fullerton et al. (0.799), and Duckitt et al. (0.720) [19, 24, 25]. Limited variables in the PMEWS might be an important cause for PMEWS inability to identify doubtful patients that need emergency care. The ROC curves showed that the use of PMEWS compared to using MEWS and social scores is stronger in predicting the need for patients to be transported by the EMS. Adding some variables to the PMEWS is suggested to increase its power to identify patients at risk.

## 5. Conclusion

EMS staff can use PMEWS $\geq 4$ to identify internal patient at risk, especially when they are in doubt about patients' transfer to the hospital. The patients with a very low PMEWS score may still have a life-threatening condition that requires special care in the prehospital environment. Thus, this system should be developed for the support of the EMS staff for decision-making about emergency internal patients in EMS responses. The optimal instrument for detection of emergency internal patient needs more studies to be illuminated.

## Conflict of Interests

The authors declare that there is no conflict of interests regarding the publishing of this paper.

## Acknowledgment

This study was supported by the School of Health Management and Information Sciences, Iran University of Medical Sciences (IUMS/ SHMIS).

## References

[1] S. A. Mulholland, B. J. Gabbe, and P. Cameron, "Is paramedic judgement useful in prehospital trauma triage?" *Injury*, vol. 36, no. 11, pp. 1298–1305, 2005.

[2] L. H. Brown, M. W. Hubble, D. C. Cone et al., "Paramedic determinations of medical necessity: a meta-analysis," *Prehospital Emergency Care*, vol. 13, no. 4, pp. 516–527, 2009.

[3] R. Brown and J. Warwick, "Blue calls—time for a change?" *Emergency Medicine Journal*, vol. 18, no. 4, pp. 289–292, 2001.

[4] A. A. Ebarhimian, N. Khalesi, G. Mohamadi, M. Tourdeh, and M. Naghipour, "Transportation management in pre-hospital emergency with physiological early warning scores," *Journal of Health Administration*, vol. 15, no. 49, pp. 1–9, 2012 (Persian).

[5] B. J. Knapp, B. L. Kerns, I. Riley, and J. Powers, "EMS-initiated refusal of transport: the current state of affairs," *The Journal of Emergency Medicine*, vol. 36, no. 2, pp. 157–161, 2009.

[6] M. Kamper, B. D. Mahoney, S. Nelson, and J. Peterson, "Feasibility of paramedic treatment and referral of minor illnesses and injuries," *Prehospital Emergency Care*, vol. 5, no. 4, pp. 371–378, 2001.

[7] C. Mann and H. Guly, "Is the emergency (999) service being misused? Retrospective analysis," *British Medical Journal*, vol. 316, no. 7129, pp. 437–438, 1998.

[8] A. Ebrahimian, H. Shabanikiya, and N. Khalesi, "The role of physiological scores for decision making in internal pre-hospital emergency situations," *Healthmed*, vol. 6, no. 11, pp. 3612–3615, 2012.

[9] J. Y. S. Ting and A. M. Z. Chang, "Path analysis modeling indicates free transport increases ambulance use for minor indications," *Prehospital Emergency Care*, vol. 10, no. 4, pp. 476–481, 2006.

[10] K. Mizumoto and E. Morita, "Evaluation of the Physiological and Operative Severity Score for the Enumeration of Mortality and Morbidity (POSSUM) scoring system in elderly patients with pressure sores undergoing fasciocutaneous flap-reconstruction," *Journal of Dermatology*, vol. 36, no. 1, pp. 30–34, 2009.

[11] K. Challen and S. W. Goodacre, "Predictive scoring in non-trauma emergency patients: a scoping review," *Emergency Medicine Journal*, vol. 28, no. 10, pp. 827–837, 2011.

[12] D. R. Prytherch, G. B. Smith, P. E. Schmidt, and P. I. Featherstone, "ViEWS-Towards a national early warning score for detecting adult inpatient deterioration," *Resuscitation*, vol. 81, no. 8, pp. 932–937, 2010.

[13] D. R. Goldhill, L. Worthington, A. Mulcahy, M. Tarling, and A. Sumner, "The patient-at-risk team: Identifying and managing seriously ill ward patients," *Anaesthesia*, vol. 54, no. 9, pp. 853–860, 1999.

[14] B. H. Cuthbertson, "Outreach critical care—cash for no questions?" *The British Journal of Anaesthesia*, vol. 90, no. 1, pp. 4–6, 2003.

[15] J. O. Jansen and B. H. Cuthbertson, "Detecting critical illness outside the ICU: the role of track and trigger systems," *Current Opinion in Critical Care*, vol. 16, no. 3, pp. 184–190, 2010.

[16] G. B. Smith, D. R. Prytherch, P. E. Schmidt, and P. I. Featherstone, "Review and performance evaluation of aggregate weighted 'track and trigger' systems," *Resuscitation*, vol. 77, no. 2, pp. 170–179, 2008.

[17] P. J. Frost and M. P. Wise, "Early management of acutely ill ward patients," *British Medical Journal*, vol. 345, no. 7874, Article ID e5677, 2012.

[18] R. Price, J. C. Bendall, J. A. Patterson, and P. M. Middleton, "What causes adverse events in prehospital care? A human-factors approach," *Emergency Medicine Journal*, vol. 30, no. 7, pp. 583–588, 2013.

[19] K. Challen and D. Walter, "Physiological scoring: an aid to emergency medical services transport decisions?" *Prehospital and Disaster Medicine*, vol. 25, no. 4, pp. 320–323, 2010.

[20] B. H. Cuthbertson, M. Boroujerdi, L. McKie, L. Aucott, and G. Prescott, "Can physiological variables and early warning

scoring systems allow early recognition of the deteriorating surgical patient?" *Critical Care Medicine*, vol. 35, no. 2, pp. 402–409, 2007.

[21] D. R. Goldhill, A. F. McNarry, G. Mandersloot, and A. McGinley, "A physiologically-based early warning score for ward patients: the association between score and outcome," *Anaesthesia*, vol. 60, no. 6, pp. 547–553, 2005.

[22] T. S. Lam, P. S. K. Mak, W. S. Siu, M. Y. Lam, T. F. Cheung, and T. H. Rainer, "Validation of a Modified Early Warning Score (MEWS) in emergency department observation ward patients," *Hong Kong Journal of Emergency Medicine*, vol. 13, no. 1, pp. 24–30, 2006.

[23] K. Challen, J. Bright, A. Bentley, and D. Walter, "Physiological-social score (PMEWS) vs. CURB-65 to triage pandemic influenza: a comparative validation study using community-acquired pneumonia as a proxy," *BMC Health Services Research*, vol. 7, article 33, 2007.

[24] J. N. Fullerton, C. L. Price, N. E. Silvey, S. J. Brace, and G. D. Perkins, "Is the Modified Early Warning Score (MEWS) superior to clinician judgement in detecting critical illness in the pre-hospital environment?" *Resuscitation*, vol. 83, no. 5, pp. 557–562, 2012.

[25] R. W. Duckitt, R. Buxton-Thomas, J. Walker et al., "Worthing physiological scoring system: Derivation and validation of a physiological early-warning system for medical admissions. An observational, population-based single-centre study," *British Journal of Anaesthesia*, vol. 98, no. 6, pp. 769–774, 2007.

# 9

# Deliberate Self-Poisoning Presenting to an Emergency Medicine Network in South-East Melbourne

**Asheq Rahman,[1,2] Catherine Martin,[1,2] Andis Graudins,[1,3] and Rose Chapman[1,2]**

[1] *Monash Health, 135 David Street, Dandenong, VIC 3175, Australia*
[2] *Australian Catholic University, 115 Victoria Parade, Fitzroy, VIC 3065, Australia*
[3] *Monash University, Clayton, VIC 3168, Australia*

Correspondence should be addressed to Asheq Rahman; asheq.rahman@monashhealth.org

Academic Editor: Seiji Morita

*Background.* Deliberate self-poisoning (DSP) comprises a small but significant proportion of presentations to the emergency department (ED). However, the prevalence and patient characteristics of self-poisoning attendances to EDs in Victoria have not been recently characterised. *Aim.* To identify and compare the characteristics of adult patients presenting to the three EDs of Monash Health following DSP. *Methods.* Retrospective clinical audit of adult DSP attendances between 1st July 2009 and 30th June 2012. *Results.* A total of 3558 cases over three years were identified fulfilling the search criteria. The mean age of patients was 36.3 years with the largest numbers aged between 18 and 30 (38%). About 30% of patients were born overseas. Forty-eight percent were discharged home, 15% were admitted to ED short stay units, and 5% required ICU admission. The median ED length of stay was 359 minutes (IQR 231–607). The most frequently reported substances in DSP were benzodiazepines (36.6%), paracetamol (22.2%), and antipsychotics (12.1%). Exposure to more than one substance for the episode of DSP was common (47%). *Conclusion.* This information may help identify the trends in poisoning substances used for DSP in Victoria, which in turn may provide clinicians with information to provide more focused and targeted interventions.

## 1. Introduction

Deliberate self-poisoning (DSP) variably accounts for 0.5 to 2% of all admissions to Emergency Departments (EDs) [1, 2]. For the purpose of this paper the term DSP was used to describe those patients who had intentionally ingested substances to cause themselves harm. Patients may have associated complex medical and mental health problems and the DSP episodes may result in a high degree of resource use and consequently cost to the health service and the community [3]. The ED is usually the initial point of contact for individuals presenting with deliberate self-harm [3–6]. In 1999, a report on adult poisoning in Victoria indicated that 4.9% of ED admissions were due to poisoning and medications were used in more than 50% of cases [2]. Although the societal burden of these admissions has been acknowledged internationally, little recent data exists on the prevalence and characteristics of patients presenting with self-poisoning to Victorian Emergency Departments.

There are very few recent Australian studies investigating the prevalence and patient characteristics of individuals presenting to the ED with DSP. Buykx et al. found that the majority of overdose patients were female in their 30s and referred for psychosocial assessment [7]. This is similar to previous studies of DSP patients. In a Victorian retrospective study from the late 1990s, Taylor et al. found that the majority of DSP presenters to their community teaching hospital were also women [1]. Single drugs such as paracetamol and antipsychotic agents were more commonly used in the repeat presenters. In another Australian retrospective study of 325 patients presenting with DSP in Queensland, the most common substances taken were benzodiazepines (39.5%), antidepressants (11.7%), or paracetamol (7.2%) [8]. Also in the mid-1990s, Buckley et al. reported that benzodiazepines, alcohol, and paracetamol figured highly in the most common substances ingested. Tricyclic antidepressant (TCA) poisoning was also common and responsible for a substantial proportion of DSP-related deaths in this study [9]. However, more recently, the same authors noted that there was a swing away from the prescribing of TCAs and a greater use of SSRI antidepressants resulting in less DSP morbidity and mortality [10]. As a result, over time, the epidemiology of substances implicated in DSP has changed and appears to parallel the marketing and frequency of prescribing of newer medications. In general, these previous studies describe more recent DSP characteristics in Queensland and New South Wales. There also have been some recent studies in Victoria examining how medications that are used to self-poison are acquired [11] and reporting on specific drugs like antidepressants [12]. However, detailed reports on DSP from Victoria are more dated and are as much as 15 to 25 years old. It is highly likely that, with the change in prescribing practice, newer prescription medications have taken the place of older drugs as preferred poisoning agents. As a result, the degree of toxicity, morbidity, and mortality may also have changed over the years.

This current study aims to describe the epidemiology of deliberate self-poisoning in adult patients presenting to the emergency departments of Monash Health, an urban health care network in South Eastern Melbourne.

## 2. Methods

*2.1. Setting.* Monash Health is one of the largest health care providers in Victoria. There are three acute hospitals with four EDs: one adult, one tertiary paediatric (Monash Medical Centre), and two mixed EDs (Dandenong and Casey Hospitals) with a total of around 171000 attendances/year. The catchment population of these three hospital areas is socioeconomically different [13].

*2.2. Data Collection.* For the purpose of this retrospective descriptive study data, all patients presenting with a triage diagnosis of overdose/poisoning/self-harm were identified in Symphony (Emergency Department clinical data system, Version 2.29, Ascribe plc, Bolton, UK) and reviewed for the presence of deliberate self-poisoning as a reason for presentation to the ED.

The extraction and recoding of the data was done in two phases. In the first phase, key words from the Triage Nurse's comments were used in Stata Statistical Software (Release 12 College Station, TX; StataCorp) to extract cases with DSP and remove cases of accidental, recreational poisoning, or drink-spiking poisoning. Manual exclusion of non-DSP cases was conducted following this and the final number of cases was 3558. In the second phase, the coding/recoding of the major classes of drugs/poisons was done according to the generic names and the codes were confirmed by using a web based free medical information system (NPS, http://www.nps.org.au/). Substances were categorized by class and any remaining drugs were grouped as others. Available patient demography, such as age, sex, marital status, country of birth, and location of the residence were included in the analysis. SEIFA (Socio Economic Indexes for Areas) Indexes rank areas in Australia according to relative socioeconomic advantage and disadvantage and an area with a lower SEIFA value indicates relatively greater disadvantage and a lack of advantage in general [14]. It might be noteworthy to mention that an area with a SEIFA value less than 1000 indicates lower relative socioeconomic advantage/disadvantage compared to other areas.

SEIFA Indexes (in particular the Index of Relative Socioeconomic Advantage and Disadvantage, IRSAD) were obtained from Australian Bureau of Statistics to assess the presence of any socioeconomic differences between the populations presenting to the three emergency departments (http://www.abs.gov.au/websitedbs/censushome.nsf/4a256353001af3ed4b2562bb00121564/seifa).

Most of the patients were from surrounding suburbs and postcodes were tabulated against frequency of patients coming from specific postcodes. As the addresses of patients were removed for the deidentification purpose, postcodes were the only locator and the Local Government Area (LGA) SIEFA scores have been used against the respective postcodes.

Relevant ED patient disposition information was obtained from electronically generated Monash Health ED Executive Report (Datasource: Health Central-Symphony) [15].

*2.3. Data Analysis.* Using Stata, descriptive statistics were generated. Differences in the occurrence and characteristics of self-poisoning presentations based on patient characteristics were assessed using different tests of significance, namely, Pearson's chi square test for comparing frequencies, ANOVA for comparing means (including application of Bonferroni, Scheffe, and Sidak test of comparison means between variables), and Kruskal Wallis for comparing median values. Statistical significance was considered at $\alpha < 0.05$.

*2.4. Inclusion Criteria.* All patients were 18 years and over presenting to the Emergency Departments of the health service with deliberate self-poisoning between the 1st July 2009 and 30th June 2012.

*2.5. Ethical Approval.* Ethical approval was sought and gained from The Australian Catholic University and the Monash Health Human Research and Ethics Committee prior to commencement of data collection.

## 3. Results

*3.1. Demography.* During the study period, there were 512,282 presentations to Monash Health ED. There were 10,548 patients presenting with poisoning of which 3558 were classified as DSP in patients >18 years. This represented 0.7% of all ED presentations. The mean age of the patients was 36.3 years and 64.6% were female. The largest numbers of patients presenting with DSP were aged between 18 and 30 (38% of the total cases) (Table 1). Both in total, and in individual groups, females were predominant. This was especially noteworthy in the 18–30 years age group where 70% were female. Around 58% of DSP presenters were single and 30% were married. Significant differences in the number of females were observed in 18–30 years and 31–40 years age

Table 1: Demographics. Age distribution of female patients according to age group (percentage of females of the total number of patients for specific age group is mentioned after the frequency).

| | Casey | Dandenong | MMC Clayton | $P$ value |
|---|---|---|---|---|
| Age group | Female | Female | Female | |
| 18–30 ≠ | 249 (68.8) | 305 (66.3) | 387 (73.3) | 0.000* |
| 31–40 ≠ | 147 (51.2) | 184 (53.6) | 202 (64.5) | 0.012* |
| 41–50 | 167 (65.0) | 175 (62.7) | 162 (65.6) | 0.774 |
| 51–60 | 74 (70.5) | 72 (67.9) | 60 (69.0) | 0.434 |
| >61 | 27 (58.7) | 44 (67.7) | 44 (60.3) | 0.081 |
| Total | **664 (62.8)** | **780 (62.3)** | **855 (68.5)** | |
| Marital status | | | | |
| Single | 436 (58.23) | 606 (55.60) | 763 (65.78) | 0.000* |
| Married/Defacto | 329 (37.9) | 335 (30.74) | 286 (24.66) | 0.105 |
| Divorced/separated | 78 (8.99) | 109 (10.2) | 70 (6.09) | 0.007* |
| Widowed | 16 (1.84) | 21 (1.93) | 17 (1.47) | 0.678 |
| Not stated/inadequately described | 9 (1.04) | 19 (1.74) | 24 (2.07) | 0.035* |
| Country of birth | | | | |
| Australia | 817 (77.3) | 834 (66.56) | 908 (72.76) | 0.064 |
| Other than Australia† | 240 (22.7) | 419 (33.44) | 340 (27.24) | 0.000* |

*Significant difference exists between hospital areas for the frequency of population (Chi square, $P < 0.05$).
≠ Significant differences exist between hospital areas among age groups, for both sexes. The information for male is not shown in the table.
†The major countries in this group were: England, India, New Zealand, Srilanka, Vietnam, and Afghanistan.

groups between the hospital areas; similar differences were observed for the males (Table 1).

The ethnic distribution of the DSP population indicated that patients who were born in Australia represented the greatest percentage of patients presenting with DSP (about 72%). However, it was not possible to identify the Aboriginal and Torres Islanders from those cases due to lack of data. Significant differences were found between hospital areas for the population who were not born in Australia. For example, Dandenong Hospital had a greater number of admissions of overseas born patients (Table 1). For patients born in countries other than Australia, England, India, New Zealand, Sri Lanka, Vietnam, and Afghanistan were the predominant countries of birth for cases with DSP. Significant main differences were found in the frequency of DSP cases for single, divorced/separated, and inadequately described groups among different hospital areas (Table 1).

In a separate analysis, we examined the postcode locations and SEIFA scores of the suburbs from which most of the patients originated; in majority, the plotted scores against postcodes for Casey and Dandenong hospitals were below 1000 and for Monash Medical Centre Clayton were above 1000. The average SEIFA score for Casey, Dandenong, and Monash Medical Centre Clayton was 984.38 (SD 32.97), 981.119 (SD 48.53), and 1043.09 (SD 59.97), respectively. The mean SEIFA scores between hospital areas were significantly different ($P = 0.0002$, one-way ANOVA). An intercomparison of mean SEIFA score (by using Bonferroni, Scheffe, and Sidak) for the three hospitals revealed that there were significant differences between Dandenong Hospital and Monash Medical Centre Clayton (Bonferroni, Scheffe, and Sidak, $P = 0.001$) and Casey hospital and Monash Medical Centre Clayton (Bonferroni and Sidak, $P = 0.002$, and Scheffe, $P = 0.003$). SEIFA scores for Dandenong and Casey areas were not different.

Around 47% of DSP patients presenting to ED were discharged home directly from the ED. This compares with 60% of patients being discharged home from the ED for all other reasons. Around 40% of the remaining DSP cases were admitted to either an ED short stay, medical, or mental health bed (Table 2). Seven percent of DSP patients were admitted to a mental health bed from the ED. A notable proportion of DSP cases (3.9%) left the ED before treatment was started. This compares to 4.7% of patients leaving prior to completion of treatment for all ED presentations [15]. There were significant differences in frequency of the major ED disposition categories between the hospital areas (Table 2). For example, more than 61% of the DSP cases remained in the same hospital campus for Dandenong, for the other two hospitals this was almost half.

Regarding the presentation of the DSP cases in the ED, no significant differences in the day or time were found between the Hospitals. However, about 50% of presentations to the ED were between 16.00 and 23.59 hours at all three sites.

The median length of stay in the Emergency Department (excluding time in the Short Stay Unit) was 359.5 minutes (IQR 231-607). Comparison of individual EDs revealed that the median length of stay was significantly longer at Monash Medical Centre compared to the other two EDs (Table 3). Around 15% of DSP patients (550 cases) were admitted to the ED Short Stay Units (SSU) of the three hospitals for longer observation periods. The median length of stay in SSU was 376.5 minutes (IQR 182-712) and was significantly different between the three hospitals. As a result, total length of stay for SSU admitted patients was 736 minutes (approximately 12.6 hours).

Table 2: Disposition from Emergency Department.

| ED disposition | Casey | Dandenong | MMC Clayton | $P$ value |
|---|---|---|---|---|
| Returning to usual residence | 657 (62.22) | 357 (28.49) | 670 (53.73) | 0.000* |
| Subcategories | | | | |
| Home | 646 (61.17) | 349 (27.85) | 652 (52.29) | |
| Mental health residential facility | 3 (0.28) | 3 (0.24) | 10 (0.80) | |
| Correctional/custodial facility | 5 (0.47) | 4 (0.32) | 2 (0.16) | |
| Residential care facility/Nursing home | 3 (0.28) | 1 (0.08) | 6 (0.48) | |
| Ward of the same Hospital Campus Subcategories | 271 (25.66) | 769 (61.37) | 429 (34.40) | 0.000* |
| ED/Short Stay Observation Unit | 48 (4.55) | 469 (37.43) | 34 (2.73) | |
| Hospital ward | 99 (9.38) | 113 (9.02) | 237 (19.01) | |
| Mental Health Bed | 96 (9.09) | 67 (5.35) | 88 (7.06) | |
| ICU | 28 (2.65) | 120 (9.58) | 70 (5.61) | |
| Left before treatment completed | 56 (5.30) | 109 (8.70) | 104 (8.34) | 0.000* |
| Subcategories | | | | |
| Left at own risk, without treatment | 29 (2.75) | 55 (4.39) | 58 (4.65) | |
| Left at own risk, after treatment started | 24 (2.27) | 49 (3.91) | 43 (3.45) | |
| Left after clinical advice regarding treatment | 3 (0.28) | 5 (0.40) | 3 (0.24) | |
| Transferred to another Hospital (not Monash Health) | 71 (6.72) | 13 (1.04) | 41 (3.29) | 0.000* |
| CCU | 1 (0.09) | 5 (0.40) | 2 (0.16) | |
| Deceased | 0 (0) | 0 (0) | 1 (0.08) | |

*Significant difference exits between hospital areas (Chi square, $P < 0.001$); for CCU and Deceased thetest was not performed due to small numbers.

Table 3: Median length of stay in hospitals.

| Department | Median length of stay across all hospitals (minutes) | Median length of stay in individual hospitals (minutes) | | | |
|---|---|---|---|---|---|
| | | Casey | Dandenong | MMC Clayton | $P$ value |
| Emergency Department ($n = 3558$) | 359.5 (IQR 231–607) | 331 (IQR 214–578) | 326 (IQR 214–537) | 408 (IQR 262–703) | 0.0001* |
| Short Stay Unit ($n = 550$) | 376.5 (IQR 182–712) | 272 (IQR 141.5–642.5) | 394.5 (IQR 187–734.5) | 258 (IQR 134–474) | 0.0184* |

*Significant difference exits between hospital areas (Kruskal Wallis, $P < 0.05$; MMC Clayton was relatively higher).

The most commonly reported class of drug involved poisoning was the benzodiazepines (36.6%), followed by paracetamol products (22.2%) and antipsychotics (12.2%). These three classes of drugs were reported in 71% of DSP cases (Table 4). Other common classes reported were the selective serotonin reuptake inhibitors (SSRIs), nonsteroidal anti-inflammatory drugs (NSAIDs), serotonin norepinephrine reuptake inhibitors (SNRIs), Opioids, anticonvulsants, tricyclic antidepressants (TCAs), Tramadol, and Lithium. Among these, SSRIs and SNRIs jointly contributed 12.6% of the total reported types of poisoning, and exposure to TCAs was low, only 1.9%. The use of more than one substance was common in DSP. In around 47% of cases, multiple substances were ingested. The frequency of intake of benzodiazepines, paracetamol, SNRI, Opioids, TCA, and miscellaneous groups was found significantly different among hospital sites (Table 4). Besides the most frequently used medications or substances for DSP cases, other substances were reported in 916 cases (25.7%). These included about 100 varying classes of toxins/medications. A list of these substances is summarised in Box 1.

## 4. Discussion

This study provides an overview of the characteristics of patients presenting to the ED following DSP in south-eastern suburbs of Melbourne, Victoria, over the last three years. Similar to previous Australian studies [7], we found that women in 18 to 30 years age group were more likely to present following DSP. One important aspect of this study was the inclusion and identification of those presenters who were from a migrant background. In some studies, migrant populations had higher rates of completed suicides [16]. In addition, similar to previous Victorian studies, we found that following DSP, about 50% of the patients presented to all EDs between the late afternoon and midnight [1]. In this study, approximately 30% of the people presenting to our network following DSP were born in countries other than Australia. While this is probably a reflection of the culturally diverse populations located in the area health service [13], we are not aware of any other studies in Australia that have reported this factor in DSP populations. Overseas-born subjects in this study were underrepresented compared to the percentage of

Table 4: Type of poisoning.

| Type | Site frequency (percent) Casey | Dandenong | MMC Clayton | $P$ value |
|---|---|---|---|---|
| Benzodiazepines | 406 (38.41) | 401 (32.00) | 496 (39.74) | 0.001* |
| Paracetamol | 229 (21.67) | 256 (20.43) | 305 (24.44) | 0.004* |
| Antipsychotic | 124 (11.73) | 147 (11.73) | 162 (12.98) | 0.079 |
| SSRI | 101 (9.56) | 97 (7.74) | 80 (6.41) | 0.261 |
| NSAID | 95 (8.99) | 87 (6.94) | 78 (6.25) | 0.434 |
| SNRI | 101 (9.56) | 52 (4.15) | 49 (3.93) | 0.000* |
| Opioids | 30 (2.84) | 54 (4.31) | 45 (3.61) | 0.033* |
| Anticonvulsant | 18 (1.70) | 24 (1.92) | 30 (2.40) | 0.223 |
| TCA | 14 (1.32) | 34 (2.71) | 19 (1.52) | 0.008* |
| Tramadol | 14 (1.32) | 26 (2.08) | 14 (1.12) | 0.069 |
| Lithium | 6 (0.57) | 8 (0.64) | 9 (0.72) | 0.738 |
| Miscellaneous groups (substances not included above) | 249 (23.56) | 369 (29.45) | 298 (23.88) | 0.000* |

*Significant difference between sites (Chi square, $P < 0.05$), number of cases may exceed the total number of patients due to ingestion of more than one poison.

(i) Antidiabetic medications (both oral and injectable)
(ii) Antihypertensive agents
(iii) Carbon monoxide
(iv) Household cleaning agents
(v) Weed killers, pesticides and head lice solutions
(vi) Fuels: petrol and kerosene
(vii) Personal and animal grooming products
(viii) Any type of medications available in the household; few examples are natural sleeping pills, multi vitamin tablets, Betadine
(ix) Medications from the country of birth for the Non-Australia born populations
(x) Alcohol

Box 1: Category of "miscellaneous poisoning substances."

those living in the community, particularly in the Dandenong and Monash Medical Centre catchment areas where 60% and 47% of the community, respectively, were born overseas [13]. This finding is notable, and a future research investigation into DSP in culturally sensitive migrant and refugee groups and comparing these with Australian born DSP groups is important to enable more focused and targeted education and preventive measures in the future.

We also assessed socioeconomic status of patients presenting to our ED with DSP by analysing the SEIFA scores of patient address postcodes. Gunnell et al. noted a strong link between socioeconomic deprivation and suicide [17], and SEIFA scores can be utilised to analyse the link between socioeconomic status and illness in Emergency Medicine research in Australia [18]. We were unable to find any current studies utilising SEIFA scores in the analysis of ED presentations for illness in any of the Victorian hospitals. As a result, it was not possible to make a comparison with other areas. However, we did not observe any significant difference in the incidence or epidemiology of DSP between our three hospital EDs despite markedly varying socioeconomic status. We found that DSP patients were more likely to need hospital admission compared to non-DSP patients, with around 40% being admitted to either SSU, a hospital ward, or ICU. The average admission rate for non-DSP patients from our EDs is closer to 30% [15]. It is important to note that around 7% of the patients in this study were admitted from the ED directly to a mental health bed. The higher admission rate for DSP patients compared to non-DSP presentations indicates an increased and potentially preventable burden on the health system [19]. It was beyond the scope of this study to explore the outcome of patients transferred to the mental health or intensive care units or the cost to the health service as a consequence of these admissions [2]. There were differences in the patient disposition categories between EDs and this happened mainly due to the difference in the process of patient disposition (e.g., more patients went from the ED to the short stay unit at Dandenong Hospital). Similarly, transfer of DSP cases to another hospital was high from Casey Hospital due to limited number of specialized facilities such as an Intensive Care Unit. In addition, the factors that related to length of stay in the hospital are also unknown. This finding may be as a result of the differences in the processes and procedures currently occurring between departments. However, examination of these factors was beyond the scope of this study and further investigation is required.

Similar to other Victorian [7] and American studies [20], we found that benzodiazepines were the most frequently ingested drugs. However, we found a difference between the use of paracetamol between our study and those conducted in the UK [20]. Paracetamol was the second most commonly used drug however in this study. However, in the UK, it is the most commonly used substance in DSP [20]. Compared to earlier studies conducted in Australia in the 1990s, we noted a change in the type of poisoning substances ingested. While benzodiazepines and paracetamol still figured highly in many DSP cases, there was an increased incidence of exposure to newer antidepressants such as the SSRIs and SNRIs [12]. There was also a significant reduction in exposure to tricyclic antidepressants compared to older Australian studies (around 10%) [9]. This most likely reflects the change in prescribing patterns for antidepressant and antipsychotic agents and it has been noted in other recent studies done in jurisdictions outside of Victoria [21]. Reasons for this change in the poisoning pattern need further investigations.

## 5. Limitations

(i) This was a retrospective study utilising a large database with limited details in the information extracted. As a result, only limited interpretations can be made in the results.

(ii) While extreme caution was taken in checking the data, there may have been missed cases due to extreme spelling mistakes in drug names, poisoning substances, and inclusion in poisoning cases in different categories.

(iii) One of the challenges with conducting this study was the inadequacies found in the triage comments. For example, a large variation existed in the spelling of drug names and the use of short hand description of the patients' history and presenting problem.

(iv) Significant difference in the level of significance may be observed due to large sample size of this study, which always may not be clinically significant.

(v) We were not able to make any major interpretation regarding poisoning severity from this data set. However, with five percent of patients requiring ICU admission, this figure is similar to other DSP studies and indirectly connotes a similar degree of severe poisoning cases as in other studies [22].

(vi) In previous studies, up to 92% of patients presenting to ED with self-harm have an existing psychiatric condition [23, 24]. We were also unable to assess this association due to limited information in the existing database.

(vii) Use of triage comments to define overdose may also be a limitation due to recall bias/unreliable information from the patients or their attendants.

## 6. Conclusions

This is the first study characterising the epidemiology of DSP in South-Eastern Melbourne, one of the fastest growing population areas in Victoria. DSP patients were more likely to be younger females and more likely to require hospital admission compared to non-DSP presentations. While the type of substances used for DSP paralleled those implicated in poisoning in other more contemporary studies, there was a change in the types of substances commonly reported in DSP in earlier Victorian studies. The high incidence of people born outside Australia and lower socioeconomic groups are two areas that require further investigation of the epidemiology of DSP in these vulnerable populations.

## Conflict of Interests

The authors declare that there is no conflict of interests regarding the publication of this paper.

## Authors' Contribution

Rose Chapman and Andis Graudins designed the study; Catherine Martin acquired the data; Asheq Rahman and Catherine Martin analysed the data; Asheq Rahman, Andis Graudins, and Rose Chapman wrote the draft; all authors approved the final paper.

## References

[1] D. M. Taylor, P. A. Cameron, and D. Eddey, "Recurrent overdose: patient characteristics, habits, and outcomes," *Journal of Accident and Emergency Medicine*, vol. 15, no. 4, pp. 257–261, 1998.

[2] V. Routley, K. Ashby, and J. Lough, "Adult poisoning overview—Victoria," *Hazard*, vol. 39, pp. 1–17, 1999.

[3] J. M. A. Sinclair, A. Gray, and K. Hawton, "Systematic review of resource utilization in the hospital management of deliberate self-harm," *Psychological Medicine*, vol. 36, no. 12, pp. 1681–1693, 2006.

[4] G. L. Carter, K. Clover, I. M. Whyte, A. H. Dawson, and C. D'Este, "Postcards from the EDge: 24-Month outcomes of a randomised controlled trial for hospital-treated self-poisoning," *British Journal of Psychiatry*, vol. 191, pp. 548–553, 2007.

[5] L. McCarthy and H. Gijbels, "An examination of emergency department nurses'attitudes towards deliberate self-harm in an Irish teaching hospital," *International Emergency Nursing*, vol. 18, no. 1, pp. 29–35, 2010.

[6] C. Martin and R. Chapman, "A mixed method study to determine the attitude of Australian emergency health professionals towards patients who present with deliberate self-poisoning," *International Emergency Nursing*, vol. 22, no. 2, pp. 98–104, 2014.

[7] P. Buykx, P. Dietze, A. Ritter, and W. Loxley, "Characteristics of medication overdose presentations to the ED: how do they differ from illicit drug overdose and self-harm cases?" *Emergency Medicine Journal*, vol. 27, no. 7, pp. 499–503, 2010.

[8] J. McGrath, "A survey of deliberate self-poisoning," *Medical Journal of Australia*, vol. 150, no. 6, pp. 317–324, 1989.

[9] N. A. Buckley, I. M. Whyte, A. H. Dawson, P. R. McManus, and N. W. Ferguson, "Self-poisoning in Newcastle, 1987–1992," *Medical Journal of Australia*, vol. 162, no. 4, pp. 190–193, 1995.

[10] N. A. Buckley and P. R. McManus, "Fatal toxicity of serotoninergic and other antidepressant drugs: analysis of United Kingdom

mortality data," *British Medical Journal*, vol. 325, no. 7376, pp. 1332–1333, 2002.

[11] P. Buykx, W. Loxley, P. Dietze, and A. Ritter, "Medications used in overdose and how they are acquired—an investigation of cases attending an inner Melbourne emergency department," *Australian and New Zealand Journal of Public Health*, vol. 34, no. 4, pp. 401–404, 2010.

[12] A. Wong, D. M. Taylor, K. Ashby, and J. Robinson, "Changing epidemiology of intentional antidepressant drug overdose in Victoria, Australia," *Australian and New Zealand Journal of Psychiatry*, vol. 44, no. 8, pp. 759–764, 2010.

[13] http://www.greaterdandenong.com/document/18464/statistical-data-for-victorian-communities.

[14] B. Pink, *An Introduction To Socio-Economic Indexes For Areas (SEIFA)*, Australian Bureau of Statistics, 2006.

[15] Southern Health Victoria, *Southern Health ED Executive Report*, Datasource: Health Central-Symphony, 2013.

[16] K. Skegg, "Self-harm," *The Lancet*, vol. 366, no. 9495, pp. 1471–1483, 2005.

[17] D. J. Gunnell, T. J. Peters, R. M. Kammerling, and J. Brooks, "Relation between parasuicide, suicide, psychiatric admissions, and socioeconomic deprivation," *British Medical Journal*, vol. 311, no. 6999, pp. 226–230, 1995.

[18] J. Greene and J. Hall, "The comparability of emergency department waiting time performance data," *Medical Journal of Australia*, vol. 197, no. 6, pp. 345–348, 2012.

[19] D. Gunnell, D. Ho, and V. Murray, "Medical management of deliberate drug overdose: a neglected area for suicide prevention?" *Emergency Medicine Journal*, vol. 21, no. 1, pp. 35–38, 2004.

[20] K. Hawton, H. Bergen, D. Casey et al., "Self-harm in England: a tale of three cities. Multicentre study of self-harm," *Social Psychiatry and Psychiatric Epidemiology*, vol. 42, no. 7, pp. 513–521, 2007.

[21] A. Graudins, R. P. Dowsett, and C. Liddle, "The toxicity of antidepressant poisoning: is it changing? A comparative study of cyclic and newer serotonin-specific antidepressants," *Emergency Medicine*, vol. 14, no. 4, pp. 440–446, 2002.

[22] M. Little, "Emergency management and resuscitation of poisoned patients: perspectives from 'down under'," *Scandinavian Journal of Trauma, Resuscitation and Emergency Medicine*, vol. 17, no. 1, article 36, 2009.

[23] C. Haw and K. Hawton, "Life problems and deliberate self-harm: associations with gender, age, suicidal intent and psychiatric and personality disorder," *Journal of Affective Disorders*, vol. 109, no. 1-2, pp. 139–148, 2008.

[24] C. Haw, K. Hawton, K. Houston, and E. Townsend, "Psychiatric and personality disorders in deliberate self-harm patients," *British Journal of Psychiatry*, vol. 178, pp. 48–54, 2001.

# 10

# Isolated T Wave Inversion in Lead aVL: An ECG Survey and a Case Report

**Getaw Worku Hassen,[1,2,3] Ana Costea,[2] Claire Carrazco,[4] Tsion Frew,[5] Anand Swaminathan,[5] Jason Feliberti,[6] Roger Chirurgi,[2] Tennyson Smith,[7] Alice Chen,[4] Sarah Thompson,[8] Neola Gushway-Henry,[8] Bonnie Simmons,[1,3] George Fernaine,[9] Hossein Kalantari,[2] and Soheila Talebi[10]**

[1] *Lutheran Medical Center, Department of Emergency Medicine, Brooklyn, NY 11220, USA*
[2] *NYMC, Metropolitan Hospital Center, Department of Emergency Medicine, New York, NY 10029, USA*
[3] *Department of Emergency Medicine, St. George's University School of Medicine, St. George's, Grenada*
[4] *School of Osteopathic Medicine, A.T. Still University, Mesa, AZ 85206, USA*
[5] *Bellevue Medical Center, Department of Emergency Medicine, New York, NY 10016, USA*
[6] *Department of Internal Medicine, NYU, New York, NY 10016, USA*
[7] *Medgar Evers College, Brooklyn, NY 11225, USA*
[8] *Lutheran Medical Center, Department of Family Practice, Brooklyn, NY 11220, USA*
[9] *Lutheran Medical Center, Department of Internal Medicine, Brooklyn, NY 11220, USA*
[10] *NYMC, Metropolitan Hospital Center, Department of Internal Medicine, New York, NY 10029, USA*

Correspondence should be addressed to Getaw Worku Hassen; getawh@yahoo.com

Academic Editor: Seiji Morita

*Background.* Computerized electrocardiogram (ECG) analysis has been of tremendous help for noncardiologists, but can we rely on it? The importance of ST depression and T wave inversions in lead aVL has not been emphasized and not well recognized across all specialties. *Objective.* This study's goal was to analyze if there is a discrepancy of interpretation by physicians from different specialties and a computer-generated ECG reading in regard to a TWI in lead aVL. *Methods.* In this multidisciplinary prospective study, a single ECG with isolated TWI in lead aVL that was interpreted by the computer as normal was given to all participants to interpret in writing. The readings by all physicians were compared by level of education and by specialty to one another and to the computer interpretation. *Results.* A total of 191 physicians participated in the study. Of the 191 physicians 48 (25.1%) identified and 143 (74.9%) did not identify the isolated TWI in lead aVL. *Conclusion.* Our study demonstrated that 74.9% did not recognize the abnormality. New and subtle ECG findings should be emphasized in their training so as not to miss significant findings that could cause morbidity and mortality.

## 1. Introduction

The electrocardiogram (ECG) is the most important initial diagnostic tool for myocardial infarction (MI). The computer is helpful in accurately identifying common pathologies on ECG. Changes in certain leads represent possible myocardial injury in specific coronary artery distributions. Therefore MI location could be inferred based on the area affected within the ECG [1, 2]. ECG changes of myocardial injury and ischemia include hyperacute T wave, ST elevation, Q wave, ST depression, T wave flattening as well as T wave inversion (TWI) [2, 3]. ST elevation has been recognized as a marker for acute myocardial infarction. ST depression and TWI are the result of myocardial ischemia except in leads V1 and V2, which may represent posterior myocardial infarction [3, 4].

Reciprocal changes such as ST depressions and TWI are well-recognized ECG changes that accompany ST elevations [5, 6] and their significance has been the subject of many

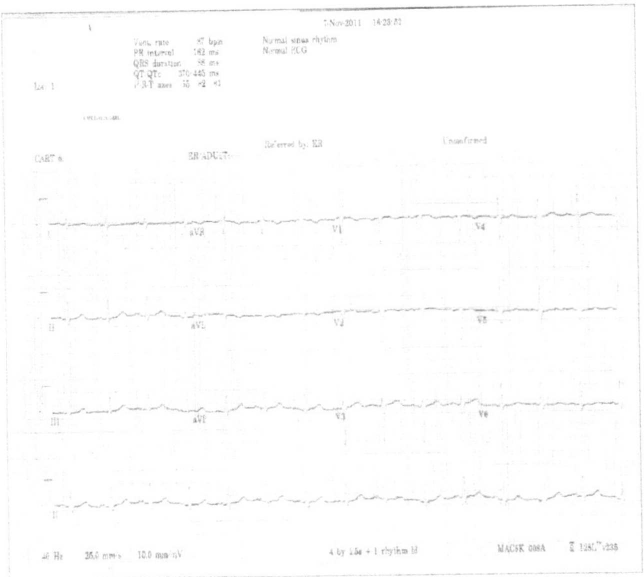

Figure 1: ECG representing isolated T wave inversion in lead aVL.

studies. These changes have been studied to localize the site of a coronary lesion [7] and also are believed to be early and sensitive markers of myocardial infarction [8]. Reciprocal changes may be the only manifestation of acute myocardial ischemia and may be present in a single lead as ST depression in lead aVL [5, 6] and TWI in lead aVL indicating a significant coronary artery lesion in left anterior descending (LAD) artery is another example [9–11]. The importance of these changes has not been emphasized and/or well recognized across all specialties.

The objective of this study was to determine the ability of physicians to identify isolated TWI in lead aVL on ECG that is read as normal by ECG computer. In addition, we sought to analyze if there is a discrepancy in interpretation in regard to a TWI in lead aVL by physicians from different specialties and a computer-generated ECG. To the best of our knowledge no such study was conducted previously.

## 2. Material and Methods

This prospective study was multicenter and multidisciplinary. The participating physicians were from the departments of Emergency Medicine (EM), Family Practice (FP), Internal Medicine (IM), and Surgery (S) of four different hospitals. These physicians had different training levels (attending physician and resident physicians of different postgraduate levels). They were grouped according to their training level: postgraduate year (PGY1–5) and attending physicians of each specialty. Institutional review boards (IRBs) of the corresponding institutions approved the study independently.

A single ECG with the isolated TWI in lead aVL that was interpreted by the computer as normal was given to all participants with a case description (Figure 1). Physicians were not allowed to consult with one other and they were given 5 minutes to perform their reading. All physicians gave their interpretations in writing after reviewing the case presentation and the corresponding ECG. The readings by all physicians and the computer interpretation were compared in regard to changes in lead aVL as well as amongst all physicians by level of education and by specialty.

Table 1: The number of physicians who did and did not identify the isolated TWI in lead aVL by specialty and training level.

| Groups | Identified TW in lead aVL | Not identified TW in lead aVL |
|---|---|---|
| EM1 | 2 | 3 |
| EM2 | 8 | 3 |
| EM3 | 2 | 10 |
| EM4 | 1 | 4 |
| EMA | 2 | 8 |
| FP1 | 5 | 9 |
| FP2 | 1 | 8 |
| FP3 | 4 | 8 |
| FPA | 1 | |
| IM1 | 6 | 30 |
| IM2 | 7 | 21 |
| IM3 | 5 | 16 |
| IM4 | | 1 |
| IMA | 3 | 2 |
| S1 | | 9 |
| S2 | | 3 |
| S3 | 1 | 4 |
| S4 | | 2 |
| S5 | | 2 |
| SA | | |

EM: Emergency Medicine; PF: Family Practice; IM: Internal Medicine; S: Surgery.

*2.1. Statistical Methods and Results.* Using generalized linear models in the statistical programming software R, a forward stepwise logistic regression analysis was performed.

## 3. Results

A total of 191 physicians participated in the study. Of the 191 physicians 43 (22.5%) were EM physicians, 91 (58.1%) were IM physicians, 36 (18.8%) were FP physicians, and 21 (11%) were surgeons (Table 1). In terms of training level, 64 (33.5%) physicians were PGY1, 51 (26.7%) physicians were PGY2, 50 (26.2%) physicians were PGY3, 8 (4.2%) physicians were PGY4, 2 (1%) physicians were PGY5, and 16 (8.4%) physicians were attending physicians. A total of 48 (25.1%) physicians identified and 143 (74.9%) physicians did not identify the isolated TWI in lead aVL. Of the 48 physicians that identified the isolated TWI in lead aVL 15 (31.3%) were EM physicians and 21 (43.8%) were IM physicians, 11 (23%) were FP physicians, and 1 (2%) physician was surgeon. In terms of training level of physicians who identified the isolated TWI in lead aVL, 13 (27.1%) were PGY1,

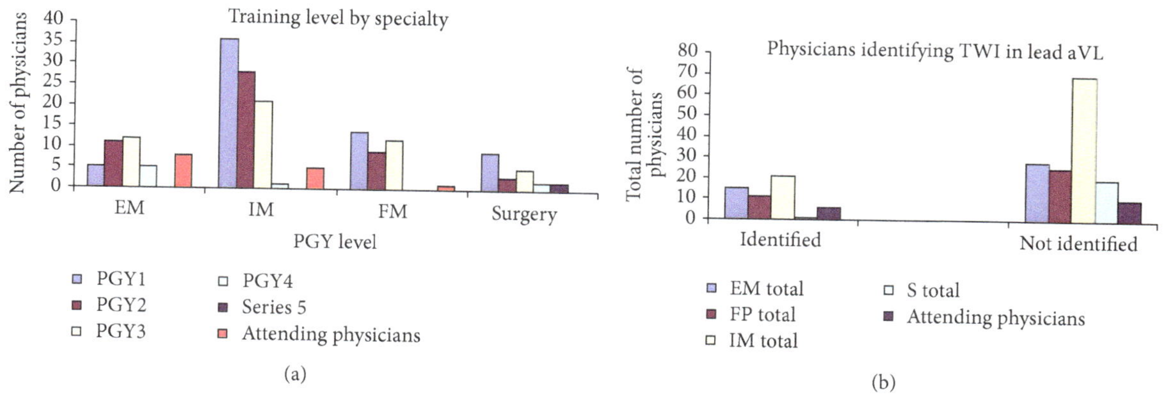


FIGURE 2: (a) Number of physicians by training level and specialties. (b) Total number of physicians who identified TWI in lead aVL on ECG by training level and specialties.

16 (33.3%) were PGY2, 12 (25%) were PGY3, 2 (4.2%) were PGY4, and 6 (12.5%) were attending physicians (Table 1 and Figures 2(a) and 2(b)). Using generalized linear models in the statistical programming software R, a forward stepwise logistic regression analysis was performed. Year of training was more significant than specialty in terms of predicting the odds of identifying TWI in lead aVL. Emergency Medicine physicians overall had the highest odds, while surgeons had the lowest odds, of identifying TWI in lead aVL. Controlling for specialty, there is an increase in odds of identification for both PGY2 and PGY3 physicians and a decrease in the odds of identification for both PGY4 and PGY5 physicians. Attending physicians have an increase in the odds of identification.

## 4. Case Report

This is the case of a 69-year-old man who presented to the emergency department (ED) with left sided chest pain for 3 days. The pain was sudden in onset, sharp in nature, and 5-6/10 in severity. He noticed the pain while walking and it radiated to the left shoulder. He took aspirin and his pain improved to 1/10, but he continued to have dull substernal chest pain without radiation. This pain was exacerbated by deep palpation and cold weather. He denied shortness of breath, dizziness, fever, chills, nausea, or vomiting. He was seen approximately 6 months ago for a nuclear stress test, which was negative. His ECG in September 2011 was sinus rhythm at 62 beats per minute, normal axis, and Q wave in lead III and upright T wave in lead aVL.

His past medical and surgical history included hypertension, benign prostate hyperplasia, gastroesophageal reflux disease (GERD), and surgery for colon cancer. He denied using alcohol or tobacco.

On presentation his vital signs were as follows: temperature 98.4 degrees Fahrenheit, respiration rate 18 breaths per minute, pulse 82 beats per minute, and blood pressure 145/80 mmHG. His physical examination was unremarkable except for mild sternal tenderness to palpation. His initial ECG showed sinus rhythm at 64 and T wave flattening in lead aVL (Figure 3(b)). The chest radiography was unremarkable. The repeat ECG showed sinus rhythm at 62 beats per minute with TWI in lead aVL along with biphasic T waves in leads V2 and V3 (Figure 3(c)). A comparative old ECG has normal T wave in lead aVL (Figure 3(a)). The patient was taken to the angiography suite and underwent a coronary angiogram. Angiography revealed a 99% mid-LAD lesion and he received a stent (Figures 4(a) and 4(b)). Laboratory results were unremarkable except for mildly elevated triglyceride levels (202 mg/dL) and white blood cell count (15, 600 $mm^3$). Cardiac troponins were within normal limits. The patient was subsequently discharged home to follow up as an outpatient. He remained symptom-free and on the follow-up clinic visit his ECG normalized with upright T waves in lead aVL (Figure 5).

## 5. Discussion

Computerized ECG analysis has been one of the most rapidly and widely adopted computer applications in medicine. A computer-assisted interpretation could be valuable especially to the noncardiologist physician [12]. It was pioneered in the 1960s and 1970s [13–15]. A system developed by Pipberger et al. was capable of automatic recognition of electrocardiographic waves by digital computer [14–16]. Two principles were used for automated ECG analysis. The first system involves pattern recognition techniques of ECG signals that have been previously recorded and stored in digital computer [16, 17]. Another program applied decision tree logic to measurements of waveform amplitude and duration [12]. Second generation programs were designed that employed statistical methods for diagnosis [18].

Clinical implementation of computerized electrocardiography occurred in the early 1970s and has continued to develop at a rapid rate. Based on the consensus standards the American College of Cardiology (ACC)/American Heart Association (AHA) requires 500 supervised ECG readings during the initial training period and 100 yearly to maintain competency in ECG reading skills [19]. The computer-assisted ECG reading is of tremendous help for noncardiologists because they do not interpret sufficient ECGs readings. In selected cases they can get immediate help from

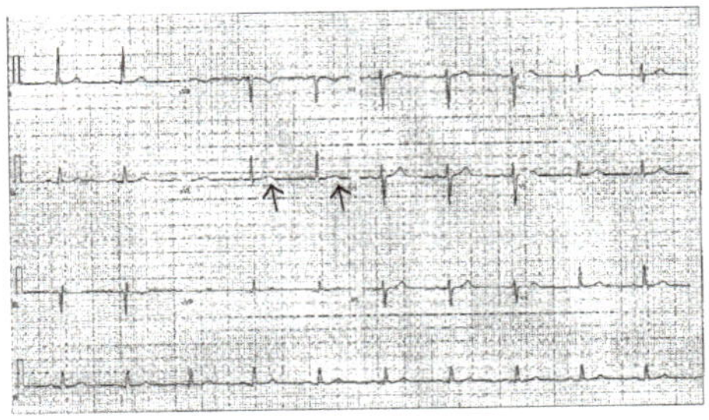

(a)

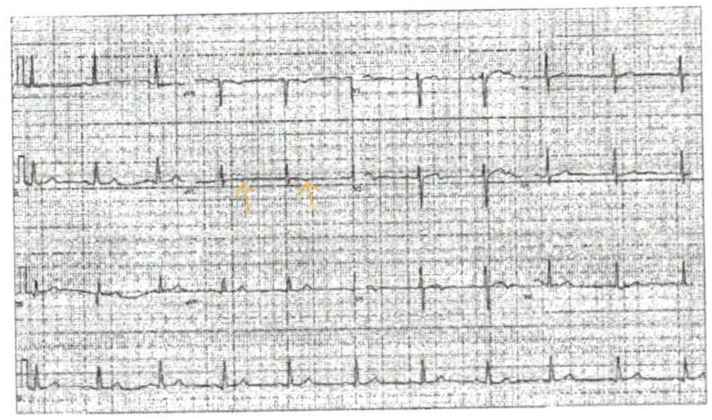

(b)

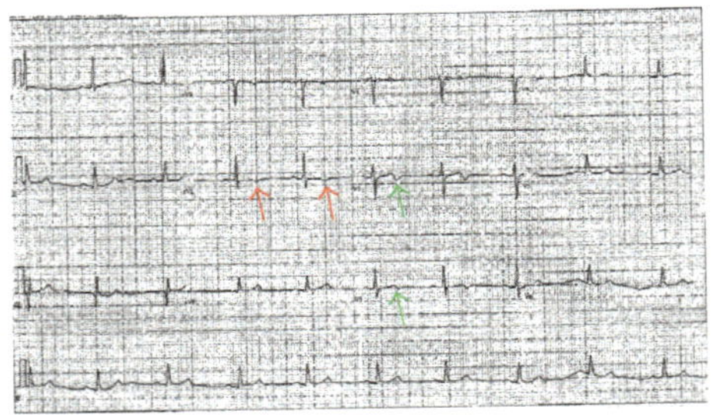

(c)

Figure 3: Dynamic T wave changes on ECG. (a) Upright T wave in lead aVL (black arrows, old ECG); (b) T wave flattening and early inversion in lead aVL (orange arrows, ECG at presentation); (c) TWI in lead aVL (red arrows, repeat ECG) and biphasic T waves in leads V2 and V3 (green arrows).

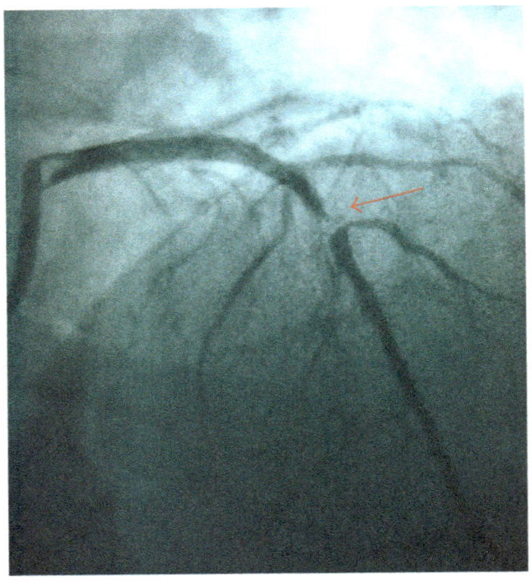

(a)

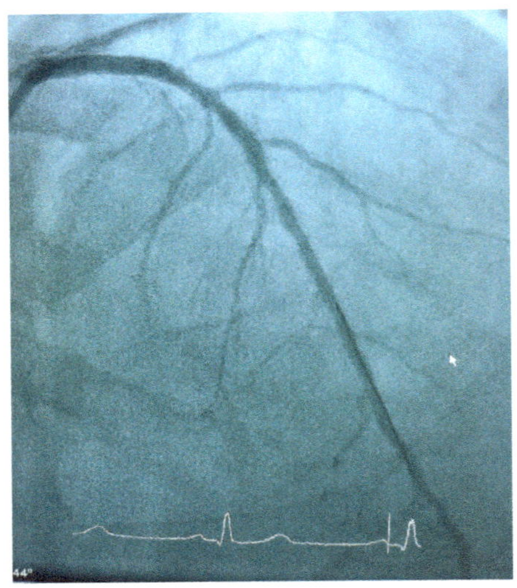

(b)

Figure 4: Coronary angiography. (a) Mid-LAD lesion (red arrow) and no proximal LAD abnormality: (b) after placement of stent.

cardiologists in interpreting the ECG. This is unfortunately not feasible on every ECG obtained routinely in medical and surgical units or in the ED. For emergency physicians ECG aids in making disposition of patients with chest pain and other cardiac complaints. Based on the ECG finding a patient can be admitted or discharged for outpatient follow-up.

Several studies have looked into patients' outcome based on ECG reading by ED physicians compared with cardiologist and computer-assisted ECG readings. Snyder et al. found significant discordance in the ECG interpretation accuracy between the ED physician and the computer-generated reading [20]. McCarthy et al. found that 1.9% of patients were discharged inappropriately of which 25% had missed ST elevations [21]. Westdrop et al. reported in their study that there was only 42% agreement between the ECG reading of the ED physicians and cardiologists with 17.5% interpretation error by the ED physician that was clinically significant [22]. Khun et al. found that 59.2% had agreement with reference standard on major abnormality, but 8.3% had serious interpretation error [23].

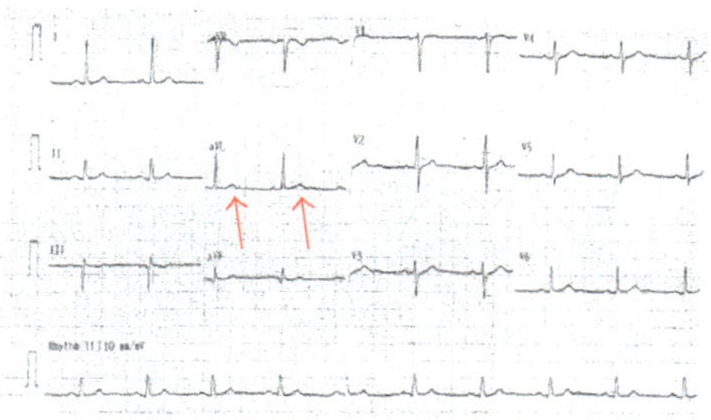

FIGURE 5: Follow-up ECG: patient returned to the cardiology office and his repeat ECG demonstrated the upright T waves in lead aVL after the stent placement.

A comparison of the different programs has been conducted [24, 25]. Systems processing ECGs have grown from 85 in 1975 to 15,000 over the years, but no consensus was found on which program is more accurate in interpreting ECGs [25]. ECGs of patients in seven common diagnoses were compared between cardiologist and different computer programs. The percentage of ECGs correctly classified by the computer programs was lower than the cardiologists [24].

Despite the sophistication and growing number of computer systems for ECG interpretation and diagnosis, can physicians solely rely on the automated ECG interpretation? The answer to this question is not simple. For instance recently detected new pathologies will not be fed into the computer system before the machines are in use. Therefore, physicians should interpret ECGs despite normal readings by the computer. For instance, Wellens and his group discovered that 75% of patients who had biphasic T wave in leads V2 and V3 (Wellens' sign) on their initial ECG and who were treated medically developed extensive anterior wall infarction within few days [1]. These observations led to a subsequent study by the same group who found critical proximal LAD lesions on coronary angiography [26]. It is recommended that patients with Wellens' sign should not undergo ergometric stress test as this can precipitate extensive MI and could lead to death [1, 26, 27]. The best management for patients with Wellens' sign is coronary angiography followed by PCI or CABG based on their angiographic findings [28, 29].

T wave changes in lead aVL might be considered nonsignificant by most physicians; however, a limited number of studies have shown the importance of T wave changes in recognition of right ventricular involvement in inferior wall MI [30, 31] and sign of mid-LAD lesion [10, 11, 32]. Farhan et al. found 14.1% of the ECGs they reviewed had TWI in lead aVL. In their study they identify isolated T wave inversion to be the only ECG variable significantly predicting mid-segment LAD lesion [32]. They demonstrated that TWI in lead aVL correlated with significant mid-LAD lesion. All ECGs with the isolated TWI in aVL were read as normal by the referring physicians [32]. ST segment changes in lead aVL are also considered as a sensitive marker for early inferior wall MI (early reciprocal change) [8]. Studies have indicated that ST segment or T wave abnormality in specific leads can signify a significant lesion of a specific coronary artery. As shown by Wellens' group there is a higher morbidity from a LAD lesion due to the involvement of larger areas of the myocardium. The accumulating evidence with regard to TWI in aVL indicates that this specific ECG finding should not be considered nonspecific and the diagnosis should not be missed as it potentially leads to significant morbidity and mortality. Unfortunately, T wave changes in lead aVL have not been emphasized and are not well recognized across all specialties.

Our survey indicated that only 25.1% of physicians identified the isolated TWI in lead aVL. The computer read the ECG as normal. The majority of physicians did not recognize the abnormality. In addition, the abnormality was not recognized uniformly across all specialties. Emergency physicians were better than other specialties in recognizing the TWI in lead aVL. A comparison between EM physicians and cardiologists might be a better comparison.

Our patient presented with symptoms suggestive of ACS. He had a recent nuclear stress test that was negative and normal ECG. He presented to the ED with symptoms suggesting ACS and significant changes on his ECG. He had two changes that signified a lesion in the LAD. The first one is Wellens' sign that signifies a proximal LAD lesion and T wave inversion in lead aVL signifying a mid-LAD lesion. The T wave changes in lead aVL suggested the following: (1) an early sign for an acute MI or a sign for a mid-LAD lesion; (2) the presence of Wellens' sign suggesting the possibility of a proximal LAD lesion. Interestingly, on literature review, in 22% of patients with biphasic T waves in leads V2 and V3 the lesions identified on angiogram were in the mid-segment of the LAD [33]. Both findings lead to the decision to take the patient for coronary angiography. Angiography revealed a 99% mid-segment LAD lesion that would go along with the TWI in lead aVL.

Dynamic ECG changes are helpful in detecting ongoing myocardial injury. Our patient's ECG showed the dynamic change from T wave flattening to mild TWI and then prominent TWI in lead aVL. TWI in lead aVL may be an early reciprocal change for acute MI and may be a sign for a mid-segment LAD lesion leading to the initiation of early therapeutic interventions. Left anterior descending artery lesion LAD supplies a larger portion of the heart and since the myocardium at risk from a LAD lesion is large that may lead to significant morbidity or mortality; therefore, it is of paramount importance to recognize subtle changes on ECG such as T wave inversion in lead aVL or Wellens' sign to make an early diagnosis and initiate appropriate treatment in a timely fashion.

The results of a recent study by our group indicated that TWI was associated with mid-LAD lesion with a sensitivity of 87.8 and positive predictive value of 81% for significant mid-LAD lesion (50% and above on coronary angiography) when evaluating angiograms for ST elevation MIs (STEMI). Patients who underwent coronary angiography for other reasons demonstrated a sensitivity of 65.2%, PPV of 83.3%, and specificity of 66.7 for significant mid-LAD lesion (70% and above on coronary angiography) [10].

Industries continue to improves the accuracy of the computer-assisted ECG reading, but as newer findings accumulate older computer programs lag behind and do not recognize findings such as Brugada syndrome, Wellens' sign, or isolated TWI in lead aVL. Therefore, physicians should not solely rely on the computer reading and should look for subtle, yet significant, findings independently of the computer reading. Health care providers should be aware of these subtle findings and it should be emphasized in their training.

One important point that needs to be emphasized is that T wave inversion in lead aVL can be a normal finding. The frequency of its presence in normal population is not known, but frequency is ranging from 10 to 20% in normal Caucasian population in Scotland [34]. In addition, the magnitude of T wave inversion may play a role to be a pathologic finding. Qualitative and quantitative description of T wave inversion have been described and may help differentiate pathological T wave inversions [35–37]. One example is the Pardee T wave in which a T wave inversion in any precordial leads of at least 0.06 mV is considered to predict changes from ischemic heart disease [38]. Other factors such as ventricular hypertrophy or bundle branch block that possibly change the polarity of T wave should be taken into consideration. The above-mentioned factors are limitations to the use of TWI in lead aVL as a sole criterion to predict CAD. The sole presence of isolated T wave inversion may not automatically predict CAD and may represent a normal finding, but the whole clinical picture, the presence of risk factors as well as patients presenting symptoms in combination with a T wave inversion of specific magnitude, may suggest ischemic heart disease.

*Limitations.* The study is limited by small sample size. In addition, the proportion of physicians in each specialty was not equally represented. This may change the final result if an equal number of physicians were included in each group. Finally, the level of training regarding ECG reading in each department and at the different sites is not obvious. Some programs may emphasize ECG reading and the residents get intensive ECG review whereas others may not have equivalent education.

## 6. Conclusion

The computer is a helpful instrument in accurately identifying common pathologies on ECG; however, certain conditions, especially newer findings, are missed by the computer. Physicians need to carefully evaluate ECGs and should not rely on the computer readings. Our study demonstrated that significant number of physicians of all specialties missed the diagnosis. Health care providers should remain alert to new ECG findings and this should be emphasized in their training.

## Conflict of Interests

The authors declare that there is no conflict of interests regarding the publication of this paper.

## Acknowledgments

The authors thank Dr. Shaw and Ms. Laura Gabbe for reviewing and editing the paper. They also thank Dr. Fahad Khan for the case.

## References

[1] C. de Zwaan, F. W. H. M. Bar, and H. J. J. Wellens, "Characteristic electrocardiographic pattern indicating a critical stenosis high in left anterior descending coronary artery in patients admitted because of impending myocardial infarction," *The American Heart Journal*, vol. 103, no. 4, pp. 730–736, 1982.

[2] J. B. Jayroe, D. H. Spodick, K. Nikus et al., "Differentiating ST elevation myocardial infarction and nonischemic causes of ST elevation by analyzing the presenting electrocardiogram," *American Journal of Cardiology*, vol. 103, no. 3, pp. 301–306, 2009.

[3] W. J. Brady, A. D. Perron, and T. Chan, "Electrocardiographic ST-segment elevation: correct identification of acute myocardial infarction AMI and non-AMI syndromes by emergency physicians," *Academic Emergency Medicine*, vol. 8, no. 4, pp. 349–360, 2001.

[4] W. J. Brady, A. D. Perron, E. A. Ullman et al., "Electrocardiographic ST segment elevation: a comparison of AMI and non-AMI ECG syndromes," *American Journal of Emergency Medicine*, vol. 20, no. 7, pp. 609–612, 2002.

[5] O. H. Kracoff, A. G. Adelman, M. Oettinger et al., "Reciprocal changes as the presenting electrocardiographic manifestation of acute myocardial ischemia," *The American Journal of Cardiology*, vol. 71, no. 15, pp. 1359–1362, 1993.

[6] O. H. Kracoff, A. G. Adelman, J.-F. Marquis, A. Caspi, H. E. Aldridge, and L. Schwartz, "Twelve-lead electrocardiogram recording during percutaneous transluminal coronary angioplasty. Analysis of reciprocal changes," *Journal of Electrocardiology*, vol. 23, no. 3, pp. 191–198, 1990.

[7] D. L. Glancy and W. Doghmi, "Use of indicative and reciprocal electrocardiographic changes to help localize the site of coronary occlusion," *Proceedings (Baylor University. Medical Center)*, vol. 14, pp. 104–105, 2001.

[8] Y. Birnbaum, S. Sclarovsky, A. Mager, B. Strasberg, and E. Rechavia, "ST segment depression in aVL: a sensitive marker for acute inferior myocardial infarction," *European Heart Journal*, vol. 14, no. 1, pp. 4–7, 1993.

[9] H. L. Farhan, K. S. Hassan, A. Al-Belushi, M. Sallam, and I. Al-Zakwani, "Diagnostic value of electrocardiographic T wave inversion in lead aVL in diagnosing coronary artery disease in patients with chronic stable angina," *Oman Medical Journal*, vol. 25, no. 2, pp. 124–127, 2010.

[10] G. W. Hassen, A. Costea, T. Smith et al., "The neglected lead on electrocardiogram: T wave inversion in lead aVL, nonspecific finding or a sign for left anterior descending artery lesion?" *The Journal of Emergency Medicine*, vol. 46, no. 2, pp. 165–170, 2014.

[11] G. W. Hassen, S. Talebi, G. Fernaine, and H. Kalantari, "Lead aVL on electrocardiogram: emerging as important lead in early diagnosis of myocardial infarction?" *The American Journal of Emergency Medicine*, vol. 32, no. 7, pp. 785–788, 2014.

[12] L. F. Staples, J. E. Gustafson, G. J. Balm, and W. A. Tate, "Computer interpretation of electrocardiograms," *American Heart Journal*, vol. 72, no. 3, pp. 351–358, 1966.

[13] C. A. Caceres, C. A. Steinberg, S. Abraham et al., "Computer extraction of electrocardiographic parameters," *Circulation*, vol. 25, pp. 356–362, 1962.

[14] H. V. Pipberger, R. J. Arms, and F. W. Stallmann, "Automatic screening of normal and abnormal electrocardiograms by means of digital electronic computer," *Proceedings of the Society for Experimental Biology and Medicine*, vol. 106, pp. 130–132, 1961.

[15] H. V. Pipberger, E. D. Freis, L. Taback, and H. L. Mason, "Preparation of electrocardiographic data for analysis by digital electronic computer," *Circulation*, vol. 21, pp. 413–418, 1960.

[16] H. V. Pipberger, "Use of digital computers in analyzing electrocardiographic data," *The Heart Bulletin*, vol. 13, pp. 44–47, 1964.

[17] F. W. Stallmann and H. V. Pipberger, "Automatic recognition of electrocardiographic waves by digital computer.," *Circulation Research*, vol. 9, pp. 1138–1143, 1961.

[18] H. V. Pipberger, D. McCaughan, D. Littmann et al., "Clinical application of a second generation electrocardiographic computer program," *The American Journal of Cardiology*, vol. 35, no. 5, pp. 597–608, 1975.

[19] A. H. Kadish, A. E. Buxton, H. L. Kennedy et al., "ACC/AHA clinical competence statement on electrocardiography and ambulatory electrocardiography. A report of the ACC/AHA/ACP-ASIM Task Force on Clinical Competence (ACC/AHA Committee to Develop a Clinical Competence Statement on Electrocardiography and Ambulatory Electrocardiography)," *Journal of the American College of Cardiology*, vol. 38, no. 7, pp. 2091–2100, 2001.

[20] C. S. Snyder, A. L. Fenrich, R. A. Friedman, C. Macias, K. O'Reilly, and N. J. Kertesz, "The emergency department versus the computer: which is the better electrocardiographer?" *Pediatric Cardiology*, vol. 24, no. 4, pp. 364–368, 2003.

[21] B. D. McCarthy, J. R. Beshansky, R. B. D'Agostino, and H. P. Selker, "Missed diagnoses of acute myocardial infarction in the emergency department: results from a multicenter study," *Annals of Emergency Medicine*, vol. 22, no. 3, pp. 579–582, 1993.

[22] E. J. Westdorp, M. C. Gratton, and W. A. Watson, "Emergency department interpretation of electrocardiograms," *Annals of Emergency Medicine*, vol. 21, no. 5, pp. 541–544, 1992.

[23] M. Kuhn, M. T. Morgan, and J. R. Hoffman, "Quality assurance in the emergency department: evaluation of the ECG review process," *Annals of Emergency Medicine*, vol. 21, no. 1, pp. 10–15, 1992.

[24] J. L. Willems, C. Abreu-Lima, P. Arnaud et al., "The diagnostic performance of computer programs for the interpretation of electrocardiograms," *The New England Journal of Medicine*, vol. 325, no. 25, pp. 1767–1773, 1991.

[25] E. Drazen, N. Mann, R. Borun, M. Laks, and A. Bersen, "Survey of computer-assisted electrocardiography in the United States," *Journal of Electrocardiology*, vol. 21, supplement, pp. S98–S104, 1988.

[26] C. de Zwaan, F. W. Bar, J. H. A. Janssen et al., "Angiographic and clinical characteristics of patients with unstable angina showing an ECG pattern indicating critical narrowing of the proximal LAD coronary artery," *American Heart Journal*, vol. 117, no. 3, pp. 657–665, 1989.

[27] T. K. Tandy, D. P. Bottomy, and J. G. Lewis, "Wellen's syndrome," *Annals of Emergency Medicine*, vol. 33, no. 3, pp. 347–351, 1999.

[28] W. E. Boden, E. W. Bough, I. Benham, and R. S. Shulman, "Unstable angina with episodic ST segment elevation and minimal creatine kinase release culminating in extensive, recurrent infarction," *Journal of the American College of Cardiology*, vol. 2, no. 1, pp. 11–20, 1983.

[29] N. E. Mead and K. P. O'Keefe, "Wellen's syndrome: an ominous EKG pattern," *Journal of Emergencies, Trauma and Shock*, vol. 2, no. 3, pp. 206–208, 2009.

[30] D. L. Rashduni and A. K. Tannenbaum, "Utility of ST segment depression in lead AVL in the diagnosis of right ventricular infarction," *New Jersey Medicine*, vol. 100, no. 11, pp. 35–37, 2003.

[31] H. Turhan, M. B. Yilmaz, E. Yetkin et al., "Diagnostic value of aVL derivation for right ventricular involvement in patients with acute inferior myocardial infarction," *Annals of Noninvasive Electrocardiology*, vol. 8, no. 3, pp. 185–188, 2003.

[32] G. W. Hassen and H. Kalantari, "Diplopia from subacute bilateral subdural hematoma after spinal anesthesia," *Western Journal of Emergency Medicine*, vol. 13, no. 1, pp. 108–110, 2012.

[33] P. Akhtar, S. N. H. Rizvi, F. Tahir, D. Saleem, J. Mulla, and T. Saghir, "Angiocardiographic findings in patients with biphasic T-wave inversion in precordial leads," *Journal of the Pakistan Medical Association*, vol. 62, no. 8, pp. 548–551, 2012.

[34] P. W. Macfarlane, A. van Oosterom, M. Janse, P. Kligfield, J. Camm, and O. Pahlm, *Specialized Aspects of ECG*, Medicine Cardiology & Angiology, Springer, London, UK, 2012.

[35] T. Chikamori, Y. L. Doi, T. Furuno, Y. Yonezawa, and T. Ozawa, "Diagnostic significance of deep T-wave inversion induced by exercise testing in patients with suspected coronary artery disease," *American Journal of Cardiology*, vol. 70, no. 3, pp. 403–406, 1992.

[36] P. M. Rautaharju, B. Surawicz, L. S. Gettes et al., "AHA/ACCF/HRS recommendations for the standardization and interpretation of the electrocardiogram: part IV: the ST segment, T and U waves, and the QT interval: a scientific statement from the American Heart Association Electrocardiography and Arrhythmias Committee, Council on Clinical Cardiology; the American College of Cardiology Foundation; and the Heart Rhythm Society. Endorsed by the International Society for Computerized Electrocardiology," *Journal of the American College of Cardiology*, vol. 53, no. 11, pp. 982–991, 2009.

[37] E. B. Hanna and D. L. Glancy, "ST-segment depression and T-wave inversion: classification, differential diagnosis, and caveats," *Cleveland Clinic Journal of Medicine*, vol. 78, no. 6, pp. 404–414, 2011.

[38] M. Kraft, W. J. French, and M. M. Laks, "Use of the computer to detect the pardee T wave. Frequent marker of coronary artery disease," *Journal of Electrocardiology*, vol. 24, supplement, pp. 50–53, 1991.

# 11

# The Global Burden of Road Injury: Its Relevance to the Emergency Physician

**Sharon Chekijian,[1] Melinda Paul,[2] Vanessa P. Kohl,[3] David M. Walker,[4] Anthony J. Tomassoni,[1] David C. Cone,[1] and Federico E. Vaca[1]**

[1] *Department of Emergency Medicine, Yale University School of Medicine, 464 Congress Avenue, Suite 260, New Haven, CT 06519, USA*
[2] *Yale University, New Haven, CT 06520, USA*
[3] *Department of Family Medicine, White Memorial Medical Center, Los Angeles, CA 90033, USA*
[4] *Division of Pediatric Emergency Medicine, Elmhurst Hospital Center, Ichahn School of Medicine at Mount Sinai School, Elmhurst, NY 11373, USA*

Correspondence should be addressed to Sharon Chekijian; sharon.chekijian@yale.edu

Academic Editor: Christian Wrede

*Background.* Road traffic crash fatalities in the United States are at the lowest level since 1950. The reduction in crash injury burden is attributed to several factors: public education and prevention programs, traffic safety policies and enforcement, improvements in vehicle design, and prehospital services coupled with emergency and acute trauma care. Globally, the disease burden of road traffic injuries is rising. In 1990, road traffic injuries ranked ninth in the ten leading causes of the global burden of disease. By 2030, estimates show that road traffic injuries will be the fifth leading causes of death in the world. Historically, emergency medicine has played a pivotal role in contributing to the success of the local, regional, and national traffic safety activities focused on crash and injury prevention. *Objective.* We report on the projected trend of the global burden of road traffic injuries and fatalities and describe ongoing global initiatives to reduce road traffic morbidity and mortality. *Discussion.* We present key domains where emergency medicine can contribute through international collaboration to address global road traffic-related morbidity and mortality. *Conclusion.* International collaborative programs and research offer important opportunities for emergency medicine physicians to make a meaningful impact on the global burden of disease.

## 1. Introduction

Deaths caused by road traffic injuries (RTI) in the United States are at their lowest number since 1950, with a nearly 10 percent decline in such fatalities between 2000 and 2009 alone [1]. Though the National Highway Traffic Safety Administration (NHSTA) cites several factors in the reduction of road traffic fatalities, including economy, unemployment, and improvements in vehicle design, success can be attributed to the attention focused on prehospital services and emergency medicine (EM) in the last half century, as well as the attention paid to injury prevention efforts within the field of EM itself.

The passage of the 1966 Traffic and Motor Vehicle Safety and Highway Safety Acts set unprecedented federal safety standards for motor vehicles and state highway safety programs [2]. In establishing such standards at federal and state levels, road safety compliance became a greater and more tangible priority. The next few decades saw an increase in federal funding, which was applied toward mass media awareness campaigns and research grants, as well as driving while intoxicated (DWI) regulations, and seatbelt and drinking-age laws [2].

With the increase in federal funding and the sense of urgency created by the 1966 publication, *Accidental Death and Disability: The Neglected Disease of Modern Society*, came the creation of emergency medical services (EMS) in the 1960s and 1970s [3]. EM, a newly recognized specialty, saw the need to bring advances to the pre-hospital care arena in cardiac and resuscitation interventions and in trauma care, helping to promote and strengthen the growth in EMS systems.

In the subsequent years following the establishment of an organized EMS system, a significant decrease was observed in RTI fatalities that would continue as an overall decrease in the decades to follow [4]. By applying scientific and research-based methods towards traffic safety aims, the United States was able to achieve great success in reducing RTIs [5]. Legislative efforts, policy making, engineering and medical advances, research initiatives, and the overall cooperation of various sectors in the United States all contributed to creating safer roads, an accomplishment so significant that it was recently recognized by the Centers for Disease Control and Prevention (CDC) as one of the top ten great public health achievements in the last decade [6].

In contrast to favorable downward trends in the US, the global burden of disease attributed to RTIs has continued to increase. In this report, we describe this worrisome trend by highlighting the escalating global disease burden of RTIs and examining global initiatives focused on RTI and fatality reduction. We conclude by identifying and suggesting four key domains where EM can make a meaningful impact with its international partners to reduce this global burden of disease.

## 2. Review

*2.1. The Global Burden of Injury.* The global burden of RTIs continues to grow and promises to overtake tropical diseases as a leading cause of death in the developing world. In 1990, RTIs ranked ninth in the ten leading causes of the global burden of disease, with respiratory infections and varying diseases in the top rankings [7]. By 2030, however, it is projected that RTIs will rank fifth in leading causes of death.

In 2004, the World Health Organization (WHO) and the World Bank combined efforts to publish the *World Report on Road Traffic Injury Prevention*, a result of a decade long discussion, to provide insight into the growing public health, economic, and social burdens caused by RTIs [5]. The report projected a rise in RTIs and fatalities, with an overwhelming and disproportionate 80% increase in low- and middle-income countries (LMIC). With an annual death toll of approximately 1.3 million people worldwide, the recent worsening of RTI statistics, and the dismal projections for the next two decades, failing to take significant, immediate action will lead to devastatingly increased death rates in an avoidable and preventable global health epidemic.

One factor in the rise of RTIs is the undeniable link between increased road travel and economic growth and prosperity. Despite the necessity of travel to fuel the economy, the weight of the monetary burdens created by RTIs is increasing [5]. According to the 2009 *Global Status Report on Road Safety*, RTIs have yielded an estimated US$518 billion in global losses, costing governments between 1% and 3% of their gross national product (GNP) [4]. This finding is disproportionally significant in low-income countries, where economic costs of RTIs exceed developmental assistance. The burden lies on national and local economies but also on individual households [5]. While mortality due to RTIs continues to decrease in higher-income countries, the projected increase in road traffic fatalities in low-income countries places monetary burdens on the global economy affecting high-, middle-, and low-income countries alike.

The social impact of global RTIs also continues to become a more tangible burden. Alongside economic costs, road traffic fatalities contribute to public health concerns, particularly among the world's younger populations. Between the ages of 5 and 44, RTIs are in the top three causes of death [5]. Not only does this affect the number of disability-adjusted life years lost (a measure combining years lost in premature death with health loss due to disability), but it also creates an added burden to families in low-income countries where the main source of household income is often from the manual labor of young hands [8]. In this way, RTIs decrease productivity and increase health costs, proving detrimental to already struggling households and economies.

Without global action, the outlook for the next few decades is far from promising. It is estimated that, despite a decrease of 30% in deaths related to RTIs in high-income countries, road traffic fatalities will continue to increase dramatically in low- and middle-income countries [5]. With such high costs for such a preventable global problem, the world has taken notice. Still, considerably more tangible day-to-day action needs to be taken.

*2.2. Major International Initiatives from Development Agencies.* The international development community has taken notice of this burgeoning toll of unintentional injury. The WHO and the World Bank, along with over 100 experts from around the world, ignited the discussion on global road safety through the 2004 *World Report on Road Traffic Injury Prevention* [5]. Their aim was to encourage governmental and societal attention to a growing burden and to fuel immediate action in the fight to decrease RTIs by presenting the facts about road traffic safety. With the *World Report on Road Traffic Injury Prevention*, the WHO and the World Bank sparked a cascade of international initiatives and campaigns toward safer roads.

The Pan American Health Organization (PAHO) organized the Pan American Conference on Road Safety just after the publication of the *World Report on Road Traffic Injury Prevention*. The conference united 16 countries in conversation in 2005 [9]. PAHO is particularly targeted toward improving public health in the Americas, working as part of the United Nations to focus especially on underresourced, more vulnerable populations. Citing the importance of consolidating efforts between countries to reduce the number of RTIs, PAHO sought to develop a pan-American road safety network to promote the adoption of the recommendations given in the *World Report on Road Traffic Injury Prevention*.

The World Bank's Global Road Safety Facility also expanded on the *World Report on Road Traffic Injury Prevention* by developing broader initiatives for combating the growing threat of RTIs [10]. Launched in 2005, its mission is to provide seed funding for the implementation of road safety programs in low- and middle-income countries.

Prior to the publication of the *World Report on Road Traffic Injury Prevention*, the United Nations General Assembly called on the WHO to coordinate the initiative to address road safety issues within the UN system [11]. Upon this appointment, the WHO established the United Nations Road Safety Collaboration (UNRSC), which initiated work in coordinating efforts between international participants in the global road safety network, developing manuals and databases and various other organizing tools to help public agencies develop interventions.

*2.3. International Programs, Associations, and Safety Campaigns.* The growing road safety crisis has been met by increased collaboration between international governments and agencies. The Global Road Safety Partnership particularly addresses the governments of LMIC, aiming to intervene in the collaboration of societal sectors (business, civil, government, etc.) at all levels (global, national, and local) to create a focus for road safety efforts [12]. The Partnership focuses on specific countries, including the Association of Southeast Asian Nations (ASEAN), Brazil, China, Hungary, India, Namibia, Poland, Romania, the Russian Federation, and South Africa, that fit particular criteria based on need and level of governmental political will to address the problem. The Bloomberg Philanthropies has also joined this important cause with the Global Road Safety Initiative. Bloomberg is targeting the ten LMICs that account for half of RTIs worldwide: Brazil, Cambodia, China, Egypt, India, Kenya, Mexico, Russia, Turkey, and Vietnam.

Alongside the Global Road Safety Partnership, the International Road Safety Academy (IRSA) Association also aims to provide support to LMICs in lowering the number of RTIs [13]. Initiated in 2004 by the Institute of Traffic Care and part of the European Road Safety Charter, its focus is encouraging improved road safety education and training, along with technological advances, to better equip future policy makers and agencies.

The International Road Federation, a not-for-profit, nongovernmental organization founded in 1948, seeks to combine the efforts of commercial and professional firms, corporations, public and governmental organizations, educational and research institutions, and national and regional road associations like the IRSA [14]. It was first established to promote the development of efficient highway systems after World War II [15]. Since then, it has aimed to improve the safety of road networks worldwide by creating a forum on road safety from a developmental and maintenance-oriented standpoint [14].

Representing the United States in this global forum, the Association for Safe International Road Travel is a nonprofit, international road safety organization that seeks to encourage safe roads through advocacy and education [16]. Founded in 1995 and still the only such organization in the United States, it encourages safer travel by providing and annually updating road travel reports for over 150 countries. It works with WHO, the UN, and the World Bank to foster conversations on international travel safety.

The Global Road Safety Forum (GRSF), founded in 2002 and part of the Task Force for Global Health, provides support for regional and global international road safety initiatives that stem from such conversations [17]. Regionally, the GRSF is conducting road safety projects in Latin America, the Caribbean, and South Asia. Internationally, the GRSF also holds forums on global road safety, encouraging open discussion of safety initiatives to raise awareness of the global burden resulting from RTIs.

One such awareness-raising initiative is the Make Roads Safe campaign, which began in 2006 in response to the *World Report on Road Traffic Injury Prevention* and in coordination with the Fédération Internationale de l'Automobile (FIA) Foundation [18]. The campaign's major initiative was the proposal of the "Decade of Action for Road Safety," declared by the United Nations General Assembly in 2010 as the years from 2011 to 2020 [19]. The goal in declaring this decade of action was to encourage cooperation between UN member nations at the global, national, and regional levels to decrease the number of road traffic fatalities by five million worldwide. The "Decade of Action" was declared immediately following the First Global Ministerial Conference on Road Safety, adopted by the UN General Assembly and held in 2009.

*2.4. Significance and Opportunities for Emergency Medicine.* The recently observed trends in global RTIs and fatalities demonstrate that current approaches to global road safety are falling short. A comprehensive injury prevention and control model is better suited to the task. To encourage action at all levels, it must be directed by those locally with influence within those same spheres. Emergency physicians have a unique opportunity to directly influence this field, as they are already participating in locally and nationally based education, EMS, acute care, and research initiatives, policymaking, and advocacy relevant to road traffic safety. Emergency physicians have learned many important lessons from the injury prevention and control activities in which they are engaged. It is therefore important that emergency physicians from those countries with longstanding experience broadly participate in assisting organizations and countries committed to global road safety and reducing the burden of injury. In turn, this promises to improve global health. Throughout their own development and evolution, US and European EM have been notably successful in making impactful contributions to national traffic safety [20]. Much of this success stems from the development and perpetual refinement of EMS, injury prevention and control, research, and policy and advocacy efforts. Each of these domains with their history of domestic success offers a highly relevant and ripe opportunity for translation to the global road safety context. Ultimately the commitment and political will must come from local physicians. We should be ready to lend support to them where it is needed in their endeavors. Without the clinical dimension and input from local physicians, the efforts of the development community will fall short. The policies need "feet on the ground" to be enacted but they also need to be informed by those who work on the frontlines. It is those who are impassioned by prevention of RTIs and trauma care in their respective countries that will ultimately make the biggest impact on reduction of traffic related morbidity and mortality. It is the synergy between already honed expertise and local political will that will serve to reduce this public health threat on a global scale.

The opportunities for collaboration are myriad. Areas with high impact potential are EMS system development, injury prevention control measures, injury prevention research, and policy and advocacy work.

*2.5. EMS System Development.* Emergency medical services (EMS) refer to the network of dispatch, ambulances, and receiving hospitals that combine to provide care for injured and ill patients. EMS system development and organization must be appropriate to the setting in order to make efficient use of existing scarce human, material, and financial resources and to facilitate future resource development and training of providers to best address global road safety. In the past, global health policy has focused on a disease specific model with interventions targeting each disease. Little attention was paid to the development of a comprehensive emergency medical system [21]. As a result, there is a great disparity among the EMS capacities of varying nations and their regions. Local system planners should reflect on best practices and components of a well-developed system within local constraints. The degree of EMS development will depend largely on available funding. In resource poor areas, we should look towards incremental progress towards the best practices.

Pre-hospital care worldwide can be organized into four categories, "unorganized pre-hospital care" where lay people or police transport patients to the hospital, basic life support systems where EMTs provide noninvasive care and transport, advanced life support systems that are staffed by highly trained paramedics that use protocols to drive their care, and finally Doc-ALS systems where physicians deliver pre-hospital care [22].

In regions that have addressed the development of EMS systems worldwide, there have been two main directions taken, the Anglo-American model based on a "scoop and run" system mainly staffed by paramedics and the Franco-German model largely staffed by physicians. In the Franco-German model, patients are treated on site and only transported to the hospital if they require further care [22]. In each particular country, the type of system that has been adopted is of utmost importance when formulating a national or regional strategy in RTI prevention. It is essential that emergency physicians worldwide take part in the dialogue that will form both the EMS and the policy backbone. They alone know the intricacies of the way their EMS systems have developed or need to develop in order to address and minimize injury morbidity and mortality.

In regions where EMS systems have yet to be developed the preference for "scoop and run" practices rather than "stay and play" should be stressed. In underresourced countries the goal should be to decrease the time to definitive care and to channel energies towards the development of trauma centers. There has been little scientific support given to increasing advanced medical care given on scene in a trauma response. In fact, if specific pre-hospital interventions such as advanced airway management, intravenous fluid administration and immobilization and splinting are examined, only immobilization and splinting are shown to be beneficial especially in areas with shorter transport times such as urban areas. In more rural areas with longer transport time, more advanced interventions may be warranted if those in the field are properly trained or have advanced training such is the case when physicians respond to calls [23]. Several studies including the OPALS study from 2008 have compared basic life support (BLS) to advanced life support (ALS) and concluded that there were no outcome improvements in morbidity or mortality [24]. Other meta-analyses have actually shown adverse outcomes in severity-matched cases in those transported by ALS units versus BLS units [25]. All of these findings must be interpreted in relation to the quality of both the EMS system and the level of training of its providers. Given these constraints, even in developed EMS systems such as Canada's, little advantage can be gained from a "stay and play" approach in traumatic injuries.

There are innumerable instances where well-meaning philanthropists have donated new, well-equipped, western style ambulances to rural areas of LMICs in areas that have no communication infrastructure to manage use of the ambulance, no trained personnel to staff it, and no medical infrastructure to accept patients that the ambulance might transport [26]. Local needs must be defined and prioritized to support the work of the doctors, community health workers, advocates and legislators. By becoming involved in the earlier stages of EMS development, local physicians can ensure that the needs of their patients are met and that their efforts are supported. Efforts are underway to define EMS needs and shortcomings at a local level. Initial needs assessment work by Razzak et al. in Pakistan found that 98% of community survey respondents were dissatisfied with the currently provided emergency medical care. Ninety-eight percent of providers felt that their facilities were not equipped to provide emergency care [27]. Further system funding, development, and expertise are sorely needed.

Many organizations offer resources to aid in the development and evolution of EMS systems: EMS, EM, and trauma professional organizations worldwide, such as ACS and NAEMT, WHO, PAHO, the UN Road Safety Organization, and the US Department of Transportation. Opportunities for interested parties to become involved in enhancing international EMS development are plentiful and include opportunities to engage in planning, policy development, teaching, oversight, and direction. In order for this collaboration to take place, local partners must first find the drive to address and ameliorate these worthy concerns. Once they do so, the international community must be ready to lend its expertise.

In many areas of the world, EM does not yet exist as a formalized specialty or the specialty is in its infancy. The development of EM is essential in the efficient and accurate delivery of care for trauma patients as well as in medical direction for the overall EMS system. In areas where the specialty of EM does not exist, there are often early proponents of the specialty from diverse backgrounds such as cardiology, internal medicine, and general surgery. Very often these early proponents either seek additional training for themselves or for the next generation of physicians entering the nascent specialty. The development of the specialty and the development of emergency medicine residency training can benefit from the collaborative expertise of more experienced partners and educators who have already advanced the specialty in their own countries and regions.

Systematic training according to ATLS training programs and guidelines ensures a protocol driven approach to complex traumatic issues and allows physicians from diverse specialties such as surgery and orthopedics to approach injuries with a consistent and comprehensive framework. These training modules devised by the American College of Surgeons (ACS) have been shown to mitigate global road fatalities, injuries, and long-term disabilities. These ACS modules include advanced trauma and life support (ATLS) [28], (http://www.facs.org/trauma/atls/), Advanced traumatic operative management (ATOM) [29], (http://www.facs.org/trauma/atom/), and Advanced Surgical Skills for Exposure in Trauma (ASSET) [30], (http://www.facs.org/trauma/education/asset.html). Moreover, the ACS has devised a strategy for the international dissemination of its educational models with over sixty countries participating voluntarily [31], (http://www.facs.org/trauma/atls/promulgation.html/). In addition, the National Association of Emergency Medical Technicians has partnered with the ACS to develop global continuing medical education for pre-hospital providers with the pre-hospital trauma and life support program or PHTLS [32], (http://www.naemt.org/education/PHTLS/whatisPHTLS.aspx).

There are many examples of recent collaborations that illustrate the efforts already undertaken in EMS development. The Department of Emergency Medicine at Emory has had significant involvement over the last several years in the area of EMS development in Ghana, Mozambique, and Georgia. Their involvement in Tbilisi, Georgia, funded by USAID, is focused on EM specialty and residency development in an area where a group of like-minded local doctors had decided to establish the first emergency department in ex-Soviet Georgia [33]. Their efforts to date have resulted in the development of a "miniresidency" certificate program that is taught by local faculty with support from the faculty at Emory.

*2.6. Injury Prevention and Control Measures.* While the field of injury prevention in low- and middle-income countries is immature compared to that in the United States, there are lessons learned in the US and other developed nations that can be effective in promoting a culture of road safety in these regions. Through a network of likeminded partners, emergency physicians and their trauma colleagues can be the vehicles through which successful programs can be adapted and implemented in other parts of the world, and there are a variety of ways in which they can promote and become involved in efforts to control injuries from road crashes (Table 1).

The WHO, in its 2004 *World Report on Road Traffic Injury Prevention*, outlines several key points that should frame any discussion on injury prevention efforts (Table 2).

While there is no "one standard approach" to injury prevention, interventions that are most effective are those encompassing a variety of strategies, including legislation, environmental modification, and public education. Interventions should reach across different sectors, build on existing networks, and involve communities. They need to be tailored to the social and physical environments of the target locales.

An example of such an intersection of multiple sectors exists in Thailand where recent attention has been paid to motorcycle crashes. Researchers have collected data to characterize the nature of motorcycle accidents, to understand the effectiveness of helmets, and to elucidate the effect of legislation on the use of motorcycle helmets. Recent efforts have culminated in a declaration by the government of Thailand that 100% crash helmet use will be targeted over the course of 2011. This federal program relies on the government's Departments of Education and Labour to educate the public and promote helmet use for all workers. It also relies on the police force for improved enforcement of a mandatory helmet law. Another example of this type of enforcement intervention can be found in work being done by the author in the Republic of Armenia in conjunction with the Department of Emergency Medicine at Yale. Car safety device usage was examined in a baseline study. An enforcement intervention followed and a second study was performed to document whether there was an improved awareness and usage in the study population. The follow-up study showed an overwhelming improvement in both areas after intervention [21].

*2.7. Injury Prevention Research.* While interventions are the mainstay of reducing traffic-related morbidity and mortality, quality research is needed to guide policy, programs, campaigns, and interventions. Substantial work is needed on research capacity development, particularly in the developing world where a paucity of trained researchers, funding, and research infrastructure persist [5]. While a number of national road traffic crash research centers exist and have made substantial progress in addressing road traffic safety, most are in the high-income countries, with national centers in Holland, Germany, and England, and regional centers in North Carolina and Michigan in the US and South Australia and Victoria in Australia. Notable exceptions are the Institute of Technology in New Delhi, India, and the Centre for Industrial and Scientific Research in South Africa, both of which have made substantial contributions to understanding road injury problems in LMICs [5].

To date, outside of these established research centers, there are few studies of a rigorous nature performed in

Table 1: Ways for EM practitioners to get involved in global road safety.

| |
|---|
| Data collection. Initiate or assist with improved injury surveillance |
| Advocacy. Working to persuade decision-makers to address injuries as a major issue and of the importance of adopting improved approaches to road traffic safety |
| Programming. Designing, implementing, monitoring, and evaluating appropriate interventions |
| Capacity building. Promoting capacity of health care systems to recognize and care for and provide rehabilitation to victims of road traffic injuries |
| Knowledge transfer. Adapt successful initiatives from the developed world to low resource settings |
| Partnering. Promote global collaboration by forming partnerships between academic institutions and foreign governments, health centers, or NGOs |
| Education. Incorporate lessons on road traffic crashes into medical school and residency curricula; educate healthcare providers and patients of safe behaviors |

Table 2: Key points for global road traffic injury prevention (WHO, 2004) [5].

| |
|---|
| Road crash injury is largely preventable and predictable; it is a human-made problem amenable to rational analysis and countermeasure |
| Road safety is a multisectorial issue and a public health issue—all sectors, including health, need to be fully engaged in responsibility, activity, and advocacy for road crash injury prevention |
| Common driving errors and common pedestrian behavior should not lead to death and serious injury—the traffic system should help users to cope with increasingly demanding conditions |
| The vulnerability of the human body should be a limiting design parameter for the traffic system and speed management is central |
| Road crash injury is a social equity issue—equal protection to all road users should be targeted for since nonmotor vehicle users bear a disproportionate share of road injury and risk |
| Technology transfer from high-income to low-income countries needs to fit local conditions and should address research-based local needs |
| Local knowledge needs to inform the implementation of local solutions |

LMICs, where the burden of RTIs is most concerning. Most articles within this body of knowledge are descriptive or simply quantify the burden of RTI in various locations [21]. Likely this is due to a lack of funding for more substantial research efforts. Little is known about the science of road injury prevention or pre-hospital treatments and interventions in LMICs. Nor do we understand attitudes and beliefs surrounding safety device usage in their populations. Attention needs to be paid to all links in trauma care such as emergency department care, surgical intervention when needed, diagnostic imaging with limited resources, and rehabilitation. Increased research support both in terms of capacity building and in funding for such research needs to be directed towards LMICs. It is the duty of EM physicians to prioritize the importance of this research to their mission to the other stakeholders and policy makers within governmental and nongovernmental organizations. It is not enough to devise a strategy. The strategy needs to be informed by useful data.

In many parts of the world where trauma care systems are underdeveloped and resources are limited, even basic descriptive epidemiological information and data are lacking. While many nations have some form of surveillance system in place for collecting road crash data, both the quality and reliability of these data vary widely, often within, as well as between, nations [34]. The development of trauma registries is of the utmost importance in strengthening the mission of road injury prevention and to allow for the development and implementation of local and regional data-driven prevention activities and efforts. Before the development of any injury prevention initiative, it is important to understand the nature and consequences of injury among the population to be targeted. Prevalence and incidence data are needed to properly and accurately inform and guide prevention activities and efforts. Disease and injury surveillance systems are indispensible in addressing the global burden of injury morbidity and mortality.

Without reliable data, it is nearly impossible to decide how to prioritize and develop effective programs. Furthermore, it is also difficult to convince local leaders, policy makers, and others that an injury problem exists and that it truly threatens the health of the entire community. Where resources are limited, it is important to collect enough data to make analysis clear and demonstrative. It is equally important to not to collect so much data that it becomes expensive and cumbersome. In order for the data to be useful and complete, a decision regarding which regions and hospitals should be included and whether or not pre-hospital systems should populate the registry needs to be made by all stakeholders including government agencies [35].

The goal of injury surveillance is to analyze modifiable risk factors and to understand populations at higher risk of injuries from road crashes. The establishment of data collection systems and hospital surveillance, development of community-based surveys, and initiation of other appropriate research can assist in evaluating the scope, characteristics, and consequences of crashes. Both the establishment of regional road crash databases (such as the Asia-Pacific Road Accident Database) and the development of international guidelines on core minimum data sets and supplementary information to be collected for all victims of injury (including road traffic victims) should help improve the quality and reliability of such surveillance data [36].

These trauma registries may exist in different stages around the world. In most LMICs, we can expect that they do not yet exist at all. The role of the local physician in the development of these registries cannot be underestimated. It takes a firm commitment to the process of collecting, entering, and maintaining records for the registry. It also takes clinical knowledge to populate the registry with accurate and pertinent information that can act as a supporting data to the mission at hand. Collaborators from regions with more experience in developing and maintaining registries can provide a shortcut for those just beginning to establish theirs. Their experience can save much frustration and unnecessary duplication of efforts.

The Queen Elizabeth Central Hospital in Blantyre, Malawi, in collaboration with trauma experts at Yale University School of Medicine, instituted a trauma registry to track and analyze all injuries for pediatric patients. This system will allow the hospital to report data that will inform future injury prevention and quality improvement efforts. Additionally, the data will be used to advocate for a national trauma registry and increased attention toward traffic injuries as a health priority. This program's success lies in its partnering of two academic centers, technology transfer via use of specialized trauma database software, and transfer of lessons learned from the management of a trauma registry at a major US trauma center.

Other efforts are underway in Mozambique in collaboration with Emory's Department of Emergency Medicine. The project has focused on training public health officials the concepts of trauma care as well and injury prevention control methods. This course was used as an impetus to start a trauma registry and laid the groundwork for future injury prevention research as well as the development of an "injury control research center."

The Fogarty International Center has been active in funding programs in injury prevention research development. In 2006, the center funded the International Research Training Program in Trauma and Injury Prevention in Colombia in collaboration with the University of Texas in order to build capacity for injury prevention research. The stated goals of the project are to "train foreign scientists and professionals in trauma and injury surveillance, prevention, control, and evaluation through an academic training and research program" [37, 38]. Felknor et al. have highlighted the importance of funding pilot projects in LMICs as a means of practical training of future injury prevention researchers in country [39].

*2.8. Policy and Advocacy.* Advocacy by stakeholders is vital to the development of policy. Emergency physicians are in a unique position to understand and therefore to advise on matters pertaining to global traffic safety, as a result of both clinical exposure and training in running and giving medical direction to EMS systems. Within the community, they are the eyes and ears of the politicians as roads, bridges, and pedestrian walkways are planned and implemented. Locally, emergency physicians, along with EMS personnel, know the most dangerous intersections and interchanges in their communities. Globally they understand the importance of systemic changes that can aim to eliminate the undue burden that road traffic injuries levy on the youngest and most productive members of society.

Areas of opportunity for effective global policy include legislation governing driving while intoxicated, traffic speed limits, mandated safety device presence, and usage in cars and two-wheeled vehicles, including child safety seats, seatbelts, and helmets. Also important is careful work with road safety engineers to eliminate hazards introduced by roads and road conditions and development and maturation of EMS systems.

A critical component to the effects of policy will continue to be enforcement. Without credible and meaningful enforcement, policies that are in place will not have the desired effect. Assurance that traffic safety policy will be effective is largely predicated on the careful coordination of the matrix between community groups, politicians, non-governmental organizations, road safety engineers, and automotive experts, with the emergency physician at the center.

An important example of collaboration in the area of policy and advocacy is the Fogarty funded "International Collaborative Trauma and Injury Research Training Grant" awarded to Johns Hopkins and Aga Khan University in Pakistan. The stated goals of the project are to "focus on using US expertise to strengthen Pakistani institutions, promote a sustainable research enterprise focused on acute care of trauma and injuries, and enable national dissemination of research evidence to influence policy and investments in Pakistan and its future." The project aims to develop trauma and injury research expertise at a public sector institution in Pakistan. This research will focus on providing data to support and inform key national priorities for trauma care and injury prevention. This will result in an increased capacity to sway policy and enact interventions based on a measurable impact. This project is a perfect illustration of a motivated group from a LMIC who is collaborating with a partner with the desired expertise in order to prioritize and realize their own national goals and agenda [38]. Stemming from this project, Waseem et al. describe the epidemiology of crashes in Punjab, Pakistan, and use their findings to point out areas for improvement in policy, legislation, and enforcement, using their pilot work to inform the national injury prevention agenda [40].

These examples highlight successful, multisectorial, multidisciplinary programs aimed at prevention of injuries from traffic accidents. EM providers can be involved in the prehospital setting, the hospital/emergency department level, or by developing programs focused on increasing access to emergency care and rehabilitation.

Advocacy on behalf of patients can take many forms. It can take persistence to ensure the establishment, updating, and optimization of EMS around the globe in order to take care of patients in their time of need. It can mean advocating for injury prevention measures and insisting that adequate resources are allocated toward enforcement. It can mean working with lawmakers and law enforcement groups to help craft culturally appropriate legislation. It can mean working with communities around the world to stress the importance of safety device usage and to ensure that they become culturally accepted and relevant. In areas where overcrowded buses or overburdened two-wheeled vehicles are employed, it can mean assisting in the long-term planning and prioritization of safe public transportation systems. As the global population grows and becomes increasingly dependent on motorized transportation, emergency physicians will have to work hard to eliminate its ill effects. Advocacy means going above and beyond daily duties as doctors to ensure that politicians know about the growing burden of disease inflicted by these inevitable changes.

## 3. Conclusions

By working on the implementation of road and traffic injury prevention measures both at home and abroad, emergency physicians can share expertise, experiences, and successes in road injury prevention, reducing the global impact of road traffic injuries. Important opportunities for transfer and translation of national successes in road injury prevention through EMS development, injury prevention research, intervention, policy, and advocacy are essential to the mission. Identification of key stakeholders in LMICs combined with intentional cooperation of international emergency physicians, global health organizations, and legislative as well as policymaking sectors can significantly strengthen the road traffic safety initiative worldwide and will result in decreased morbidity and mortality attributed to traffic related injury.

## Conflict of Interests

The authors declare that there is no conflict of interests regarding the publication of this paper.

## References


[1] National Highway Traffic Safety Administration, *Highlights of 2009 Motor Vehicle Crashes*, U.S. Department of Transportation, 2010.

[2] The National Road Safety Foundation, "Legislative Timeline," 2011, http://www.nationalroadsafety.org/page.php?id=28.

[3] American College of Emergency Physicians, "EMS: Where We've Been and Where We're Going. EMS Week Planning Guide," 2006, http://www.dsf.health.state.pa.us//health/lib/health/ems/week04/2004_planning_kit_final.pdf.

[4] World Health Organization, "Global Status Report on Road Safety: Time for Action," 2009, http://www.un.org/ar/roadsafety/pdf/roadsafetyreport.pdf.

[5] World Health Organization, "World Report on Road Traffic Injury Prevention," 2004, http://www.who.int/violence_injury_prevention/publications/road_traffic/world_report/en/.

[6] R. Koppaka, "Ten great public health achievements—United States, 2001–2010," *Morbidity and Mortality Weekly Report*, vol. 60, no. 19, pp. 619–623, 2011.

[7] World Health Organization, "2nd Global Status Report on Road Safety," 2011, http://www.who.int/entity/violence.../global_status_report/flyer_en.pdf.

[8] C. Murray, T. Vos, R. Lozano et al., "Disability-adjusted life years (DALYs) for 291 diseases and injuries in 21 regions, 1990–2010: a systematic analysis for the Global Burden of Disease Study 2010," *The Lancet*, vol. 380, no. 9859, pp. 2197–2223, 2012.

[9] Pan American Health Organization, "PanAmerican Conference on Road Safety: The Health Sector Answers to the Challenge of Safer Roads in America," 2005, http://www.bvsde.paho.org/bvsacd/cd51/respuestaseng.pdf.

[10] The World Bank, "World Bank Global Road Safety Facility Strategic Plan," 2009, http://siteresources.worldbank.org/EXTTOPGLOROASAF/Resources/2582212-1265307800361/GRSF_strategic_plan.pdf.

[11] United Nations Road Safety Collaboration, "Terms of Reference of the United Nations Road Safety Collaboration," 2011, http://www.who.int/roadsafety/about/en/.

[12] Global Road Safety Partnership, July 2011, http://www.grsproadsafety.org/.

[13] International Road Safety Academy Association, July 2011, http://www.irsa-association.eu/.

[14] International Road Federation, July 2011, http://www.irfnet.org/.

[15] International Road Federation, "Fifty Years of Service," 1997, http://www.irfnet.org/about.php.

[16] Association for Safe International Road Travel, July 2011, http://www.asirt.org/.

[17] Global Road Safety Forum, July 2011, http://www.globalroadsafety.org/.

[18] "Make Roads Safe: The Campaign for Global Road Safety," July 2011, http://www.makeroadssafe.org/.

[19] World Health Organization, "Decade of Action: Saving Millions of Lives," 2011, http://www.who.int/violence_injury_prevention/publications/road_traffic/decade_booklet/en/index.html.

[20] F. E. Vaca, R. Sayegh, M. J. Mello, and S. W. Hargarten, "Historical parallel evolution of injury prevention and control science and emergency medicine," *Academic Emergency Medicine*, vol. 16, no. 11, pp. 1049–1053, 2009.

[21] World Health Organization, "Prehospital Trauma Care Systems," 2005, http://www.who.int/violence_injury_prevention/publications/services/39162_oms_new.pdf.

[22] J. Tintinalli, *EMS: A Practical Global Guidebook*, People's Medical Publishing House, Shelton, Conn, USA, 2010.

[23] R. M. Smith and A. K. Conn, "Prehospital care—scoop and run or stay and play?" *Injury*, vol. 40, supplement 4, pp. S23–S26, 2009.

[24] I. G. Stiell, L. P. Nesbitt, W. Pickett et al., "The OPALS Major Trauma study: impact of advanced life-support on survival and morbidity," *Canadian Medical Association Journal*, vol. 178, no. 9, pp. 1141–1152, 2008.

[25] M. Liberman, D. Mulder, and J. Sampalis, "Advanced or basic life support for trauma: meta-analysis and critical review of the literature," *Journal of Trauma*, vol. 49, no. 4, pp. 584–599, 2000.

[26] S. Chekijian and N. Truzyan, "Practices, attitudes and perceptions toward road traffic safety in Yerevan, Reublic of Armenia," *Annals of Advances in Automotive Medicine*, vol. 56, pp. 191–200, 2012.

[27] J. A. Razzak, A. A. Hyder, T. Akhtar, M. Khan, and U. R. Khan, "Assessing emergency medical care in low income countries: a pilot study from Pakistan," *BMC Emergency Medicine*, vol. 8, article 8, 2008.

[28] The American College of Surgeons Trauma Programs, "Advanced Trauma Life Support," October 2013, http://www.facs.org/trauma/atls/.

[29] The American College of Surgeons Trauma Programs, "Advanced Trauma Operative Management," October 2013, http://www.facs.org/trauma/atom/.

[30] The American College of Surgeons Trauma Programs, "Advanced Surgical Skills for Exposure in Trauma (ASSET) Course," October 2013, http://www.facs.org/trauma/education/asset.html.

[31] The American College of Surgeons Trauma Programs, "ATLS International Promulgation," October 2013, http://www.facs.org/trauma/atls/promulgation.html/.

[32] National Association of Emergency Medical Technicians Programs, October 2013, http://www.naemt.org/education/PHTLS/whatisPHTLS.aspx.

[33] Department of Emergency Medicine, Emory University, "Selected Core Projects," Website Project List, December 2012, http://www.em.emory.edu/services/international_health/section_activities/core_projects.html.

[34] World Health Organization, "Injury Surveillance Guidelines," 2001, http://whqlibdoc.who.int/publications/2001/9241591331.pdf.

[35] B. C. Nwomeh, W. Lowell, R. Kable, K. Haley, and E. A. Ameh, "History and development of trauma registry: lessons from developed to developing countries," *World Journal of Emergency Surgery*, vol. 1, no. 1, article 32, 2006.

[36] Transport Division (TD), "Asia-Pacific Road Accident Database (APRAD) User Manual," 2001, http://www.unescap.org/publications/detail.asp?id=457.

[37] National Institutes of Health, "International research training program in trauma and injury prevention," Project Reporter, December 2012, http://projectreporter.nih.gov/project_info_description.cfm?aid=7780441&icde=0.

[38] National Institutes of Health, "International collaborative trauma and injury research training," Project Reporter, December 2012, http://projectreporter.nih.gov/project_info_description.cfm?aid=8087708&icde=8373934.

[39] S. A. Felknor, G. L. Delclos, D. Gimeno et al., "Funding of pilot projects in Latin America: a tool for capacity building in occupational health research," *International Journal of Occupational and Environmental Health*, vol. 12, no. 4, pp. 408–414, 2006.

[40] H. Waseem, L. Carenzo, J. Razzak, and R. Naseer, "Epidemiology of major incidents: an EMS study from Pakistan," *International Journal of Emergency Medicine*, vol. 4, no. 1, article 48, 2011.

# 12

# Which Dermatological Conditions Present to an Emergency Department in Australia?

**Julia Lai-Kwon,[1] Tracey J. Weiland,[2,3] Alvin H. Chong,[1] and George A. Jelinek[2,3]**

[1] *Department of Medicine (Dermatology), St. Vincent's Hospital, Melbourne, VIC, Australia*
[2] *Emergency Practice Innovation Centre, St. Vincent's Hospital, 41 Victoria Parade Fitzroy, Melbourne, VIC 3065, Australia*
[3] *Faculty of Medicine Dentistry and Health Sciences, The University of Melbourne, VIC, Australia*

Correspondence should be addressed to George A. Jelinek; george.jelinek@svhm.org.au

Academic Editor: Rade B. Vukmir

*Background/Objectives.* There is minimal data available on the types of dermatological conditions which present to tertiary emergency departments (ED). We analysed demographic and clinical features of dermatological presentations to an Australian adult ED. *Methods.* The St. Vincent's Hospital Melbourne (SVHM) ED database was searched for dermatological presentations between 1 January 2009 and 31 December 2011 by keywords and ICD-10 diagnosis codes. The lists were merged, and the ICD-10 codes were grouped into 55 categories for analysis. Demographic and clinical data for these presentations were then analysed. *Results.* 123 345 people presented to SVHM ED during the 3-year period. 4817 (3.9%) presented for a primarily dermatological complaint. The most common conditions by ICD-10 diagnosis code were cellulitis ($n$ = 1741, 36.1%), allergy with skin involvement ($n$ = 939, 19.5%), boils/furuncles/pilonidal sinuses ($n$ = 526, 11.1%), eczema/dermatitis ($n$ = 274, 5.7%), and varicella zoster infection ($n$ = 161, 3.3%). *Conclusion.* The burden of dermatological disease presenting to ED is small but not insignificant. This information may assist in designing dermatological curricula for hospital clinicians and specialty training organisations as well as informing the allocation of dermatological resources to ED.

## 1. Introduction

Dermatology is primarily an outpatient specialty in Australia. However, up to 5–8% of all emergency department (ED) presentations may be due to dermatological complaints [1]. Despite this, there have been few studies that have characterised the types of patients who present to ED with dermatological conditions, with the most focused on paediatric rather than adult ED presentations [2–4]. The variability in the types of presentations between countries has also been described previously, highlighting the importance of country-specific data [5]. However, Australian data is limited, with only one retrospective study from South Australia found on a review of the literature [6]. We conducted a three-year retrospective study on patients with dermatological conditions presenting to the St. Vincent's Hospital ED in Melbourne, Australia, in order to gather demographic and clinical data on patients who present, and the types of dermatological conditions with which they present. This may better inform Junior Medical Officers and ED physicians of dermatology curriculum design as well as assist with dermatological resource allocation to ED.

## 2. Methods

*2.1. Data Selection.* St. Vincent's Hospital Melbourne (SVHM) ED is an adult tertiary facility which sees approximately 40,000 patients per year. The hospital is situated on the fringe of the city's Central Business District and serves a culturally diverse and socially disadvantaged population. All ED visits between 1 January 2009 and 31 December 2011 were extracted from the hospital database. A keyword search was performed in the "Presenting Complaint" and "Triage Notes" fields of the Victorian Emergency Minimum Dataset (VEMD) at St. Vincent's Hospital Melbourne, as well as an ICD-10 (International Statistical Classification of Diseases, 10th Revision) diagnosis code search in the

Table 1: Demographic data for dermatological presentations compared to nondermatological presentations to ED.

| | Dermatological presentations | Other ED presentations | $P$ value |
|---|---|---|---|
| Age (years) (mean, median) | 44.2<br>39.0 | 47.8<br>44.0 | <0.001 |
| Triage category 1 | 6 (0.1%)° | 1245 (1.1%)* | |
| Triage category 2 | 187 (3.9%)° | 9837 (8.3%)* | |
| Triage category 3 | 778 (16.2%)° | 45140 (38.2%)* | <0.001 |
| Triage category 4 | 3261 (67.7%)* | 53646 (45.4%)° | |
| Triage category 5 | 585 (12.1%)* | 8193 (6.9%)° | |
| Time to ED doctor (min) (median, IQR) | 56.0<br>19–117 | 31.0<br>8–82 | <0.001 |

*Overrepresented according to adjusted standardised residuals.
°Underrepresented according to adjusted standardised residuals.

primary, secondary, and tertiary diagnostic fields in order to identify dermatological presentations. Keywords and ED ICD-10 diagnoses were selected by consultation between researchers (see Appendices A and B in the Supplementary Material). The ICD-10 codes were selected from a list of available ICD-10 diagnoses in the ED and therefore did not include all possible dermatological diagnoses as listed in the full ICD-10 manual. In cases where there was any doubt as to whether the presentation was primarily a skin complaint, the cases were reviewed by the consultant dermatologist (AC). These lists were then merged, and traumatic skin injuries, burns (excluding sunburn), postoperative wound complications, and repeat presentations were excluded. In order to handle the data more efficiently, the 91 ICD-10 codes were grouped into 55 diagnostically related categories. The grouping of diagnoses was determined by consensus between researchers. The demographic and clinical data for these presentations were then analysed.

*2.2. Data Analysis.* Epidemiological data was summarised using frequencies and percentages for nominal data and means and interquartile ranges (IQR) for continuous data using Microsoft Excel 2010. Inferential comparisons of continuous data were made using the Mann-Whitney $U$ test, and comparison of categorical data was made using Pearson's chi-squared test.

This study received approval from the Hospital Research Ethics Committee at SVHM (LRR 146/12, 10/10/2012).

## 3. Results

Over the 3-year period, there were 123 345 presentations to the ED. Of these, 4,817 had a primarily dermatological complaint (3.9%). The majority (52.9%) were male, and 7 patients did not have their gender recorded (Table 1).

The most common skin complaints by ICD-10 diagnosis code were cellulitis ($n = 1741$, 36.1%), allergy with skin involvement ($n = 939$, 19.5%), boils/furuncles/pilonidal sinuses ($n = 526$, 11.1%), eczema/dermatitis ($n = 274$, 5.7%), and varicella zoster infections ($n = 161$, 3.3%) (Table 2).

Table 2: Top 20 skin complaints seen at SVHM ED by ICD-10 diagnostic code.

| Complaint | $N$ | % of total cases |
|---|---|---|
| Cellulitis | 1741 | 36.1 |
| Allergy with skin involvement | 939 | 19.5 |
| Boils/ furuncles/ pilonidal sinuses | 536 | 11.1 |
| Eczema/dermatitis | 274 | 5.7 |
| Varicella zoster | 161 | 3.3 |
| Nonspecific skin infections | 135 | 2.8 |
| Unlisted | 109 | 2.3 |
| Nonspecific viral infections with rash | 98 | 2.0 |
| Skin lump unspecified | 82 | 1.7 |
| Nonspecific rashes | 79 | 1.6 |
| Sebaceous cyst | 71 | 1.5 |
| Impetigo | 69 | 1.4 |
| Drug rash | 55 | 1.1 |
| Psoriasis | 46 | 1.0 |
| Superficial thrombosis/thrombophlebitis | 41 | 0.9 |
| Ingrown nail of finger/toe | 37 | 0.8 |
| *Candida* infections | 31 | 0.6 |
| Skin neoplasms | 30 | 0.6 |
| Pruritus | 30 | 0.6 |
| Scabies | 27 | 0.6 |

## 4. Discussion

A significant proportion of ED presentations (3.9%) is due to skin complaints, which is slightly higher than previously reported [5–8]. This may be due to our broad definition of dermatological complaints, which included conditions such as cellulitis and boils/furuncles/pilonidal sinuses which are often excluded as they are typically managed by General Medical or Surgical units.

Patients who presented with skin complaints were generally younger than other patients presenting to ED and their presentations were less urgent, with around two-thirds of dermatological patients triaged as category 4 and the second least urgent category in the five-category triage scale used in a number of countries. This was higher than nondermatological ED presentations, where less than half of the patients were category 4. All six category 1 dermatological patients presented with anaphylaxis with a component of skin involvement such as urticaria or angioedema. This highlights the fact that the majority of skin complaints that present to ED do not require immediate emergency care and could often be managed in outpatient settings. This has been previously recognised in the literature [9]. As a result of their lower urgency, patients with skin complaints waited longer to be seen by a doctor than other ED patients.

Patients with a diverse range of skin complaints presented during the three-year period. Cellulitis was the most common condition (36.1%), consistent with previous studies [7, 10]. However, the prevalence of cellulitis may be misleading, as multiple studies have reported high rates of misdiagnosis of cellulitis in ED due the lack of familiarity with more specific dermatological diagnoses such as lipodermatosclerosis and contact dermatitis. In a retrospective study of 196 inpatient dermatology consults [11], a third of patients consulted for cellulitis had a cutaneous mimicker. Similarly, David et al. [12] demonstrated a misdiagnosis rate of 28% for cellulitis cases following review by a Dermatologist and Infectious Diseases specialist. Misdiagnosis of cellulitis may result in inappropriate and costly antibiotic use. In our study, the high rates of cellulitis may also be partly explained by the lower socioeconomic patient population, with a significant proportion of patients being homeless or affected by drugs or alcohol, placing them at higher risk of cellulitis.

A similar study of dermatological presentations to ED was conducted at the Royal Adelaide Hospital in 2011 [6]. Interestingly, the top three diagnoses were similar for both centres, with eczema being the fourth most common diagnosis at St. Vincent's and the fifth most common at the Royal Adelaide Hospital. However, chronic ulcers, which accounted for 3.7% of ED presentations to the Royal Adelaide Hospital, did not feature in the top ten ED diagnoses at St. Vincent's Hospital. This is despite the high prevalence of pyoderma gangrenosum as a discharge diagnosis (13.9% of admissions under Dermatology). On retrospective analysis of their initial ED diagnosis, six pyoderma gangrenosum cases were classified as "nonspecific skin infection," two as "cellulitis of the lower limb," two as "nonspecific rash," and one each as "atopic dermatitis," "drug rash," "dermatitis," "decubitus ulcer," and "skin and subcutaneous disorder not otherwise specified." This reflects the difficulty in making definitive dermatological diagnoses in ED due to time restraints and perhaps limited dermatological experience but also the lack of a specific ICD-10 code in ED for chronic ulcerating conditions.

This study may inform the development of evidence-based dermatological curricula for a number of clinician groups involved in ED dermatological assessment and management. It also provides data on the burden of dermatological presentations to ED which may guide resource allocation in this setting. The significant nonspecific diagnosis rate amongst dermatological ED presentations supports the development of a dermatological consulting service in the ED, a concept which has been previously described [7]. Whilst this role is traditionally filled by the on-call dermatological registrar, a dedicated service would be mutually beneficial to both the ED and Dermatology units. Dermatology registrars would receive increased exposure to common initial dermatological presentations, which is often limited in a tertiary hospital environment, as well as provide diagnostic support to their ED colleagues, limiting unnecessary investigations and treatments. However, given that dermatological presentations account for only 4% of ED presentations, such a service may not be an effective use of health care resources.

Other potential options include the use of a teledermatology referral service within the ED. This has been previously studied in Queensland, where a store-and-forward photography system accompanied by relevant history and examination findings was a rapid and accurate diagnostic tool for dermatological presentations to ED [13]. Whilst this study used photos taken with a camera, a Swedish study used multimedia messaging systems (MMS) from mobile phone cameras as an easier way of transmitting information from the bedside, which would be more practical in the ED setting [14]. It was reported that the diagnostic accuracy and adequacy of management decisions made via MMS referrals were similar to store-and-forward teledermatology systems. Such a system could be particularly useful in rural centres where access to dermatology services may be limited, a possibility previously studied in third world countries [15]. However, there are several limitations to an MMS referral system, including poor picture quality, privacy and consent issues surrounding the storage of photos on private cameras, and the inability of a single photo to substitute for a comprehensive skin examination. Hospitals should therefore consider the suitability of teledermatology services for dermatology ED consultations as a means of improving the accuracy of skin-related ED diagnoses but be aware of its limitations.

*4.1. Limitations.* The study was limited by incomplete demographic information in the Victorian Emergency Minimum Dataset. The ED coding system may have also resulted in inaccuracies as it required ED doctors to search for specific keywords relating to their intended diagnosis. Coding inaccuracies may have resulted from inaccurate or broad keyword searches. Coding unavailability, such as an appropriate ICD-10 code for chronic ulcers, also resulted in the inappropriate classification of some dermatological conditions which may have concealed their true prevalence.

## 5. Conclusion

The burden of dermatological presentations to EDs in Australia may be somewhat larger than previously thought but overall remains small compared to other conditions. Cellulitis, allergy with skin involvement, and boils/furuncles/pilonidal sinuses were the most common presenting conditions. It is important that junior doctors receive appropriate training in the initial investigation and management of these common dermatological presentations. The study will have implications for curriculum design for ED doctors as well as inform them of decisions regarding dermatological resource allocation to ED and highlight the importance of an accessible dermatology consulting service via teledermatology.

## Conflict of Interests

The authors declare that there is no conflict of interests regarding the publication of this paper.

## References


[1] A. T. Trott, "Rash," in *Emergency Medicine: An Approach to Clinical Problem Solving*, G.C. Hamilton, A. Sanders, and G.S. Strange, Eds., pp. 185–206, Saunders, Philadelphia, Pa, USA, 2003.

[2] N. Kramkimel, V. Soussan, A. Beauchet et al., "High frequency, diversity and severity of skin diseases in a paediatric emergency department," *Journal of the European Academy of Dermatology and Venereology*, vol. 24, no. 12, pp. 1468–1475, 2010.

[3] O. M. Dolan, E. A. Bingham, J. F. T. Glasgow, G. Burrows, and J. R. Corbett, "An audit of dermatology in a paediatric accident and emergency department," *Journal of Accident and Emergency Medicine*, vol. 11, no. 3, pp. 158–161, 1994.

[4] S. Auvin, A. Imiela, B. Catteau, V. Hue, and A. Martinot, "Paediatric skin disorders encountered in an emergency hospital facility: a prospective study," *Acta Dermato-Venereologica*, vol. 84, no. 6, pp. 451–454, 2004.

[5] J. Y. Kim, H. H. Cho, J. S. Hong et al., "Skin conditions presenting in emergency room in Korea: an eight-year retrospective analysis," *Journal of the European Academy of Dermatology and Venereology*, vol. 27, no. 4, pp. 479–485, 2013.

[6] A. Wallett and S. Sidhu, "Management pathway of skin conditions presenting to an Australian tertiary hospital emergency department," *Australasian Journal of Dermatology*, vol. 53, no. 4, pp. 307–310, 2012.

[7] M. L. Martínez-Martínez, E. Escario-Travesedo, M. Rodríguez-Vázquez, J. M. Azaña-Defez, M. C. Martín De Hijas-Santos, and L. Juan-Pérez-García, "Dermatology consultations in an emergency department prior to establishment of emergency dermatology cover," *Actas Dermo-Sifiliograficas*, vol. 102, no. 1, pp. 39–47, 2011.

[8] E. Wang, B. L. Lim, and K. Y. Than, "Dermatological conditions presenting at an emergency department in Singapore," *Singapore Medical Journal*, vol. 50, no. 9, pp. 881–884, 2009.

[9] E. K. Symvoulakis, K. Krasagakis, I. D. Komninos et al., "Primary care and pattern of skin diseases in a mediterranean island," *BMC Family Practice*, vol. 7, article 6, 2006.

[10] A. Baibergenova and N. H. Shear, "Skin conditions that bring patients to emergency departments," *Archives of Dermatology*, vol. 147, no. 1, pp. 118–120, 2011.

[11] J. Bauer and M. Maroon, "Dermatology inpatient consultations: a retrospective study," *Journal of the American Academy of Dermatology*, vol. 62, no. 3, pp. 518–519, 2010.

[12] C. V. David, S. Chira, S. J. Eells et al., "Diagnostic accuracy in patients admitted to hospitals with cellulitis," *Dermatology Online Journal*, vol. 17, no. 3, article 1, 2011.

[13] J. Muir, C. Xu, S. Paul et al., "Incorporating teledermatology into emergency medicine," *Emergency Medicine Australasia*, vol. 23, no. 5, pp. 562–568, 2011.

[14] A. Börve, A. Holst, A. Gente-Lidholm, R. Molina-Martinez, and J. Paoli, "Use of the mobile phone multimedia messaging service for teledermatology," *Journal of Telemedicine and Telecare*, vol. 18, no. 5, pp. 292–296, 2012.

[15] J. Frühauf, R. Hofman-Wellenhof, C. Kovarik et al., "Mobile teledermatology in sub-Saharan Africa: a useful tool in supporting health workers in low-resource centres," *Acta Dermato-Venereologica*, vol. 93, no. 1, pp. 122–123, 2013.

# 13

# Urinary Tract Infections due to Multidrug-Resistant Enterobacteriaceae: Prevalence and Risk Factors in a Chicago Emergency Department

**Thana Khawcharoenporn,[1,2] Shawn Vasoo,[1] and Kamaljit Singh[1]**

[1] *Division of Infectious Diseases, Faculty of Medicine, Thammasat University, Pathum Thani 12120, Thailand*
[2] *Section of Infectious Diseases, Rush University Medical Center, Chicago, IL 60612, USA*

Correspondence should be addressed to Thana Khawcharoenporn; thanak30@yahoo.com

Academic Editor: Chak W. Kam

*Background.* Selection of empiric antibiotics for urinary tract infections (UTIs) has become more challenging because of the increasing rates of multidrug-resistant Enterobacteriaceae (MDRE) infections. *Methods.* This retrospective study was conducted to determine antibiotic resistance patterns, risk factors, and appropriate empiric antibiotic selection for MDRE UTIs. Adult patients seen in the Emergency Department (ED) with Enterobacteriaceae UTIs during 2008-2009 were identified from review of microbiology records. MDRE were defined as organisms resistant to at least 3 categories of antibiotics. *Results.* There were 431 eligible patients; 83 (19%) had MDRE UTIs. Resistance rates for individual antibiotics among MDRE UTIs were significantly greater than non-MDRE UTIs: levofloxacin, 72% versus 14%; TMP-SMX, 77% versus 12%; amoxicillin-clavulanate, 35% versus 4%; nitrofurantoin, 21% versus 12%, and ceftriaxone, 20% versus 0%. All Enterobacteriaceae isolates were susceptible to ertapenem (MIC $\leq$ 2 mg/L). Independent risk factors for MDRE UTI were prior fluoroquinolone use within 3 months (adjusted odds ratio (aOR) 3.64; $P = 0.001$), healthcare-associated risks (aOR 2.32; $P = 0.009$), and obstructive uropathy (aOR 2.22; $P = 0.04$). *Conclusion.* Our study suggests that once-daily intravenous or intramuscular ertapenem may be appropriate for outpatient treatment of ED patients with MDRE UTI.

## 1. Introduction

Enterobacteriaceae are the most common cause of urinary tract infections (UTIs) in both community and healthcare settings. Selection of empiric antibiotic therapy for UTIs is therefore often based on the institutional susceptibility profiles of the Enterobacteriaceae [1]. Recent guidelines from the Infectious Diseases Society of America recommended that empiric antibiotic therapy for UTIs should be based on local resistance data, drug availability, and antibiotic intolerance/allergy history of treated patients [1, 2]. For uncomplicated cystitis, nitrofurantoin or trimethoprim-sulfamethoxazole (TMP-SMX, if local resistance $\leq$ 20%) can be used empirically, while fluoroquinolones, ceftriaxone, aminoglycosides, and carbapenems are appropriate for pyelonephritis and complicated UTIs.

The increase in rates of antibiotic resistance among Enterobacteriaceae has posed challenges in choosing empiric regimens, especially when infections due to multidrug-resistant Enterobacteriaceae (MDRE) are suspected or endemic [3]. In the past decade, emerging resistance among the Enterobacteriaceae due to extended-spectrum beta-lactamases (ESBL) has been reported worldwide, including in Chicago [4]. In addition, other mechanisms of resistance among urinary pathogens including *Klebsiella pneumoniae* carbapenemases (KPC) and New Delhi metallo-beta-lactamases (NDM)-1 have also been increasingly described [5, 6]. Infections caused by these MDRE require timely and appropriate antibiotic therapy to improve patients' survival [7].

The treatment of UTIs in the Emergency Department (ED) poses a unique challenge as patients often present with a spectrum of illness severity and comorbidities. Some patients have had recurrent UTIs with multiple antibiotic exposures, failed empiric outpatient treatment, or healthcare-associated (HA) infection (including MDRE) risks [8]. As a consequence, patients are more likely to have urine cultures obtained to guide therapy; however, initial empiric antibiotic selection is frequently based on inpatient antibiograms which may overestimate antibiotic resistance. The objective of this study was to determine prevalence of patterns of antibiotic resistance, risk factors, and appropriate empiric therapy for MDRE UTIs among ED patients.

## 2. Methods

*2.1. Study Design, Setting, and Population.* This is a structured, retrospective, observational study. All patients aged ≥ 12 who were evaluated at Rush University Medical Center (RUMC) ED from 1 August 2008 to 31 March 2009 with positive urine cultures were eligible for the study. RUMC is a 613-bed tertiary academic center in Chicago with over 48,000 ED visits annually. Patients were identified by daily review of urine specimens sent to the microbiology laboratory during the study period. In RUMC ED, urine cultures are performed in the majority of patients suspected of UTI or in those with positive urinalysis for leukocyte esterase and/or nitrite. Patients who had urine cultures with significant enterobacteriaceae growth $\geq 10^4$ CFUs/mL were included for chart review. Only the first episode of the positive urine culture per patient was included in our analysis. The study was approved by the institutional review board of RUMC.

*2.2. Study Protocol and Definitions.* Chart review was performed exclusively using our electronic medical record system (Epic; Wisconsin, USA) by two independent reviewers (T. Khawcharoenporn and S. Vasoo). These reviewers were trained in data abstraction procedure. The collected data included ethnicity, demographics, pregnancy status, underlying medical comorbidities, relevant surgical history including urological procedure and obstructive uropathy, prior UTI, prior antibiotic use within 3 months, UTI diagnoses, empiric treatments, causative bacteria, and antibiotic susceptibility. Healthcare-associated risks were defined as presence of chronic indwelling urinary catheters, healthcare exposure including hospital stay for at least 48 hours, nursing home or long-term care facility residence, regular hemodialysis clinic visits, or undergoing urological procedures within the past 3 months [9, 10]. The diagnosis of UTI (cystitis, pyelonephritis, and urosepsis) was determined solely by the treating physician. Patients with asymptomatic bacteriuria or urinary tract colonization were excluded from the study. Identification and antibiotic susceptibilities of causative bacteria were determined using MicroScan Walkaway (Siemens, CA). The minimum inhibitory concentration (MIC) breakpoints for resistance were based on Clinical Laboratory Standards Institute criteria: levofloxacin, ≥8 mg/L; TMP-SMX, ≥4/76 mg/L; nitrofurantoin, ≥128 mg/L; gentamicin, ≥16 mg/L; amikacin, ≥64 mg/L; ampicillin, ≥32 mg/L; amoxicillin-clavulanate, ≥32/16 mg/L; piperacillin-tazobactam, ≥128/4 mg/L; ceftriaxone, ≥64 mg/L; cefepime, ≥32 mg/L, and ertapenem, ≥8 mg/L [11]. MDRE isolates were defined as isolates that were resistant or intermediate susceptible to ≥3 of the following antimicrobial categories: (1) penicillins ± beta-lactamase inhibitors (PBI); (2) cephalosporins either ceftriaxone or cefepime; (3) carbapenems; (4) fluoroquinolones; (5) gentamicin or amikacin; (6) TMP-SMX; and (7) nitrofurantoin [12, 13]. Enterobacteriaceae isolates that did not meet the criteria were considered to be non-MDRE. Results of interest included the prevalence of each Enterobacteriaceae, antibiotic resistance rates, resistance patterns of and risk factors for MDRE UTIs.

*2.3. Statistical Analysis.* All analyses were performed using SPSS, version 15.0 (SPSS, Chicago, Illinois). Categorical variables were compared using Pearson's $\chi^2$ or Fisher's exact test as appropriate. Continuous variables were compared using Mann Whitney $U$ test. All $P$ values were 2-tailed; $P$ values less than 0.05 were considered statistically significant. Risk factors for MDRE UTI were identified by comparison of variables between the patients infected with MDRE and non-MDRE bacteria. Variables that were present inmore than 10% of patients at a significance level of $P$ less than 0.20 or that had a prior clinical significance (e.g., recent antibiotic use and healthcare-associated risks including presence of indwelling catheters and resident of a long-term care facility) [12, 14, 15] were entered into stepwise backward logistic regression models. Significant variables that were thought to be covariates were grouped, and only one variable from each group was chosen for model entry. The model's overall robustness was confirmed by Hosmer-Lemeshow goodness-of-fit statistic. Adjusted odd ratios (aORs) and 95% confidence intervals (CIs) were calculated to determine independent risk factors for MDRE UTI.

## 3. Results

*3.1. Patient Characteristics.* There were 676 patients with positive urine cultures identified during the study period; 184 who had asymptomatic bacteriuria or urinary tract colonization were excluded. Of the remaining 492 patients, 61 had UTIs due to non-Enterobacteriaceae bacteria (24 *Enterococcus* spp., 18 *Pseudomonas aeruginosa*, 15 *Staphylococcus aureus*, 3 *Staphylococcus saprophyticus*, and one *Stenotrophomonas maltophilia*) and were excluded. The study population consisted of 431 patients with Enterobacteriaceae UTIs. Demographics, comorbidities, types of UTIs, and history of antibiotic use are summarized in Table 1. The median age was 44 years (range 14–101 years) and the majority of patients were female (81%) and African American (52%). Obstructive uropathy was present in 59 (14%) patients and was secondary to urinary tract calculi, cervical cancer, bladder cancer, vaginal cancer, benign prostate hypertrophy, and ureteropelvic junction obstruction. Prior antibiotic use within the last 3 months was documented for 114 of 431 patients (27%) and fluoroquinolones were the most commonly used antibiotic (12%). Lower UTIs were diagnosed in 280 (65%) patients. Eighty-three patients (19%) had MDRE UTIs, while 348 patients (81%) had non-MDRE UTIs. Of these 431 patients with Enterobacteriaceae UTIs, 306 (71%) were treated as outpatients and 125 (29%) were hospitalized.

TABLE 1: Characteristics of patients with urinary tract infections caused by multidrug-resistant (MDR) and non-MDR Enterobacteriaceae.

| Characteristics | All patients ($N$ = 431) | MDR group ($N$ = 83) | Non-MDR group ($N$ = 348) | $P^a$ |
|---|---|---|---|---|
| Median age (IQR) (years) | 44 (27–68) | 61 (33–82) | 41 (26–62) | **<0.001** |
| Male gender | 80 (19) | 22 (26) | 58 (17) | **0.04** |
| Ethnicity | | | | |
| African American | 226 (52) | 38 (46) | 188 (54) | 0.18 |
| Caucasian | 96 (22) | 20 (24) | 76 (22) | 0.66 |
| Hispanic | 93 (22) | 22 (27) | 71 (20) | 0.22 |
| Asian | 6 (1) | 2 (2) | 4 (1) | 0.33 |
| Other | 10 (2) | 1 (1) | 9 (3) | 0.70 |
| Pregnancy | 19 (4) | 1 (1) | 18 (5) | 0.14 |
| Comorbidities | | | | |
| Diabetes mellitus | 87 (20) | 25 (30) | 62 (18) | **0.01** |
| Renal transplant | 34 (8) | 5 (6) | 29 (8) | 0.48 |
| Obstructive uropathy | 59 (14) | 24 (29) | 35 (10) | **<0.001** |
| Healthcare-associated risks[b] | 143 (33) | 51 (61) | 92 (26) | **<0.001** |
| Prior urinary tract infection | 172 (40) | 53 (64) | 119 (34) | **<0.001** |
| Prior antibiotic use within 3 months | | | | |
| Any antibiotics | 114 (27) | 40 (48) | 74 (21) | **<0.001** |
| Fluoroquinolones | 50 (12) | 27 (33) | 23 (7) | **0.02** |
| Cephalosporins | 38 (9) | 13 (16) | 25 (7) | **0.01** |
| Penicillins | 31 (7) | 11 (13) | 20 (6) | **<0.001** |
| Vancomycin | 26 (6) | 8 (10) | 18 (5) | 0.11 |
| TMP-SMX | 18 (4) | 8 (10) | 10 (3) | **0.006** |
| Nitrofurantoin | 14 (3) | 5 (6) | 9 (3) | 0.09 |
| Clindamycin | 11 (3) | 3 (4) | 8 (2) | 0.13 |
| Carbapenems | 6 (1) | 3 (4) | 3 (1) | 0.25 |
| Macrolides | 5 (1) | 2 (2) | 3 (1) | 0.45 |
| Type of urinary tract infection | | | | 0.45 |
| Lower tract disease | 280 (65) | 51 (61) | 229 (66) | |
| Upper tract disease | 151 (35) | 32 (39) | 119 (34) | |

Data are in number (%) unless otherwise indicated.
[a]Compared between MDR and non-MDR groups.
[b]Defined as presence of chronic indwelling urinary catheters, healthcare exposure including hospital stay for at least 48 hours, nursing home or long-term care facility residence, regular hemodialysis clinic visits or urological procedures within the past 3 months.
IQR: interquartile range; TMP-SMX: trimethoprim-sulfamethoxazole.

*3.2. Prevalence and Antibiotic Resistance of Enterobacteriaceae.* There were 451 non-duplicate Enterobacteriaceae isolates recovered from the 431 patients (some of these patients had UTIs caused by more than 1 organism in the same episode). The distribution of the bacteria in patients with and without MDRE UTIs is shown in Table 2. The majority of uropathogens were *Escherichia coli* [323 (72%)], *Klebsiella* spp. (66 (15%)), and *Proteus* spp. (32 (7%)). *Klebsiella* spp. was significantlymore common in patients with non-MDRE UTIs than those with MDRE UTIs (17% versus 5%; $P = 0.002$), while *Serratia* spp. and *Providencia* spp. were only identified in patients with MDRE UTIs. Rates of antibiotic resistance for Enterobacteriaceae are summarized in Table 3. The overall resistance rate for TMP-SMX, levofloxacin and nitrofurantoin was 24%, 17% and 14%, respectively. Antibiotic resistance rates for MDRE UTIs were significantly greater than non-MDRE UTIs for the majority of tested antibiotics including levofloxacin, 72% versus 14%; TMP-SMX, 77% versus 12%; gentamicin, 47% versus 1%; amoxicillin-clavulanate, 35% versus 4%; nitrofurantoin, 21% versus 12% and ceftriaxone, 20% versus 0%. All of the Enterobacteriaceae isolates were ertapenem susceptible (MIC $\leq$ 2 mg/L).

TABLE 2: Distribution of 451 unique Enterobacteriaceae bacteria with and without multidrug resistance (MDR) isolated from 431 study patients.

| Enterobacteriaceae bacteria | All isolates ($N = 451$) | MDR isolates ($N = 86$) | Non-MDR isolates ($N = 365$) | $P^a$ |
|---|---|---|---|---|
| *Escherichia coli* | 323 (72) | 65 (76) | 258 (71) | 0.37 |
| *Klebsiella* spp. | 66 (15) | 4 (5) | 62 (17) | **0.002** |
| *Proteus mirabilis* | 32 (7) | 5 (6) | 27 (7) | 0.61 |
| *Citrobacter* spp. | 17 (4) | 5 (6) | 12 (3) | 0.27 |
| *Enterobacter* spp. | 9 (2) | 3 (3) | 6 (2) | 0.38 |
| *Serratia* spp. | 2 (0.4) | 2 (2) | 0 (0) | — |
| *Providencia* spp. | 2 (0.4) | 2 (2) | 0 (0) | — |

Data are in number (%) unless otherwise indicated.
[a]Compared between MDR and non-MDR isolates.

3.3. *Resistance Pattern of MDRE.* Among the 86 unique MDRE isolates, 21 (24%) isolates were ESBL producers. In regards to resistance pattern by antibiotic categories, the three most common patterns were combined PBI, fluoroquinolone and TMP-SMX resistance [18/86 (21%)], combined PBI, TMP-SMX and aminoglycoside resistance [11/86 (13%)] and combined PBI, fluoroquinolone, TMP-SMX and aminoglycoside resistance [8/86 (9%)].

3.4. *Risk Factor for MDRE UTIs.* Risk factors associated with MDRE UTIs were analyzed by comparing patients with and without MDRE UTIs. By univariate analysis [Table 1], age, male gender, diabetes mellitus, obstructive uropathy, healthcare-associated risks, prior UTI, and prior use of any antibiotics, penicillins, cephalosporins, fluoroquinolones, or TMP-SMX within 3 months were associated with MDRE UTIs. In the multivariate logistic regression analysis [Table 4], independent risk factors for MDRE were prior fluoroquinolone use within 3 months (aOR 3.64; 95% CI 1.74–7.64; $P = 0.001$], healthcare-associated risks (aOR 2.32; 95% CI 1.23–4.37; $P = 0.009$), and obstructive uropathy (aOR 2.22; 95% CI 1.04–4.78; $P = 0.04$).

Based on in vitro antibiotic susceptibility testing, 61 of the 431 (13%) patients received empiric treatment with an antibiotic that tested nonsusceptible. Of these 61 patients, 31 (51%) received levofloxacin. Patients with MDRE UTIs were significantly more likely to receive a nonsusceptible antibiotic compared to those with non-MDRE UTIs (39% versus 8%; $P$ less than 0.001).

## 4. Discussion

Our study found that the Enterobacteriaceae are the major causes of UTIs (88%) among ED patients and *E. coli* remains the most common pathogen in both MDRE and non-MDRE UTIs. We found a surprisingly high prevalence of MDRE UTIs among ED patients, 19% overall, and the prevalence of ESBL-associated UTIs was 4.6% of all UTIs which is comparable to the results of previous studies [4, 16]. A Chicago study of outpatient UTIs reported an increase in prevalence of ESBL-producing *E. coli* UTIs from 0.2% in 2003 to 3.0% in 2008 [4]. High rates of MDRE UTIs have also been reported in other US cities and overseas [16]. In the Americas, studies have focused mainly on the prevalence of ESBL-associated UTIs which are a subset of MDRE UTIs. The prevalence of ESBL community onset UTI has been as high as 30% in some Latin America countries [17].

Among non-MDRE UTIs, all tested antibiotics in this study, except ampicillin, were suitable for empiric treatment while the appropriate empiric therapy for MDRE UTIs was limited to carbapenems (100% susceptible) and amikacin (99% susceptible). In an outpatient setting like the ED, ertapenem is a particularly attractive option for treatment of MDRE UTIs due to its convenient once daily dosing. The drug can be administered intravenously or intramuscularly at other facilities near patients' residence or, if applicable, by trained family members. The efficacy of ertapenem 1 g daily was found to be comparable to once daily ceftriaxone in two well-designed studies that looked at the microbiologic eradication rates in patients with complicated urinary tract infections [18, 19]. The drug has a good safety profile and rarely causes hypersensitivity reactions or antibiotic-associated diarrhea. In addition, ertapenem is stable to hydrolysis by several types of beta-lactamases including ESBLs and concentrates well in the urine [20]. We found that ceftriaxone, another once daily antibiotic that is commonly used to treat UTIs, cannot be recommended for the treatment of MDRE UTIs given the high rate of resistance (20%). Amikacin demonstrated high level of in vitro susceptibility and could be used for a short course empiric therapy while awaiting the urine culture result. However, the risk of nephrotoxicity and ototoxicity, particularly in the elderly whose creatinine levels may underestimate the true glomerular filtration rate, should be borne in mind. In addition, clinicians are generally reluctant to use even a single dose of aminoglycoside in patients with active kidney disease or in patients receiving concomitant nephrotoxic drugs and prefer to reserve amikacin for the treatment of multidrug-resistant *Pseudomonas aeruginosa*. Unfortunately, there are few oral options for the treatment of MDRE UTIs and we found that oral antibiotic therapy is best guided by formal susceptibility results from urine cultures. Fosfomycin

TABLE 3: Antibiotic resistance rates among 451 unique Enterobacteriaceae bacteria with and without multidrug resistance (MDR) isolated from 431 study patients.

| Antibiotics | All isolates ($N$ = 451) | MDR isolates ($N$ = 86) | Non-MDR isolates ($N$ = 365) | $P^a$ |
|---|---|---|---|---|
| Ampicillin | 55% | 99% | 45% | **<0.001** |
| Amoxicillin-clavulanate | 10% | 35% | 4% | **<0.001** |
| Piperacillin-tazobactam | 2% | 9% | 1% | **<0.001** |
| Cefuroxime | 8% | 38% | 1% | **<0.001** |
| Ceftriaxone | 4% | 20% | 0% | **<0.001** |
| Cefepime | 3% | 17% | 0% | **<0.001** |
| Ertapenem | 0% | 0% | 0% | 1.00 |
| Levofloxacin | 17% | 72% | 4% | **<0.001** |
| Gentamicin | 10% | 47% | 1% | **<0.001** |
| Amikacin | 1% | 2% | 0.3% | 0.10 |
| Trimethoprim-sulfamethoxazole | 24% | 77% | 12% | **<0.001** |
| Nitrofurantoin | 14% | 21% | 12% | **0.04** |
| ESBL resistance pattern | 5% | 24% | 0% | **<0.001** |

[a]Compared between MDR and non-MDR isolates.
ESBL: extended-spectrum beta-lactamase.

TABLE 4: Risk factors associated with multidrug-resistant Enterobacteriaceae-associated urinary tract infections.

| Risk factors | Univariate analysis | | Multivariate analysis | |
|---|---|---|---|---|
| | OR (95% CI) | $P$ | aOR (95% CI) | $P$ |
| Age | 1.02 (1.01–1.04) | **<0.001** | 1.01 (1.00–1.02) | 0.14 |
| Male gender | 1.80 (1.03–3.17) | **<0.001** | 0.84 (0.41–1.69) | 0.62 |
| Diabetes mellitus | 1.99 (1.16–3.42) | **0.01** | 1.40 (0.75–2.63) | 0.29 |
| Obstructive uropathy | 3.64 (2.02–6.56) | **<0.001** | 2.22 (1.04–4.78) | **0.04** |
| Prior urinary tract infection | 3.40 (2.06–5.60) | **<0.001** | 1.73 (0.97–3.08) | 0.06 |
| Healthcare-associated risks[a] | 4.44 (2.68–7.32) | **<0.001** | 2.32 (1.23–4.37) | **0.009** |
| Prior penicillin use within 3 months | 2.51 (1.15–5.46) | **0.02** | 0.66 (0.25–1.71) | 0.39 |
| Prior cephalosporin use within 3 months | 2.40 (1.17–4.92) | **0.01** | 0.78 (0.32–1.89) | 0.59 |
| Prior fluoroquinolone use within 3 months | 6.81 (3.65–12.72) | **<0.001** | 3.64 (1.74–7.64) | **0.001** |
| Prior TMP-SMX use within 3 months | 3.61 (1.38–9.44) | **0.006** | 1.16 (0.35–3.84) | 0.81 |

[a]Defined as presence of chronic indwelling urinary catheters, healthcare exposure including hospital stay for at least 48 hours, nursing home or long-term care facility residence, regular hemodialysis clinic visits or urological procedures within the past 3 months.
aOR: adjusted odds ratio; CI: confidence interval; OR: odds ratio; TMP-SMX: trimethoprim-sulfamethoxazole.

represents a promising option as it is active against ESBLs and is well tolerated with excellent urinary penetration [20], although this antibiotic was not assessed in our study.

One of the significant findings of our study is the importance of identifying patients with risk factors for MDRE UTIs in order to guide empiric drug selection. Common risk factors for MDRE-associated infections are not well-defined since most studies focus on particular subgroups of MDRE including ESBLs, KPC and NDM-1-associated infections or specific organism types, such as *E. coli* and *Klebsiella* spp. Previously-reported risk factors associated with infections caused by ESBL-producing Enterobacteriaceae include length of hospital and intensive care unit stay, presence of central venous or arterial catheters, emergency abdominal surgery, prior administration of antibiotic, especially second and third generation cephalosporins, prior residence in a long-term care facility, presence of a urinary catheter, ventilatory assistance, and chronic hemodialysis [21]. Poor functional status, ICU stay, and receipt of antibiotics, particularly fluoroquinolones, broad spectrum cephalosporins, and carbapenems were independently associated with KPC-associated infections [22], while risk factors for NDM-1-associated infections were travel and/or undergoing medical procedures in the Indian subcontinent [6]. We identified prior fluoroquinolone use within 3 months, healthcare-associated risks, including presence of chronic indwelling urinary catheters, healthcare exposure including hospital stay for at least 48 hours, nursing home or long-term care facility residence, regular hemodialysis clinic visits or recent urological procedures within the past 3 months, and obstructive uropathy as independent risk factors associated with MDRE UTIs. Most of these risk factors were consistent with previously reported ESBL-associated risks. However, we also identified hitherto unreported risk factors for MDRE UTIs including prior fluoroquinolone use, recent urological procedures, and obstructive uropathy. As recent fluoroquinolone use has been reported to be associated with quinolone-resistant UTIs [23], it is not surprising that we identified it as a risk factor for MDRE UTI given the well-recognized "collateral damage" associated with fluoroquinolone use [24]. Urological procedures and obstructive uropathy are risk factors for recurrent UTIs which likely result in multiple prior antibiotic exposures and could explain the increased risk of MDRE UTIs among patients with these characteristics.

In this study, we found that the majority of the MDRE isolates (76%) did not have an ESBL resistance pattern. Among the non-ESBL isolates, fluoroquinolone resistance was a common component of multidrug resistance. These findings correspond with the high rate of fluoroquinolone resistance reported in this study. Although fluoroquinolones are recommended for empiric therapy of complicated UTIs due to the previously reported low rates of resistance in the United States [1, 2, 25], our data suggests that fluoroquinolones are not appropriate empiric therapy in our ED for patients with risk factors for MDRE UTIs. In addition, our findings emphasize the importance of local antibiotic resistance patterns and risk factors assessment to guide appropriate therapy.

Limitations of our study include the retrospective chart review nature of the study and the limited generalizability of our findings to other settings with different local susceptibility patterns and patient populations. In addition, the study was not designed to evaluate clinical and microbiological outcomes in patients receiving either active or inactive (based on in vitro susceptibility testing) antibiotic therapy. However, our findings suggest the need for research on uropathogen susceptibility pattern to direct appropriate therapy in each individual ED setting.

Regularly updated surveillance of local microbial prevalence and resistance patterns are needed to guide the empiric therapy for UTIs. In our ED setting, ertapenem may be appropriate therapy for outpatients with suspected or proven MDRE UTI. We suggest that all patients with risk factors for MDRE UTIs should have urine cultures performed to direct therapy.

## Conflict of Interests

Drs. Shawn Vasoo and Thana Khawcharoenporn have no conflict of interests to declare.

## Acknowledgments

Dr. Kamaljit Singh is on the Visiting Speakers Board for Forest Pharmaceuticals and is a Scientific Advisory Board Member of Quidel Corporation. The results of this study were presented as a poster in the 52nd Interscience Conference on Antimicrobial Agents and Chemotherapy 2012, San Francisco, USA.

## References

[1] K. Gupta, T. M. Hooton, K. G. Naber et al., "International clinical practice guidelines for the treatment of acute uncomplicated cystitis and pyelonephritis in women: a 2010 update by the infectious diseases society of America and the European society for microbiology and infectious diseases," *Clinical Infectious Diseases*, vol. 52, no. 5, pp. e103–e120, 2011.

[2] T. M. Hooton, S. F. Bradley, D. D. Cardenas et al., "Diagnosis, prevention, and treatment of catheter-aassociated urinary tract infection in adults: 2009 international clinical practice guidelines from the infectious diseases society of America," *Clinical Infectious Diseases*, vol. 50, no. 5, pp. 625–663, 2010.

[3] G. V. Sanchez, R. N. Master, J. A. Karlowsky, and J. M. Bordon, "In vitro antimicrobial resistance of urinary *Escherichia coli* isolates among U.S. outpatients from 2000 to 2010," *Antimicrobial Agents and Chemotherapy*, vol. 56, no. 4, pp. 2181–2183, 2012.

[4] C. Qi, V. Pilla, J. H. Yu, and K. Reed, "Changing prevalence of *Escherichia coli* with CTX-M-type extended-spectrum $\beta$-lactamases in outpatient urinary E. coli between 2003 and 2008," *Diagnostic Microbiology and Infectious Disease*, vol. 67, no. 1, pp. 87–91, 2010.

[5] N. Gupta, B. M. Limbago, J. B. Patel, and A. J. Kallen, "Carbapenem-resistant enterobacteriaceae: epidemiology and prevention," *Clinical Infectious Diseases*, vol. 53, no. 1, pp. 60–67, 2011.

[6] K. K. Kumarasamy, M. A. Toleman, T. R. Walsh et al., "Emergence of a new antibiotic resistance mechanism in India, Pakistan, and the UK: a molecular, biological, and epidemiological study," *The Lancet Infectious Diseases*, vol. 10, no. 9, pp. 597–602, 2010.

[7] D. L. Paterson, W.-C. Ko, A. Von Gottberg et al., "Antibiotic therapy for *Klebsiella pneumoniae* bacteremia: implications of production of extended-spectrum $\beta$-lactamases," *Clinical Infectious Diseases*, vol. 39, no. 1, pp. 31–37, 2004.

[8] F. M. Abrahamian, G. J. Moran, and D. A. Talan, "Urinary tract infections in the emergency department," *Infectious Disease Clinics of North America*, vol. 22, no. 1, pp. 73–87, 2008.

[9] T. C. Horan, M. Andrus, and M. A. Dudeck, "CDC/NHSN surveillance definition of health care-associated infection and criteria for specific types of infections in the acute care setting," *The American Journal of Infection Control*, vol. 36, no. 5, pp. 309–332, 2008.

[10] 10. American Thoracic Society and Infectious Diseases Society of America, "Guidelines for the management of adults with hospital-acquired, ventilator-associated, and healthcare-associated pneumonia," *American Journal of Respiratory and Critical Care Medicine*, vol. 171, no. 4, pp. 388–416, 2005.

[11] Clinical and Laboratory Standards Institute, "Performance standards for antimicrobial susceptibility testing. Nineteenth informational supplement. Approved standard M100-S19," *Clinical and Laboratory Standards Institute*, Wayne, Pa, USA.

[12] K. Cohen-Nahum, L. Saidel-Odes, K. Riesenberg, F. Schlaeffer, and A. Borer, "Urinary tract infections caused by multi-drug resistant proteus mirabilis: risk factors and clinical outcomes," *Infection*, vol. 38, no. 1, pp. 41–46, 2010.

[13] A.-P. Magiorakos, A. Srinivasan, R. B. Carey et al., "Multidrug-resistant, extensively drug-resistant and pandrug-resistant bacteria: an international expert proposal for interim standard definitions for acquired resistance," *Clinical Microbiology and Infection*, vol. 18, no. 3, pp. 268–281, 2012.

[14] G. A. Jacoby, "Epidemiology of extended-spectrum beta-lactamases," *Clinical Infectious Diseases*, vol. 27, no. 1, pp. 81–83, 1998.

[15] C. Gudiol, F. Tubau, L. Calatayud et al., "Bacteraemia due to multidrug-resistant gram-negative bacilli in cancer patients: risk factors, antibiotic therapy and outcomes," *Journal of Antimicrobial Chemotherapy*, vol. 66, no. 3, pp. 657–663, 2011.

[16] D. J. Diekema, B. J. BootsMiller, T. E. Vaughn et al., "Antimicrobial resistance trends and outbreak frequency in United States hospitals," *Clinical Infectious Diseases*, vol. 38, no. 1, pp. 78–85, 2004.

[17] P. H. A. Bours, R. Polak, A. I. M. Hoepelman, E. Delgado, A. Jarquin, and A. J. Matute, "Increasing resistance in community-acquired urinary tract infections in Latin America, five years after the implementation of national therapeutic guidelines," *International Journal of Infectious Diseases*, vol. 14, no. 9, pp. e770–e774, 2010.

[18] F. Jimenez-Cruz, A. Jasovich, J. Cajigas et al., "A prospective, multicenter, randomized, double-blind study comparing ertapenem and ceftriaxone followed by appropriate oral therapy for complicated urinary tract infections in adults," *Urology*, vol. 60, no. 1, pp. 16–22, 2002.

[19] K. M. Tomera, E. A. Burdmann, O. G. Pamo Reyna et al., "Ertapenem versus ceftriaxone followed by appropriate oral therapy for treatment of complicated urinary tract infections in adults: results of a prospective, randomized, double-blind multicenter study," *Antimicrobial Agents and Chemotherapy*, vol. 46, no. 9, pp. 2895–2900, 2002.

[20] V. Prakash, J. S. Lewis II, M. L. Herrera, B. L. Wickes, and J. H. Jorgensen, "Oral and parenteral therapeutic options for outpatient urinary infections caused by enterobacteriaceae producing ctx-m extended-spectrum $\beta$-lactamases," *Antimicrobial Agents and Chemotherapy*, vol. 53, no. 3, pp. 1278–1280, 2009.

[21] G. A. Jacoby and L. S. Munoz-Price, "The new beta-lactamases," *The New England Journal of Medicine*, vol. 352, no. 4, pp. 380–391, 2005.

[22] M. J. Schwaber, S. Klarfeld-Lidji, S. Navon-Venezia, D. Schwartz, A. Leavitt, and Y. Carmeli, "Predictors of carbapenem-resistant *Klebsiella pneumoniae* acquisition anions hospitalized adults and effect of acquisition on mortality," *Antimicrobial Agents and Chemotherapy*, vol. 52, no. 3, pp. 1028–1033, 2008.

[23] L. Johnson, A. Sabel, W. J. Burman et al., "Emergence of fluoroquinolone resistance in outpatient urinary *Escherichia coli* isolates," *The American Journal of Medicine*, vol. 121, no. 10, pp. 876–884, 2008.

[24] D. L. Paterson, ""Collateral damage" from cephalosporin or quinolone antibiotic therapy," *Clinical Infectious Diseases*, vol. 38, supplement 4, pp. S341–S345, 2004.

[25] G. G. Zhanel, T. L. Hisanaga, N. M. Laing et al., "Antibiotic resistance in outpatient urinary isolates: final results from the North American Urinary Tract Infection Collaborative Alliance (NAUTICA)," *International Journal of Antimicrobial Agents*, vol. 26, no. 5, pp. 380–388, 2005.

# 14

# Knowledge and Confidence of a Convenience Sample of Australasian Emergency Doctors in Managing Dental Emergencies: Results of a Survey

**Hossein Samaei,[1] Tracey Joy Weiland,[2,3] Stuart Dilley,[1,3] and George Alexander Jelinek[2,3]**

[1] *Department of Emergency Medicine, St. Vincent's Hospital, Melbourne, VIC 3065, Australia*
[2] *Emergency Practice Innovation Centre, St. Vincent's Hospital, Melbourne, VIC 3065, Australia*
[3] *Department of Medicine, Dentistry and Health Sciences, The University of Melbourne, Melbourne, VIC 3010, Australia*

Correspondence should be addressed to Tracey Joy Weiland; tracey.weiland@svha.org.au

Academic Editor: Jeffrey R. Avner

*Background.* We aimed to determine Australasian Specialist Emergency Physicians' and Emergency Physicians in Training (Trainees') level of knowledge of common dental emergencies. We also explored confidence in managing dental emergencies; predictors of confidence and knowledge; and preferences for further dental education. *Methods.* A questionnaire was distributed electronically (September 2011) and directly (November 2011) to Fellows and Trainees of the Australasian College for Emergency Medicine. It explored demographics, confidence, knowledge of dental emergencies, and educational preferences. *Results.* Response rate was 13.6% (464/3405) and college members were proportionally represented by region. Fewer than half (186/446; 42%) had received dental training. Sixty-two percent (244/391, 95% CI 57.5–67.1) passed (>50%) a knowledge test. More than 60% incorrectly answered questions on dental fracture, periodontal abscess, tooth eruption dates, and ulcerative gingivitis. Forty percent (166/416) incorrectly answered a question about Ludwig's Angina. Eighty-three percent (360/433) were confident in the pharmacological management of toothache but only 26% (112/434) confident in recognizing periodontal disease. Knowledge was correlated with confidence ($r = 0.488$). Interactive workshops were preferred by most (386/415, 93%). *Conclusions.* The knowledge and confidence of Australasian Emergency Physicians and Trainees in managing dental emergencies are varied, yet correlated. Interactive training sessions in dental emergencies are warranted.

## 1. Introduction

Patients presenting to the emergency department (ED) with dental problems account for 0.3 to 4% of ED visits [1–4]. In one United Kingdom (UK) study [5], dental problems were the second most common reason (after drug reactions) patients telephoned the ED for advice. The most common dental conditions presenting to ED were dental pain, dental infections, dental and maxillofacial trauma, and postdental treatment-related complications such as haemorrhage and dry socket [2, 6–8].

Emergency department medical staff may have difficulty making a specific diagnosis for dental presentations, and often manage these patients symptomatically [9]. This may be because they have had little training in dental emergencies and little exposure to these conditions. A survey of newly graduated physicians working in hospitals in Bahrain, Ireland, Kuwait, and the UK reported that 97% had not received any dental education prior to graduation [10]. In a large study from the United States involving 1030 pediatricians and family physicians, most respondents had less than two hours of preventive dental education during their whole medical training [11]. A further study from England showed that only 6% of ED medical staff had received any dental training in medical school [12].

In a cross sectional, nationwide survey that included 118 doctors working at Welsh emergency departments, knowledge for the management dental trauma was found to be partial, with greater knowledge associated with experience and training [13].

In a small US study of 72 physicians and directors, knowledge was poor for dental fractures, and good for luxations and avulsions. Specialist qualification in paediatric emergencies was found to be associated with great knowledge in managing dental trauma [14].

Some studies suggest that emergency physicians with inadequate training and insufficient knowledge had difficulty with diagnosis, investigation, management, and appropriate referral of dental conditions [1, 15].

An assessment of Australasian ED staff knowledge and confidence is lacking and to our knowledge there are no known studies of factors that predict knowledge and confidence in dental emergencies. An understanding of these factors may permit the targeting of relevant educational resources. In addition, awareness of emergency doctors' views about preferred activities which can improve these weaknesses may enable decision makers to consider suitable teaching methods to improve knowledge and confidence.

We aimed to determine specialist emergency physicians' (fellows') and emergency physicians in training (trainees') knowledge of common dental emergencies. Secondary aims were to assess respondent's self-rated confidence in managing dental emergencies, to determine predictors of knowledge and confidence in managing dental emergencies, to determine the degree of correlation between knowledge and confidence and to determine attitudes towards further education in dental emergencies.

## 2. Methods

*2.1. Study Design and Ethics.* This cross sectional survey was approved by St. Vincent's Hospital Melbourne's Ethics Committee and by the Scientific Committee of the Australasian College for Emergency Medicine (ACEM).

*2.2. Inclusion and Exclusion Criteria.* Participants eligible for inclusion in the study were doctors registered with ACEM including Emergency Physicians ("fellows" or "FACEM"), advanced trainees, and provisional trainees. Doctors not registered with ACEM were excluded.

*2.3. Tool Development and Validation.* A questionnaire was designed based on dentistry exam multiple choice questions [16–18], emergency medicine textbooks [19–21], and internet teaching sites. Face validity was ensured using iterative feedback from six ED consultants, two dentists, a researcher, and an emergency medicine trainee after which minor changes were made to the original survey. To ensure content validity, a sample of six emergency physicians and five trainees rated relevance of survey items on a four-point scale. This enabled the identification of items not to be centrally relevant to the topic, items requiring revision in formatting or wording, and items requiring no alteration.

The final questionnaire (see the appendix) comprised 40 items including nine demographic items, 11 items about confidence in diagnosis and management of some of the most frequent dental presentations, 15 multiple choice questions assessing participants' knowledge of common dental emergencies, and five questions regarding desired further training in dental emergencies. The survey incorporated graded responses using Likert scales for attitudinal questions, binary response formats for demographics, and multicategory format (demographics, knowledge questions, and further training in dental emergencies). Some open-ended questions were also included.

*2.4. Survey Distribution.* The electronic survey, formatted using online SurveyMonkey software, was distributed in September, 2011, by email by the ACEM. Electronic surveys were delivered via hyperlink to the online questionnaire embedded in the email. Due to the rules of the ACEM who distributed the survey on behalf of the authors, only one reminder was sent (October 2011). For ethical and privacy reasons the authors were restricted from making direct contact with potential respondents via electronic means. For these reasons, the authors were limited in maximizing the response rate. The electronic survey remained open until January, 2012.

Although not permitted to send more than one reminder, the authors were able to disseminate a paper based version of the survey to conference registrants at the ACEM Annual Scientific Meeting in Sydney, November, 2011. This conference would not have been attended by all those eligible for the study; however the use of a paper based survey was used both to maximize recruitment and to minimise bias that may have occurred due to limited internet access (which can occur in remote or rural areas) and preference for paper based surveys over electronic formats. Paper surveys were collected in a box to preserve anonymity.

All participants (via electronic recruitment and face-to-face) received an invitation to participate and a comprehensive information form outlining participant rights, the length of the survey, and the purpose of the study which was to assess Australasian emergency doctors' knowledge and confidence for dental emergencies. Survey commencement was taken as implied consent and survey completion took approximately 15 minutes.

*2.5. Primary Outcome.* The primary outcome was the proportion of respondents obtaining a pass mark on the knowledge test. A pass mark was defined *a priori* by a panel of emergency physicians and registrars as >50% total score (at least 8/15) and was calculated by summing correct answers on the knowledge test for those participants who answered all questions.

*2.6. Sample Size.* Based on an ACEM membership of 3405 (1392 FACEM, 2013 Trainees) at the time of survey distribution (personal communication, Jane Macaulay, 9/9/11), a sample size of 346 was required in order to estimate the proportion of respondents passing the knowledge test within a 5% margin of error (assuming a 50% response distribution) at a 95% confidence level. This equates to a 50% pass rate for the knowledge portion of the survey. This figure was chosen as it provides the most conservative estimate of sample size required (i.e., maximizing the number required). Further power analyses indicated that a sample size of 346 would be sufficient to detect a difference in two proportions of 15 percentage points (50% versus 65%) with power at 80% and criterion for significance set at 0.05. For multiple regression analyses, we adhered to the rule of thumb for sample size; that is, number of cases = 50 + (8 × number of predictors).

*2.7. Data Analysis.* Quantitative data were analysed using IBM SPSS Statistics 20.0 (Chicago, IL). For each survey summary statistics (%, 95% confidence interval (CI)) were calculated for the entire sample and by the demographic variables. Arithmetic mean (95% CI) was used to summarize the total number of correct knowledge items across that sample. All data reported were adjusted for missing data on an item by item basis.

Representation of membership per state and membership type was calculated by comparing the confidence intervals (CI) of the percentages of all members of ACEM to the percentages of respondents to the survey. If the CI overlapped, we considered that they were adequately represented.

Negatively worded survey items from the confidence section were reverse scored. Exploratory inferential analyses on confidence and attitudinal items were undertaken after collapsing Likert Scales to binary scales (strongly disagree/disagree/neutral versus agree/strongly agree). Fisher's exact test was used for 2 × 2 contingency tables and Pearson's Chi Square (linear by linear association) was used to identify linear trends for ordinal data (4 × 2 contingency tables).

A total score for overall confidence was calculated by summing collapsed items for confidence. Similarly, a total score was calculated for each participant that completed all items in the knowledge test. Each item was identified as being either correct or incorrect ("incorrect/do not know") prior to summing. To ensure validity of derived total scores, internal consistency of these items was verified using Cronbach's alpha ($r = 0.805$).

Since the primary outcome (proportion of respondents obtaining a pass mark on the knowledge test) was based on a panel determining that a pass mark be defined as 50% or more, further sensitivity analyses were undertaken comparing mean total knowledge score by Fellow (yes/no), received formal training in dental emergencies (yes/no), attended workshops in dental emergencies (yes/no), ED type and number of patients seen per year (0–25, 26–50, 51+). Data were analysed using independent samples $t$-test and ANOVA in situations where there were 3+ categories.

Multiple regression ("enter" method) was then used to identify (demographic) predictors of knowledge score and all predictors of total confidence. For total knowledge, 11 demographic predictors were assessed: FACEM (no/yes); ED type (adult/other); whether formal education in dental emergencies had been received (yes/no); whether the respondent had participated in a conference workshop on dental emergencies (yes/no), and the number of patients seen annually (continuous); access to specialized dental service coded as six dummy variables (none; onsite dentist 24/7; onsite dentist, limited; dentist on call; refer to dental hospital; refer to private dentist). For confidence, these same predictors were included in the model with the addition of total knowledge score.

For multiple regression, variance inflation factor (VIF) was used to indicate the presence or absence of multicollinearity with a criterion of VIF <5 set for retention of variables. Other assumptions (outliers, linearity, homoscedasticity, and independence of residuals) were assessed by inspecting the residuals scatterplot and the normal probability plot of regression standardised residuals. Pearson's correlation was used to explore an association between knowledge score and total confidence score.

For all inferential tests, alpha was set at 0.05 and two tailed tests of significance were used.

Table 1: Distribution of respondents by region [number (percentage; 95% CI)].

| | Survey respondents | ACEM members |
|---|---|---|
| VIC | 143 (31.8; 27.6–36.2) | 772 (22.7; 21.3–24.1) |
| NSW | 106 (23.6; 19.9–27.7) | 820 (24.1; 22.7–25.6) |
| QLD | 65 (14.4; 11.5–18.0) | 705 (20.7; 19.4–22.1) |
| WA | 44 (9.8; 7.3–12.9) | 321 (9.4; 8.5–10.5) |
| NZ | 37 (8.2; 6.0–11.2) | 337 (9.9; 8.9–11.0) |
| SA | 25 (5.6; 3.8–8.1) | 214 (6.3; 5.5–7.2) |
| TAS | 12 (2.7; 1.5–4.7) | 78 (2.3; 1.8–2.9) |
| NT | 7 (1.6; 0.7–3.2) | 44 (1.3; 1.0–1.7) |
| ACT | 5 (1.1; 0.4–2.7) | 51 (1.5; 1.1–2.0) |
| Overseas | 6 (1.3; 0.5–3.0) | 63 (1.9; 1.5–2.4) |
| Total | **450 (100.0)*** | **3405 (100.0)** |

*14 respondents did not specify their region.

## 3. Results

*3.1. Participation.* Four hundred and ten respondents were recruited via the online survey during the study period and 56 via the paper-based survey. Two participants were not registered with ACEM and were therefore excluded resulting in 464 participants commencing the survey from an eligible pool of 3405 ACEM members (13.6%). Of these, 14 completed the demographics section of the survey only and were excluded from all further analyses. There were no significant differences according to demographics in respondents that commenced the survey ($n = 464$) and those that completed all elements of the survey ($n = 391$).

*3.2. Demographics.* Respondents were from a total of 117 hospitals, and two respondents were fulltime locums. The distribution of respondents by region is comparable to the membership of ACEM (Table 1) except for a slight preponderance of Victorian respondents and fewer respondents from Queensland proportional to the ACEM membership. Respondents identified working mainly at EDs that receive both adults and children (adult: 108/449, 24.1%; paediatric only: 13/449, 2.9%; mixed: 328/449, 73.1%). Data for paediatric and mixed hospitals were collapsed for subsequent analyses.

Approximately one fifth of participants (85/447, 19.0%) had not completed the primary exam and almost half the respondents (204/434, 47.0%) had not yet completed the fellowship exam. This was substantially less than the proportion of trainees registered with ACEM at the time of the study

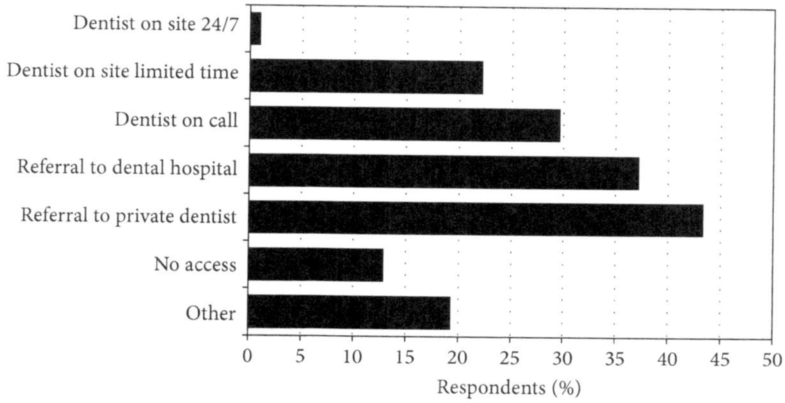


FIGURE 1: Percentage of respondents according to access to dental services from ED (more than one response accepted).

(2013/3405, 59.1%). Of respondents who had completed the fellowship, 16.6% (72/434) obtained the fellowship during or prior to 2000; 16.4% (71/434) between 2001 and 2005; and 20.0% (87/434) after 2005.

One hundred and eighty six respondents (41.7%) reported having received some formal training in dental emergencies, while 121/447 (27.1%) indicated participating in either a conference or workshop specifically on dental emergencies. Respondents indicated having limited access to a dentist in ED (Figure 1).

*3.3. Knowledge of Dental Emergencies.* In total, 391 respondents completed all knowledge test items. For those participants, the mean (95% CI) total score out of a possible 15 was 8 (7.8–8.3; range 1–14). A total of 244/391 (62.4%, 95% CI 57.5–67.1) participants completing all items achieved a pass (>50%) in the knowledge test. Knowledge of dental emergencies varied considerably across topics (Table 2). The majority of respondents obtained 6–10 items correctly not adjusted for missing data; 284/417, 68.1%, (95% CI 63.5–72.4) with the remainder fairly evenly distributed in the 1–5 range (68/417, 16.3%, 95% CI 13.1–20.2) and the 11–15 range (65/417, 15.6%, 95% CI 12.4–19.4).

Sensitivity analyses indicated that those that had attended formal education and workshops in dental emergencies, and those that were fellows obtained significantly higher total confidence scores compared to their counterparts. There were no significant differences according to ED type and number of patients seen per year (data not shown).

*3.4. Confidence in Dental Emergency Related Tasks.* Confidence for tasks relating to the management of dental emergencies ranged from 26.6% of participants (95% CI 22.7–30.8%, 119/448) reporting confidence in recognition of periodontal disease to 82.9% (95% CI 79.1–86.1, 372/449) for pharmacological management of toothache (Figure 2). Receipt of formal dental education was significantly associated with confidence for all tasks apart from pharmacological management of toothache and managing a dental abscess (Table 3).

TABLE 2: Percentage (95% CI) of participants answering knowledge item correctly.

| Item | % Correct (95% CI); numerator/denominator |
|---|---|
| Acute necrotizing ulcerative gingivitis knowledge | **7.0** (4.9–9.9); 29/413 |
| Tooth eruption dates | **18.1** (14.7–22.1); 75/415 |
| Periodontal abscess knowledge | **25.3** (21.3–29.7); 104/411 |
| Dental fracture knowledge | **38.6** (34.1–43.4); 160/414 |
| Dry socket management | **52.9** (48.1–57.7); 217/410 |
| Ludwig's angina knowledge | **59.7** (54.9–64.3); 246/412 |
| Reimplantation of a deciduous avulsed tooth? | **59.7** (54.9–64.3); 247/414 |
| Full dentition description | **60.2** (55.4–64.8); 251/417 |
| Dry socket knowledge | **70.3** (65.7–74.5); 291/414 |
| Aphthous stomatitis knowledge | **70.5** (66.0–74.7); 292/414 |
| Causes of oral pain | **70.9** (66.4–75.8); 295/416 |
| Antibiotics for dental pain | **75.2** (70.9–79.2); 313/416 |
| Tooth avulsion knowledge | **81.6** (77.6–85.1); 338/414 |
| Naming of teeth | **83.9** (80.1–87.2); 350/417 |
| Tooth avulsion advice | **89.4** (86.1–92.1 ); 372/416 |

Confidence varied significantly by hospital type for several tasks: performing local anesthetic block for toothache ($P = 0.026$; adult hospitals: 26/108, 24.1%, 95% CI 16.9–33.0; other hospitals: 122/341; 35.8%, 95% CI 30.9–41.0); recognizing significant complications of abscess ($P = 0.036$; adult: 75/108, 69.4%, 95% CI 60.2–77.4; other: 269/339, 79.4%, 95% CI 74.7–83.3); and managing the completely avulsed tooth ($P = 0.036$; adult: 47/108, 43.5%, 95% CI 34.6–52.9; other: 188/340; 55.3%, 95% CI 50.0–60.5). Confidence also varied significantly by recency of graduation as a specialist, with more senior graduates more confident in many areas (Figure 3). Total confidence score was positively correlated with total knowledge score ($r = 0.488$, $P < 0.001$). Significant linear relationships existed between confidence for most tasks explored and year fellowship obtained, with a trend toward

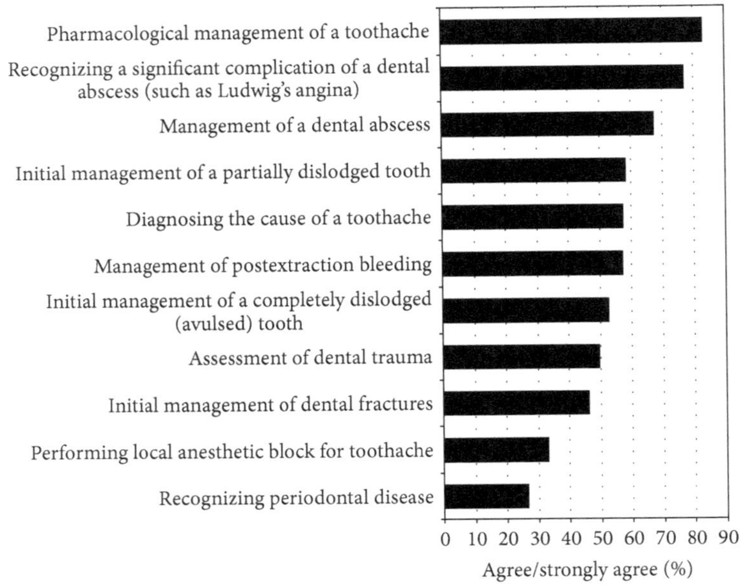


Figure 2: Practitioner confidence in specific topics of dental emergencies.

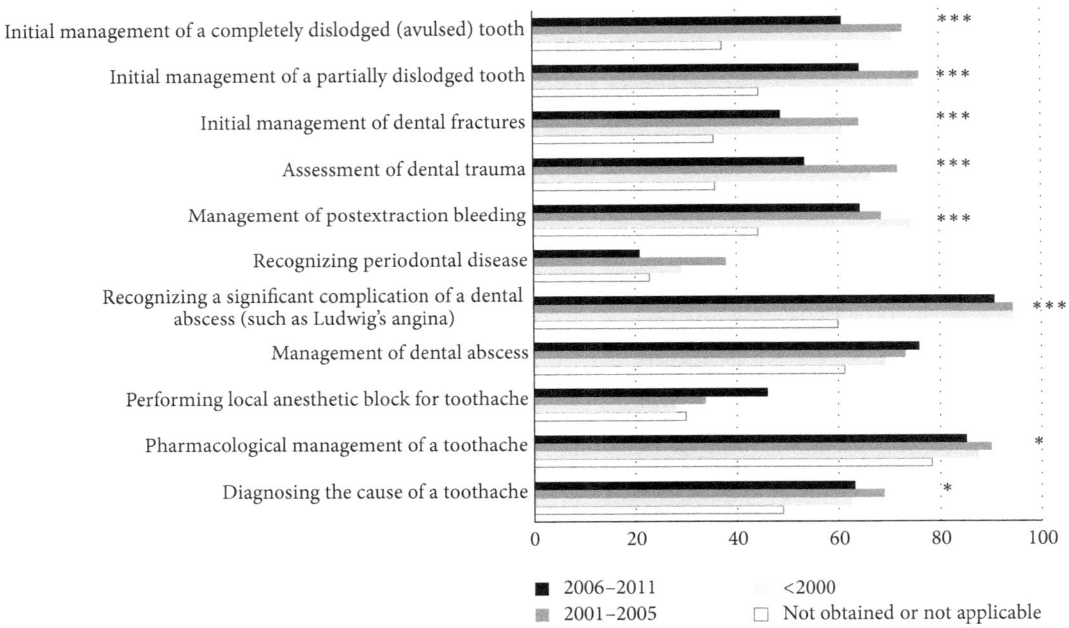


Figure 3: Practitioner confidence (agreed/strongly agreed) in specific skills relating to dental emergencies according to year the Fellowship was obtained. *denotes $P < 0.05$. ***denotes $P < 0.001$.

a greater level of confidence and earlier attainment of the fellowship (Figure 3).

*3.5. Predictors of Knowledge and Confidence.* A significant model emerged for predictors of knowledge ($F_{(11,348)} = 6.722$, $P < 0.001$; adjusted $R$ square = 0.149) and also for predictors of total confidence score ($F_{(12,350)} = 23.545$, $P < 0.001$; Adjusted $R$ square = 0.428). For knowledge, the strongest predictor was being a FACEM, whereas the strongest predictor of confidence was receipt of formal education. Other significant predictors of knowledge were having attended a conference workshop in dental emergencies and having received formal training in dental emergencies (Table 4). Other significant predictors for confidence were being a FACEM having attended a conference workshop in dental emergencies, having a dentist on call, total score on the knowledge test, and number of patients seen (Table 4).

*3.6. Attitudes towards Knowledge and Training in Dental Emergencies.* The majority of respondents (393/405, 97.0%,

TABLE 3: Participants who agreed/strongly agreed to being confident in specific skills according to receipt of formal education and participation in workshops and conferences.

| Item/skill | Received formal education | | | Participated in a conference or workshop on dental emergencies | | |
|---|---|---|---|---|---|---|
| | Yes | No | $P$ value[†] | Yes | No | $P$ value[†] |
| Diagnosing the cause of a toothache | 134/186<br>72.0%<br>65.2–78.0 | 123/259<br>47.5%<br>41.5–53.6 | **<0.001** | 84/121<br>69.4%<br>60.7–77.0 | 174/325<br>53.5%<br>48.1–58.9 | **0.003** |
| Pharmacological management of a toothache | 175/185<br>94.6%<br>90.2–97.2 | 193/280<br>74.2%<br>63.3–47.9 | **<0.001** | 106/121<br>87.6%<br>80.4–92.5 | 264/325<br>81.2%<br>76.6–85.1 | 0.121 |
| Performing local anesthetic block for toothache?* | 81/149<br>54.4%<br>46.4–62.2 | 105/297<br>35.4%<br>30.1–41.0 | **<0.001** | 68/148<br>45.9%<br>38.1–54.0 | 53/299<br>17.7%<br>13.8–22.5 | **<0.001** |
| Management of a dental abscess? | 141/186<br>75.8%<br>69.2–81.4 | 159/280<br>61.2%<br>50.9–62.5 | **0.001** | 87/121<br>71.9%<br>63.3–79.2 | 215/326<br>66.0%<br>60.6–70.9 | 0.257 |
| Recognizing a significant complication of a dental abscess (such as Ludwig's angina) | 158/185<br>85.4%<br>79.6–89.8 | 185/259<br>71.4%<br>65.6–76.6 | **0.001** | 106/121<br>87.6%<br>80.4–92.5 | 238/324<br>73.5%<br>68.4–78.0 | **0.001** |
| Recognizing periodontal disease?* | 56/119<br>47.9%<br>38.3–56.0 | 129/325<br>39.7%<br>34.5–45.1 | 0.192 | 50/118<br>42.4%<br>33.8–51.4 | 70/257<br>27.2%<br>22.2–33.0 | **<0.001** |
| Management of postextraction bleeding? | 128/186<br>68.8%<br>61.8–75.1 | 122/254<br>48.0%<br>42.0–54.2 | **<0.001** | 83/119<br>69.7%<br>61.0–77.3 | 169/323<br>52.3%<br>46.9–57.7 | **0.001** |
| Assessment of dental trauma?* | 129/220<br>58.6%<br>52.0–65.0 | 60/224<br>26.8%<br>21.4–33.0 | **<0.001** | 88/222<br>39.6%<br>33.4–46.2 | 33/223<br>14.8%<br>10.7–20.1 | **<0.001** |
| Initial management of dental fractures? | 118/185<br>63.8%<br>56.6–70.4 | 87/257<br>33.9%<br>28.3–39.8 | **<0.001** | 89/119<br>74.8%<br>66.3–81.8 | 116/324<br>35.8%<br>30.8–41.2 | **<0.001** |
| Initial management of a partially dislodged tooth? | 143/186<br>76.9%<br>70.3–82.4 | 115/256<br>44.9%<br>39.0–51.1 | **<0.001** | 99/121<br>81.8%<br>73.9–87.7 | 160/322<br>49.7%<br>44.3–55.1 | **<0.001** |
| Initial management of a completely dislodged (avulsed) tooth? | 123/234<br>52.6%<br>46.2–59.1 | 62/211<br>29.4%<br>23.6–35.9 | **<0.001** | 88/235<br>37.4%<br>31.5–43.8 | 33/211<br>15.6%<br>11.3–21.2 | **<0.001** |

[†]Inferential analyses conducted using Fisher's exact test.
*Negatively worded items reverse coded before collapsing.

95% CI 94.8–98.4) agreed or strongly agreed that it was important for emergency trainees to have practical knowledge about dental emergencies. Less than one percent (3/408; 0.7%, 95% CI 0.2–2.2) agreed or strongly agreed that there was too much attention on dental emergencies in the current emergency medicine training program.

There were no significant attitudinal differences according to year of fellowship, receipt of formal education, or participation in workshops or conferences on dental emergencies.

*3.7. Continuing Professional Development.* The preferred format of future continuing professional development (CPD) activities relating to dental emergencies revealed a strong preference for interactive workshops (386/415, 93.0%, 95% CI 90.1–95.1), watching visual presentations (357/415, 86.0%, 95% CI 82.3–89.1), didactic lectures (333/415, 80.2%, 95% CI 76.1–83.8), and case-based conferences (331/415, 79.8%, 95% CI 75.6–83.4). Fewer respondents indicated a desire for CPD obtained through the internet (318/415, 76.6%, 95% CI 72.3–80.5), textbooks (295/415, 71.1%, 95% CI 66.5–75.2), and listening to audio presentations (293/415, 70.6%, 95% CI 66.0–74.8). Other suggested CPD methods included a short rotation at an acute dental clinic or dental hospital ED, bedside teaching with a dentist or maxillofacial surgeon, a course, and on the job teaching.

When asked to indicate the preferred frequency of live education programs (e.g., lectures and workshops) on dental emergencies, the modal responses were annually (200/405; 49.4%, 95% CI 44.5–54.2) and every six months (115/405; 28.4%, 95% CI 24.2–33.0). The most commonly preferred duration of live education programs ranged between half

TABLE 4: Predictors of knowledge and confidence in dental emergencies.

| | Knowledge | | | Confidence | | |
|---|---|---|---|---|---|---|
| | *P* | Beta | 95% CI | *P* | Beta | 95% CI |
| (Constant) | <0.001 | 3.223 | 1.713–4.733 | <0.001 | −3.990 | −5.550-2.431 |
| ED type (adult/other) | 0.609 | 0.153 | −0.433–0.738 | 0.310 | 0.299 | −0.280–0.878 |
| Received formal education in dental emergencies | **0.023** | 0.592 | −0.082–1.102 | **<0.001** | 1.827 | 1.320–2.333 |
| Participated in conference or workshop specifically about dental emergencies | **0.002** | 0.926 | 0.337–1.516 | **<0.001** | 1.064 | 0.486–1.643 |
| Number of dental patients seen annually | 0.512 | −0.001 | −0.004–0.002 | **0.026** | 0.003 | 0.000–0.006 |
| Fellow (no/yes) | **<0.001** | 1.438 | 0.927–1.949 | **<0.001** | 1.114 | 0.590–1.638 |
| No access* | 0.417 | 0.357 | −0.508–1.222 | 0.830 | −0.092 | −0.932–0.749 |
| Dentist on site 24/7* | 0.945 | 0.117 | −3.223–3.457 | 0.342 | 1.314 | −1.405–4.033 |
| Dentist on site (limited)* | 0.209 | 0.382 | −0.214–0.978 | 0.100 | 0.497 | −0.096–1.089 |
| Dentist on call* | 0.841 | −0.058 | −0.631–0.514 | **0.004** | 0.824 | 0.261–1.386 |
| Refer to dental hospital* | 0.274 | 0.308 | −0.245–0.862 | 0.787 | 0.076 | −0.477–0.629 |
| Refer to private dentist* | 0.228 | 0.328 | −0.206–0.863 | 0.843 | 0.054 | −0.479–0.586 |
| Total knowledge score | N/A | N/A | N/A | **<0.001** | 0.421 | 0.315–0.527 |

*Option when asked "What access does your ED have to specialist dental services?"

a day (160/404, 39.6%, 95% CI 35.0–44.5) and 2 hours (139/404, 34.4%, 95% CI 29.9–39.2).

## 4. Discussion

Patients with dental problems present to the ED [3, 22] mostly on weekends and outside normal working hours, when dentists might not be available. One third of Australian adults do not visit the dentist because of expenses [1, 23]. An adequate understanding of dental disease and trauma is important for ED physicians to be able to diagnose, treat, and refer patients with dental emergency efficiently [24]. Poor knowledge can result in premature referral, where management is possible by the emergency doctor but is not provided, or late referral in situations when a tooth- or life-threatening problem exists.

To our knowledge, this is the first study to assess the knowledge and confidence of Australasian Emergency Physicians and Trainees' with respect to dental emergencies. We have demonstrated that knowledge and confidence vary considerably and that they are intimately related. Both are enhanced by seniority and experience working in emergency medicine and by participation in teaching programs or educational activities. Clinicians who scored well on the knowledge score were justifiably confident in their ability to manage dental emergencies.

We found knowledge to be better in some areas than others. More than 70% of respondents correctly answered questions relating to common dental conditions such as tooth avulsion, antibiotics treatment, and treatment of dry sockets. Less than half the surveyed doctors however correctly answered questions about dental abscesses, dental fractures, and ulcerative gingivitis. A previous study [10] of 30 new graduates reported that "no physician" showed a high level of knowledge with respect to managing tooth avulsion. This contrasts with more than 80% of all respondents in our study who correctly answered this knowledge question.

While confidence is not an indicator for competence, it may affect the decisiveness of management. In our study, the range of confidence varied from 27% (95% CI 22.7–30.8) in recognition of periodontal disease to 83% (95% CI 79.1–86.1) for pharmacological management of toothache. Almost 70% of FACEMs and 37% of trainees in our study were confident in managing tooth avulsion which conflicts with a recent UK study [4] among 120 ED physicians with only 20% of them confident in managing dental avulsion injuries. Surprisingly, doctors' self-rated confidence was high in managing dental fractures and abscesses despite their lack of knowledge in these areas. They did however recognize their lack of knowledge in recognizing periodontal disease.

Confidence and knowledge were moderately strongly correlated, and knowledge was a significant predictor of confidence suggesting that the two are intimately related. It is possible that being a FACEM may increase confidence generally, but clearly education plays an important part in both knowledge and confidence since being a FACEM, having received formal training in dental emergencies, and having attended a conference workshop in dental emergencies were significant predictors of both.

These findings suggest that specific education in dental emergencies may be beneficial for doctors working in EDs. Virtually all respondents agreed that it was important for emergency trainees to have practical knowledge of dental emergencies. Interactive workshops were the most highly valued educational format, supported by visual presentations, lectures, and case-based conferences. This is unsurprising since interactive workshop which was most preferred format of future CPD in our study, has significant effect on professional practice based on a Cochrane Database Systemic Review [25]. Most members of the ACEM feel that such training should be provided once or twice a year, for a two hour to half day period. The ACEM may consider offering more sessions on dental emergencies at their annual scientific meetings, potentially involving dental practitioners with particular background, and expertise in dental emergencies.

An interesting finding of the recent UK study [7] showed that only 3.9% of ED physicians would choose to be seen and treated by another ED doctor if they had a traumatic dento-facial injury. Seventy-two percent preferred to be treated by a maxillofacial surgeon and 23.5% by a dentist [4]. While this may be a reflection of attitudes towards emergency clinicians dealing with dental injuries, it is also likely that survey respondents are aware of the "system" and the likely referral to specific dental or faciomaxiallary clinicians for definitive care.

The data from this study reinforce anecdotal evidence that access to dental services in emergency situations is very limited. This lack of access makes it even more important that emergency clinicians have adequate knowledge to manage dental emergencies. Referral off-site to other providers may delay treatment, increase morbidity, and inconvenience patients. Emergency clinicians should be able to manage most of the common emergencies in the ED.

Many dental emergencies rely on the clinician's ability to provide adequate pain relief, including local anesthetic blockade. Although this skill is a procedure for which a high level of competence is expected among ACEM members, only one third of respondents reported that they could confidently use local anesthetics in toothache. Regional anaesthesia techniques, including dental anaesthesia, were rated as one of the most requested education procedures by ACEM fellows in a national learning need analysis [26]. This analysis suggested that high quality and well explained videos and regular workshops could help members improve this core competency, as suggested by respondents to our survey. Our finding that only 17% of members without formal education could perform local anesthetics compared with 46% with some kind of formal education, supports the value of such educational activities.

## 5. Limitations

This study is not without limitation. The overall response rate was low which is not uncommon for survey research and may be lower among this cohort due to the possibility of eligible participants being asked to complete multiple survey-based research projects via the ACEM (Dr Andrew Gosbell, personal communication), thereby resulting in survey fatigue. The distribution of respondents by region was however comparable to the eligible study population, except for a slight preponderance of Victorian respondents and fewer respondents from Queensland. This suggests the sample was reasonably representative of ACEM members. Further demographic information about the total ACEM population was not available to the authors and therefore restricted further assessment of representativeness. The use of ACEM as the organization distributing the email to potential participant was an ethical requirement for the study due to privacy laws but is likely to have resulted in the use of correct email addresses as ACEM is the professional body that manages specialist status in Australasia for emergency physicians.

We attempted to minimise selection bias by recruiting participants through the two methods described: an online survey and by direct distribution of the survey to eligible registrants at the ACEM Annual Scientific Meeting. The direct recruitment approach was used in order to enroll eligible doctors whose participation in the study through completion of the online questionnaire was unlikely due to internet access barriers or a bias against online survey completion. We cannot exclude the possibility of responder bias; those more interested in dental emergencies may have been more likely to respond to the survey. If such effect were present this may have produced an overestimate the actual knowledge and confidence of ACEM members.

We cannot exclude the possibility of responder bias; those more interested, competent, or confident in dental emergencies may have been more likely to respond to the survey, and those less comfortable with their knowledge may have been less inclined to respond. The possible survey fatigue among the target group may have biased participation to those who are more engaged and possibly therefore more likely to have been involved in educational and other college activities; this might also have resulted in higher test scores.

We attempted to minimise measurement bias by establishing face validity and content validity of the tool, given the absence of a previously validated tool on dental emergencies. Additionally, we undertook further validation of the internal consistency of the knowledge component and confidence component of the tool using Cronbach's alpha. Although the multiple choice questions that comprised the knowledge assessment in this survey were reviewed by several ED consultants and registrars, it was not an exhaustive examination of dental emergencies, assessing just a few key presentations and therefore may not extrapolate well to other dental emergencies not included in the survey. Further, although the pass mark of 50% was set *a priori* by a panel of emergency physicians, this cutoff may be deemed by some as somewhat arbitrary; however the findings of sensitivity analyses were in line with the expectation that seniority and exposure to education and training would result in higher total scores.

We did not instruct participants to avoid consulting educational materials to improve performance. The anonymous nature of the survey, however, may have minimised any such Hawthorne Effect.

## 6. Conclusions

The knowledge and confidence of Australasian ED doctors with respect to dental emergencies is varied, being good in some areas but in need of improvement in others. Seniority in the ED is associated with both confidence and knowledge. However, formal interactive education is also associated with confidence and knowledge, and importantly, is desired by the majority of specialist and trainee emergency physicians in Australasia. The use of designated training workshops on dental emergencies is therefore warranted.

## Appendix

The appendix contains the questionnaire items presented to respondents. It includes four parts. Part one requests demographic information. Part two requests respondents to rate their confidence in dental emergencies. Part three requests respondents to complete a multiple choice knowledge test of dental emergencies. Part four requests respondents to provide suggestions for further training in dental emergencies.

*Part One (demographics)*

(1) In which region do you usually work?

QLD
NSW
VIC
ACT
SA
WA
NT
TAS
New Zealand

(2) Which year did you pass the primary exam?

...

(3) Which year did you pass the fellowship exam?

...

(4) In which hospital do you primarily work (The hospital will be de-identified prior to publication)?

(5) The ED in which you work is:

Adult ED
Paediatric ED
Mixed ED

(6) Have you had any formal education about dental emergencies during your emergency training?

Yes
no

(7) Have you ever participated in any conference or workshop specifically about dental emergencies?

Yes
no

(8) How many patients do you see approximately each year with a tooth-related complaint (pain, abscess, trauma, etc)?

(9) What access does your ED have to specialist dental services? (you can choose more than one option)

No access
Dentist on site (24/7)
Dentist on site (limited time)
Dentist on call
referral to dental hospital
referral to private dentist
Other-please specify...

*Part Two (your confidence in dental emergencies).* Please rate your agreement to the following statements about your confidence in dental emergencies:

(1) I am confident in diagnosing the cause of a toothache?

□ Strongly Disagree
□ Disagree
□ Neutral
□ Agree
□ Strongly Agree

(2) I am confident in the pharmacological management of a toothache?

□ Strongly Disagree
□ Disagree
□ Neutral
□ Agree
□ Strongly Agree

(3) I *am not* confident in performing local anesthetic block for toothache?

□ Strongly Disagree
□ Disagree
□ Neutral
□ Agree
□ Strongly Agree

(4) I am confident in the management of a dental abscess?

□ Strongly Disagree
□ Disagree
□ Neutral
□ Agree
□ Strongly Agree

(5) I am confident in recognizing a significant complication of a dental abscess (such as Ludwig's angina)

□ Strongly Disagree
□ Disagree
□ Neutral
□ Agree
□ Strongly Agree

(6) I *am not* confident in recognizing periodontal disease?

- □ Strongly Disagree
- □ Disagree
- □ Neutral
- □ Agree
- □ Strongly Agree

(7) I am confident in the management of post-extraction bleeding?

- □ Strongly Disagree
- □ Disagree
- □ Neutral
- □ Agree
- □ Strongly Agree

(8) I *am not* confident in the assessment of dental trauma?

- □ Strongly Disagree
- □ Disagree
- □ Neutral
- □ Agree
- □ Strongly Agree

(9) I am confident in the initial management of dental fractures?

- □ Strongly Disagree
- □ Disagree
- □ Neutral
- □ Agree
- □ Strongly Agree

(10) I am confident in the initial management of a partially dislodged tooth?

- □ Strongly Disagree
- □ Disagree
- □ Neutral
- □ Agree
- □ Strongly Agree

(11) I *am not* confident in the initial management of a completely dislodged (avulsed) tooth?

- □ Strongly Disagree
- □ Disagree
- □ Neutral
- □ Agree
- □ Strongly Agree

*Part Three (knowledge test of dental emergencies).* In the following questions, choose the single best answer. If you are not sure about the correct answer, please choose the last option (e)

(1) Full dentition in an adult and in a child consists of:

(a) 28 permanent teeth, 20 deciduous teeth
(b) 32 permanent teeth, 20 deciduous teeth
(c) 28 permanent teeth, 16 deciduous teeth
(d) 32 permanent teeth, 16 deciduous teeth
(e) I am not sure

(2) What is the name of the left upper fourth tooth from the midline in the adult dentition?

(a) Incisor
(b) Canine
(c) Premolar
(d) Molar
(e) I am not sure

(3) Regarding eruption date of teeth, which one of the following statements is *incorrect*?

(a) At about 6 years of age, the first permanent teeth begin to erupt
(b) Between approximately 6 and 12 years age, children have a mix of permanent and deciduous teeth
(c) The first permanent molars (upper and lower) and lower incisors are the first permanent teeth to erupt
(d) By the age of 12 most children have all their permanent teeth
(e) I am not sure

(4) Which one of the following is incorrect about Aphthous Stomatitis?

(a) The lesions are tender
(b) The condition is self limiting
(c) An antibiotic is usually given to prevent secondary infection
(d) It may occur following oral trauma
(e) I am not sure

(5) What is the most common source of oral pain?

(a) Maxillary sinusitis
(b) Dental caries
(c) Cracked tooth
(d) Root canal pain
(e) I am not sure

(6) When would you consider re-implantation of a primary (deciduous) avulsed tooth?

(a) Always
(b) Never
(c) Depends on the age of child
(d) Depends on the child's cooperation
(e) I am not sure

(7) Which one of the following is *incorrect* regarding dental fracture?

(a) In Ellis class III fracture the pulp is involved
(b) Ellis class II fracture is more serious in children because of less dentin to protect the pulp after exposure to the oral cavity
(c) The most common dental fracture involves pulp exposure
(d) pulp exposure is a true dental emergency and a dentist should be notified immediately
(e) I am not sure

(8) Which of the following statements is incorrect regarding tooth avulsion?

(a) Foreign bodies on the root may be gently removed with forceps
(b) Remove any blood from the tooth with alcohols/anti-septic irrigation
(c) The tooth must not be allowed to dry out, it may be stored in milk for a short period
(d) A permanent tooth should be replaced into its socket as soon as possible, ideally within 2 hours
(e) I am not sure

(9) After an accidental injury, a 30 year old patient calls the ED for advice about an avulsed front tooth. The first advice that you give to the patient is:

(a) Wrap the tooth in a tissue and see a dentist
(b) scrub and clean the tooth and put it back in the socket
(c) Wash the tooth in the running warm water, then clean the root of the tooth with gauze, put it in the socket, see a dentist as soon as possible
(d) Wash it in the running cold water, do not touch the root of the tooth, put it in the socket and if not possible, store in milk, see a dentist as soon as possible
(e) I am not sure

(10) You generally give an antibiotic to a patient with dental pain in all following situations *except*?

(a) Pain not responding to analgesia
(b) Systemic symptom (e.g., fever)
(c) Regional lymphadenopathy
(d) Facial swelling
(e) I am not sure

(11) A patient presents to ED 2 days after a routine tooth extraction, complaining of pain in the same site where the tooth was extracted. The pain is much worse than the original toothache. On examination the patient is afebrile and there is food debris in the socket. What is the most likely diagnosis?

(a) Osteomyelitis
(b) Alveolar osteitis (dry socket)
(c) Retained root
(d) Incorrect extraction
(e) I am not sure

(12) Regarding "acute necrotizing ulcerative gingivitis", which one of the following statements is *incorrect*?

(a) The diagnostic triad includes pain, ulcerated interdental papillae, and gingival bleeding
(b) The most important predisposing factor is human immunodeficiency virus (HIV)
(c) Unusual emotional stress is one of the contributing factors
(d) The peak age of incidence is early 40's
(e) I am not sure

(13) The following statements are correct about "periodontal abscess" *except*:

(a) The tooth is usually mobile
(b) It usually causes extra-oral swelling
(c) The tooth is tender to percussion
(d) There is swelling of adjacent gingiva
(e) I am not sure

(14) How do you manage a patient with alveolar osteitis (dry socket)?

(a) Give analgesia and send him to see the same dentist who extracted the tooth
(b) Start antibiotic and analgesia and send him to his dentist
(c) Check the socket for any discharge or infection and then irrigate the socket, pack the socket with sterile gauze soaked in local anesthetic, then send him to see a dentist
(d) Give chlorhexidine mouthwash and prescribe antibiotic and analgesia and send him to see a dentist
(e) I am not sure

(15) Which one of the following statements is incorrect regarding Ludwig's angina?

(a) The most serious immediate sequela is airway obstruction
(b) Hemolytic streptococcus is most commonly responsible for the infection

(c) A site of discrete fluctuance can often be found
(d) It is bilateral swelling involving the submandibular, submental and sublingual spaces
(e) I am not sure

*Part Four (suggestions about further training in dental emergencies).* Please enter your agreement/disagreement (where applicable) with the following statements:

(1) It is important for emergency trainees to have practical knowledge about dental emergencies:

□ Strongly Disagree
□ Disagree
□ Neutral
□ Agree
□ Strongly Agree

(2) There is too much attention on dental emergencies in the current emergency medicine training program:

□ Strongly Disagree
□ Disagree
□ Neutral
□ Agree
□ Strongly Agree

(3) Which of the following types of education about dental emergencies would you undertake [please choose as many as you want and prioritise them with number (1-2-3...)]:

(i) didactic lectures
(ii) interactive workshops
(iii) case-based conferences
(iv) textbook
(v) internet
(vi) listening to audio presentations
(vii) watching visual presentations
(viii) other

(4) How frequently should there be live educational program (lectures, workshops ...) about dental emergencies available for ED trainees?

Never
every 6 months
every year
every 18 months
every 2 years
every 5 years

(5) What is the optimal duration for a live educational program (lectures, workshops...) on dental emergencies?

1 hour
2 hours
Half day
Full day
Multi-day
Other-(please specify)...

## Conflict of Interests

The authors report no conflict of interests.

## References


[1] T. Skapetis, T. Gerzina, and W. Hu, "Review article: management of dental emergencies by medical practitioners: recommendations for Australian education and training," *Emergency Medicine Australasia*, vol. 23, no. 2, pp. 142–152, 2011.

[2] C. Lewis, H. Lynch, and B. Johnston, "Dental complaints in emergency departments: a national perspective," *Annals of Emergency Medicine*, vol. 42, no. 1, pp. 93–99, 2003.

[3] C. Quiñonez, D. Gibson, A. Jokovic, and D. Locker, "Emergency department visits for dental care of nontraumatic origin," *Community Dentistry and Oral Epidemiology*, vol. 37, no. 4, pp. 366–371, 2009.

[4] C. Trivedy, N. Kodate, A. Ross et al., "The attitudes and awareness of emergency department (ED) physicians towards the management of common dentofacial emergencies," *Dental Traumatology*, vol. 28, no. 2, pp. 121–126, 2012.

[5] R. Crouch, A. Patel, S. Williams, and J. Dale, "An analysis of telephone calls to an inner-city accident and emergency department," *Journal of the Royal Society of Medicine*, vol. 89, no. 6, pp. 324–328, 1996.

[6] A. B. Douglass and J. M. Douglass, "Common dental emergencies," *The American Family Physician*, vol. 67, no. 3, pp. 511–516, 2003.

[7] G. Roberts, C. Scully, and R. Shotts, "ABC of oral health: dental emergencies," *British Medical Journal*, vol. 321, no. 7260, pp. 559–562, 2000.

[8] A. Kingon, "Solving dental problems in general practice," *Australian Family Physician*, vol. 38, no. 4, pp. 211–216, 2009.

[9] A. Pennycook, R. Makower, A. Brewer, C. Moulton, and R. Crawford, "The management of dental problems presenting to an accident and emergency department," *Journal of the Royal Society of Medicine*, vol. 86, no. 12, pp. 702–703, 1993.

[10] M. Abu-Dawoud, B. Al-Enezi, and L. Andersson, "Knowledge of emergency management of avulsed teeth among young physicians and dentists," *Dental Traumatology*, vol. 23, no. 6, pp. 348–355, 2007.

[11] O. M. Sánchez, N. K. Childers, L. Fox, and E. Bradley, "Physicians' views on pediatric preventive dental care," *Pediatric Dentistry*, vol. 19, no. 6, pp. 377–383, 1997.

[12] I. H. Nasr, A. Papineni Mcintosh, S. Mustafa, and A. Cronin, "Professional knowledge of accident and emergency doctors on the management of dental injuries," *Community Dental Health*, vol. 30, no. 4, pp. 234–240, 2013.

[13] H. L. Needleman, K. Stucenski, P. W. Forbes, Q. Chen, and A. M. Stack, "Massachusetts emergency departments' resources and physicians' knowledge of management of traumatic dental injuries," *Dental Traumatology*, vol. 29, no. 4, pp. 272–279, 2013.

[14] K. K. Patel and P. Driscoll, "Dental knowledge of accident and emergency senior house officers," *Emergency Medicine Journal*, vol. 19, no. 6, pp. 539–541, 2002.

[15] P. J. McCann, M. P. Sweeney, J. Gibson, and J. Bagg, "Training in oral disease, diagnosis and treatment for medical students and doctors in the United Kingdom," *British Journal of Oral and Maxillofacial Surgery*, vol. 43, no. 1, pp. 61–64, 2005.

[16] K. F. M. Fan and J. Jones, *MCQs for Dentistry*, Pastest, Cheshire, UK, 2nd edition, 2010.

[17] D. Hammond, *EMQs for Dentistry*, PasTest, Cheshire, UK, 2007.

[18] D. Hammond, *Best of Fives for Dentistry*, Pastest, Cheshire, UK, 2nd edition, 2009.

[19] P. Cameron, G. Jelinek, A.-M. Kelly, L. Murray, and A. Brown, *Textbook of Adult Emergency Medicine*, Churchill Livingstone, 3rd edition, 2009.

[20] J. Marx, R. Hockberger, and R. Walls, *Rosen's Emergency Medicine*, Mosby, St. Louis, Mo, USA, 7th edition, 2010.

[21] J. E. Tintinalli, J. S. Stapczynski, O. J. Ma, D. Cline, R. Cydulka, and G. Meckler, "Tintinalli's emergency medicine: a comprehensive study guide," in *Chapter 240: Oral and Dental Emergencies*, pp. 1572–1583, McGraw-Hill, New York, NY, USA, 7th edition, 2011.

[22] T. E. Ladrillo, M. H. Hobdell, and A. C. Caviness, "Increasing prevalence of emergency department visits for pediatric dental care, 1997–2001," *The Journal of the American Dental Association*, vol. 137, no. 3, pp. 379–385, 2006.

[23] Commonwealth of Australia, "Healthier future for all Australians—final report of the national health and hospitals reform commission—June 2009," Tech. Rep. P3-5499, NHHRC, Canberra, Australia, 2009.

[24] P. Klokkevold, "Common dental emergencies. Evaluation and management for emergency physicians," *Emergency Medicine Clinics of North America*, vol. 7, no. 1, pp. 29–63, 1989.

[25] M. A. Thomson O'Brien, N. Freemantle, A. D. Oxman, F. Wolf, D. A. Davis, and J. Herrin, "Continuing education meetings and workshops: effects on professional practice and health care outcomes," *Cochrane Database of Systematic Reviews*, no. 2, Article ID CD003030, 2001.

[26] A. W. Dent, T. J. Weiland, and D. Paltridge, "Australasian emergency physicians: a learning and educational needs analysis. Part Four. CPD topics desired by emergency physicians," *Emergency Medicine Australasia*, vol. 20, no. 3, pp. 260–266, 2008.

# 15

# Validation of the Diagnostic Score for Acute Lower Abdominal Pain in Women of Reproductive Age

**Kijja Jearwattanakanok,[1] Sirikan Yamada,[2] Watcharin Suntornlimsiri,[3] Waratsuda Smuthtai,[4] and Jayanton Patumanond[5]**

[1] *Department of Surgery, Nakornping Hospital, Chiang Mai 50180, Thailand*
[2] *Division of Gastrointestinal Surgery and Endnoscopy, Department of Surgery, Faculty of Medicine, Chiang Mai University, Chiang Mai 50200, Thailand*
[3] *Department of Obstetrics & Gynecology, Nakornping Hospital, Chiang Mai 50180, Thailand*
[4] *Department of Emergency Medicine, Nakornping Hospital, Chiang Mai 50180, Thailand*
[5] *Clinical Epidemiology Unit, Clinical Research Center, Faculty of Medicine, Thammasat University, Pathum Thani 12120, Thailand*

Correspondence should be addressed to Jayanton Patumanond; j.patumanond@yahoo.com

Academic Editor: Marco L. A. Sivilotti

*Background.* The differential diagnoses of acute appendicitis obstetrics, and gynecological conditions (OB-GYNc) or nonspecific abdominal pain in young adult females with lower abdominal pain are clinically challenging. The present study aimed to validate the recently developed clinical score for the diagnosis of acute lower abdominal pain in female of reproductive age. *Method.* Medical records of reproductive age women (15–50 years) who were admitted for acute lower abdominal pain were collected. Validation data were obtained from patients admitted during a different period from the development data. *Result.* There were 302 patients in the validation cohort. For appendicitis, the score had a sensitivity of 91.9%, a specificity of 79.0%, and a positive likelihood ratio of 4.39. The sensitivity, specificity, and positive likelihood ratio in diagnosis of OB-GYNc were 73.0%, 91.6%, and 8.73, respectively. The areas under the receiver operating curves (ROC), the positive likelihood ratios, for appendicitis and OB-GYNc in the validation data were not significantly different from the development data, implying similar performances. *Conclusion.* The clinical score developed for the diagnosis of acute lower abdominal pain in female of reproductive age may be applied to guide differential diagnoses in these patients.

## 1. Background

Abdominal pain is one of the most common chief complaints of emergency department patients. It was the main symptom of 12.1% to 20.4% of noninjury visits to emergency departments of USA, and 16.8% to 17.8% of them were in severe conditions [1]. It is difficult to diagnose the causes of abdominal pain in some patients. Diagnosis of acute appendicitis, for example, was less accurate in young adult females than in males. The accuracies of diagnosis of acute appendicitis in young adult females were 71.7% to 75.3%, while the accuracies in male were 88.6% to 90.0% [2]. Diagnosis of acute lower abdominal pain in young adult females was particularly difficult due to overlapping symptoms of obstetrics and gynecological conditions with those of acute appendicitis. Negative appendectomies often occurred mostly from missed diagnoses of obstetrics and gynecological conditions [3].

CT scan improved accuracy in diagnosing appendicitis and can detect other causes of abdominal pain in female patients [4]. The use of CT scan can reduce negative appendectomies [5]. However, the universal use of CT scan for diagnosing appendicitis may not be cost-effective in global budget scheme reimbursement for healthcare [6].

Although ultrasound is not as accurate as CT scan, it also showed benefit in diagnosing acute lower abdominal pain [7, 8], especially for pregnant women and children, whom

Table 1: The scoring scheme for appendicitis and obstetrics-gynecological conditions (OB-GYNc) and the criteria used to guide diagnosis of abdominal pain caused by appendicitis, obstetrics, and gynecological conditions (OB-GYNc) or nonspecific abdominal pain (NSAP).

| Predictors | Assigned score | | Suggested diagnoses | Criteria |
|---|---|---|---|---|
| | Appendicitis score | OB-GYN score | | |
| Guarding or rebound tenderness | 1.9 | 0 | Appendicitis | Appendicitis score > OB-GYN score and appendicitis score >0 |
| Pregnancy | −1.7 | 2.4 | | |
| Leukocytosis (WBC ≥10,000/$\mu$L) | 1.5 | 0 | OB-GYNc | OB-GYN score ≥ appendicitis score and OB-GYN score >0 |
| Neutrophil ≥75% | 1.3 | 1.6 | | |
| RLQ tenderness | 1.5 | 0 | | |
| LLQ tenderness | 0 | 1.9 | NSAP | Appendicitis score ≤0 and OB-GYN score ≤0 |
| Diarrhea | −1.4 | −2.3 | | |
| Constant | −1.5 | 0 | | |

RLQ: right lower quadrant; LLQ: left lower quadrant.

radiation is relatively contraindicated. However, ultrasound alone had low sensitivity in the diagnosis of appendicitis. Its sensitivity was not more than unaided-clinical judgment [9].

Clinical prediction rules, through which clinical findings were systematically applied to predict difficult clinical conditions [10], may be another approach for the diagnosis of acute lower abdominal pain in females of reproductive age. Alvarado's score, although intentionally developed for early diagnosis of acute appendicitis [11], has been studied for admission criteria [12] or criteria for CT scan [13]. However, appendicitis scores were not adequately applicable to abdominal pain in females of reproductive age, because they could not detect obstetrics and gynecological causes. We, therefore, developed a clinical scoring for the diagnosis of acute lower abdominal pain in these particular patients [14]. In this study, we aimed to validate our clinical scoring with patients in a different time period.

## 2. Method

*2.1. The Scoring System.* The score is comprised of simple clinical findings, laboratory results, and a constant. Item scores were assigned for guarding or rebound tenderness, pregnancy (either by clinical or urine pregnancy test), tenderness at right lower quadrant of abdomen, tenderness at left lower quadrant of abdomen, leukocytosis (white cell count ≥ 10,000/$\mu$L), predominate neutrophil ≥75% in complete blood count, and a constant. The assigned scores and algorithm for diagnostic prediction were shown (Table 1). The item scores had both positive and negative values, which reflected an increase or a decrease in probabilities of the corresponding diagnoses when presenting with those clinical findings.

*2.2. Validation Data.* The setting hospital is Nakornping Hospital, a tertiary care hospital in Chiang Mai, Thailand. Validation data were extracted from the medical records of female patients aged 15–50 years who were admitted to surgical department or obstetrics and gynecology department during January and July 2009 with a chief complaint of acute lower abdominal pain within 14 days. Patients were classified into three groups upon their final professional diagnoses, which were (1) acute appendicitis (ICD10 code K-35); (2) obstetrics and gynecological conditions (OB-GYNc), including ectopic pregnancy (ICD10 code O-00), pelvic inflammatory disease (ICD10 code N70), and complicated ovarian cyst (ICD10 code N83); and (3) nonspecific abdominal pain (NSAP) (ICD10 code A09, K57, and R10 or other causes of abdominal pain). Study variables were age, marital status, duration of pain, presence of shifting of pain, nausea and vomiting, pregnancy, abnormal vaginal bleeding, presence of fever, systolic blood pressure, site of abdominal pain, presence of guarding or rebound tenderness from abdominal examination, result of complete blood count, and urine pregnancy test. Item scores were calculated and diagnostic prediction was performed for each patient. Final professional diagnoses in the medical records were considered as the reference standard for testing of the score accuracy.

*2.3. Statistical Analysis.* Patients' characteristics of the development data and the validation data were summarized. Score predicted diagnosis of each patient was compared with final professional diagnosis. Diagnostic indices were calculated in the validation data. The abilities to discriminate appendicitis and OB-GYNc, in terms of areas under the receiver operating curves of the two data sets, were compared with the test for equality of two ROC curves. The positive likelihood ratios for the diagnosis of appendicitis and OB-GYNc of the development data and the validation data were tested with chi-squared for homogeneity test. The probability curves of appendicitis score and OB-GYN score were estimated from logistic regression postestimation function on actual rates of appendicitis and OB-GYNc in the development data and validation data.

*2.4. Ethics.* The study was approved by the Ethical Committee of Nakornping Hospital and the Ethical Committee of the Faculty of Medicine, Chiang Mai University.

## 3. Results

The patients' characteristics of the derivation data and the validation data were similar (Table 2). Appendicitis was the most common diagnosis in both data sets (70.5% in

TABLE 2: Demographic and clinical characteristics of patients in the development data set and validation data set.

| Characteristics | Development ($n$ = 542) | Validation ($n$ = 302) |
|---|---|---|
| Age (year) | | |
| Mean (SD) | 29.9 (10.7) | 29.4 (10.3) |
| Single (%) | 51.1 | 56.0 |
| Duration of pain (hr) | | |
| Mean (SD) | 35.4 (41.4) | 36.9 (47.2) |
| Shifting of pain (%) | 29.3 | 16.6 |
| Nausea and vomiting (%) | 43.4 | 42.7 |
| Abnormal vaginal bleeding (%) | 5.7 | 4.6 |
| Diarrhea (%) | 8.5 | 8.9 |
| Temperature ≥37.5°C (%) | 28.3 | 35.3 |
| Pulse rate (/min) | | |
| Mean (SD) | 89.6 (16.1) | 89.7 (14.7) |
| Systolic blood pressure (mmHg) | | |
| Mean (SD) | 119.6 (16.6) | 122.2 (16.6) |
| RLQ tender (%) | 91.9 | 91.7 |
| LLQ tender (%) | 12.7 | 18.5 |
| Guarding/rebound tenderness (%) | 55.7 | 54.0 |
| Hematocrit (%) | | |
| Mean (SD) | 37.0 (4.9) | 36.5 (4.6) |
| WBC (/$\mu$L) | | |
| Mean (SD) | 13266.1 (4928.0) | 12811.3 (4639.4) |
| Neutrophil (%) | | |
| ≥75 (%) | 56.9 | 62.3 |
| Pregnant/positive pregnancy test (%) | 10.5 | 12.6 |

development data and 65.2% in validation data). The final diagnoses of patients were shown (Table 3).

When comparing the score-predicted diagnoses and the final professional diagnoses in patients from the validation data, the score correctly diagnosed 24 of 33 NSAP patients (72.7%), 181 of 203 appendicitis patients (89.2%), and 46 of 66 OB-GYNc patients (69.7%). The overall accuracy of the score was 83.1% (251/302) (Table 4). The score had a sensitivity of 91.9%, a specificity of 79.0%, and a positive likelihood ratio of 4.39 for diagnosis of appendicitis. For the diagnosis of OB-GYNc, the score had a sensitivity of 73.0%, a specificity of 91.6%, and a positive likelihood ratio of 8.73, respectively. The diagnostic indices and their 95% confidence intervals were displayed (Table 5).

When using the criteria in Table 1 for prediction of diagnoses, the performance of the score in discrimination of appendicitis in terms of ROC analysis and positive likelihood ratio in the validation data were not significantly different from those in the development data. The area under ROC curve for the discrimination of appendicitis and "nonappendicitis" was 0.855 in the validation data and 0.796 in the development data ($P$ = 0.068). The positive likelihood ratios for diagnosis of appendicitis in the validation data and the development data were 4.39 and 2.97, respectively ($P$ = 0.100). The areas under ROC curves for the discrimination of OB-GYNc and "non-OB-GYNc" were not different in the validation data and the development data (0.823 and 0.808; $P$ = 0.706). The ROC areas of the development data reported in this study were different from those reported in our previous study because in previous study we reported the ROC areas of individual scores (appendicitis score for appendicitis and OB-GYN score for OB-GYNc), not as the whole algorithm like in this study. Similarly, the positive likelihood ratios for diagnosis of OB-GYNc were not significantly different in the validation data and the development data (8.73 and 12.94; $P$ = 0.244) (Table 6). The estimate probability curves from actual rates in the development data and the validation data of appendicitis diagnosis from appendicitis score and OB-GYNc from OB-GYN score were shown (Figure 1).

## 4. Discussion

The present study was the second part of the previous study in clinical prediction rule for the diagnosis of acute lower abdominal pain in females of reproductive age [14]. In general, clinical prediction rule studies are comprised of derivation, validation, and impact studies, with an increase in the level of evidences in each phase [15]. Validation study is important before applying such clinical prediction rule into clinical practice because the results of prediction may not necessarily be reproducible in other settings or in the other time periods [16]. In this validation study, we found no significant differences in the prediction of diagnoses between the validation data and the development data. This could be explained simply by the fact that we conducted the study at the same setting as in the development of the diagnostic score;

TABLE 3: Final professional diagnosis of patients in the development data and validation data.

| Diagnoses | Development ($n$ = 542) $n$ (%) | Validation ($n$ = 302) $n$ (%) |
|---|---|---|
| Appendicitis | 382 (70.5) | 197 (65.2) |
| OB-GYNc | 97 (17.9) | 63 (20.9) |
| Ectopic pregnancy | 48 | 34 |
| Pelvic inflammatory disease | 7 | 5 |
| Complicated ovarian cyst | 42 | 24 |
| NSAP | 63 (11.6) | 42 (13.9) |
| Abdominal pain without specific diagnosis | 31 | 20 |
| Enteritis/colitis | 21 | 15 |
| Diverticulitis | 5 | 4 |
| Urinary tract infection | 2 | 3 |
| Radiation enteritis | 2 | |
| Twisted omentum | 1 | |

TABLE 4: Diagnosis suggested by the scoring system and final professional diagnosis in the validation data.

| Diagnosis suggested by scoring system | Final professional diagnosis | | | Total | Correct diagnosis (%) |
|---|---|---|---|---|---|
| | NSAP | Appendicitis | OB-GYNc | | |
| NSAP | 24 | 4 | 5 | 33 | 72.7 |
| Appendicitis | 10 | 181 | 12 | 203 | 89.2 |
| OB-GYNc | 8 | 12 | 46 | 66 | 69.7 |
| Total | **42** | **197** | **63** | **302** | **83.1** |

TABLE 5: Diagnostic indices (and 95% confidence interval) of the scoring system for appendicitis (versus nonappendicitis) and OB-GYNc (versus non-OB-GYNc) in the validation data (based on final professional diagnosis).

| Diagnostic indices | Appendicitis (versus nonappendicitis) | OB-GYNc (versus non-OB-GYNc) |
|---|---|---|
| Sensitivity (%) | 91.9 (87.1–95.3) | 73.0 (60.3–83.4) |
| Specificity (%) | 79.0 (70.0–86.4) | 91.6 (87.4–94.8) |
| Receiver operating characteristic area | 0.855 (0.811–0.898) | 0.823 (0.765–0.881) |
| Positive likelihood ratio | 4.39 (3.02–6.37) | 8.73 (5.59–13.62) |
| Negative likelihood ratio | 0.10 (0.06–0.17) | 0.29 (0.20–0.44) |
| Positive predictive value (%) | 89.2 (84.1–93.1) | 69.7 (57.1–80.4) |
| Negative predictive value (%) | 83.8 (75.1–90.5) | 92.8 (88.7–95.7) |

TABLE 6: Areas under receiver operating characteristic curves (AuROC) and positive likelihood ratios (and 95% confidence intervals) of the scoring system for appendicitis and OB-GYNc in the development and validation data.

| Diagnosis | Development | Validation | $P$-value |
|---|---|---|---|
| Appendicitis | | | |
| AuROC | 0.796 (0.751–0.841) | 0.855 (0.811–0.898) | 0.068 |
| Positive likelihood ratio | 2.97 (2.26–3.92) | 4.39 (3.02–6.37) | 0.100 |
| OB-GYNc | | | |
| AuROC | 0.808 (0.750–0.865) | 0.823 (0.765–0.881) | 0.706 |
| Positive likelihood ratio | 12.94 (7.91–21.17) | 8.73 (5.59–13.62) | 0.244 |

patients' characteristics and patterns of clinical practices were unlikely to be different from time to time.

Clinical scoring for the diagnosis of abdominal pain has been extensively studied for appendicitis [17–22]. There were relatively fewer studies for obstetrics and gynecological conditions [23–25]. However, those studied were applied for the diagnosis of only single disease (appendicitis, ectopic pregnancy, pelvic inflammatory disease, or adnexal torsion). The present diagnostic score has an advantage in inferring differential diagnosis of more than one condition, resembling

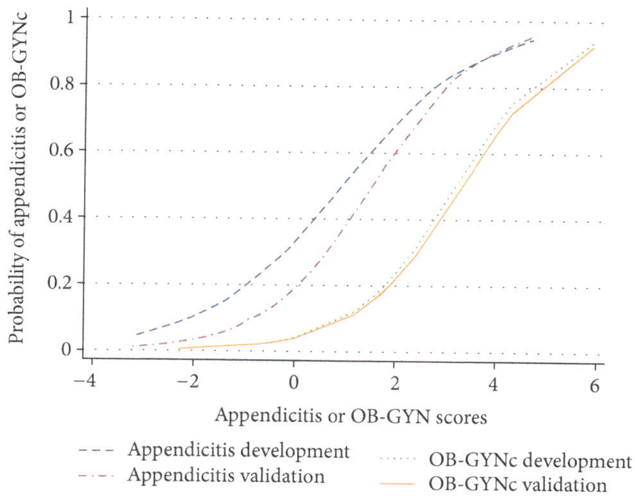


Figure 1: Estimated probabilities of appendicitis (dash and dash-dotted lines) and OB-GYNc (dot and solid lines) from actual rates of final diagnoses in development data set and validation data set.

routine clinical approach to patients. The main advantage of this score is triaging. It can guide emergency room physicians whether to admit the patients, and what specialties to consult. For example, a patient with appendicitis score and OB-GYN score equal to or less than zero, which diagnosis of NSAP is likely; this patient can probably be admitted to the observation room or discharged from emergency room and appointed to followup in the next 24 hours for a case with mild symptoms. The probability of appendicitis in this case would be approximately 20% or less; and the probability of OB-GYNc is very low (Figure 1). In addition, score-predicted probability in Figure 1 can also be applied for selective management. Patients with appendicitis score of 0–2 or OB-GYN score of 2–4, whose probabilities of appendicitis or OB-GYNc are approximately 20% to 60%, would be appropriate candidates for further investigations, such as ultrasound or CT, prior to admission. By triaging and selective management, the time spent in emergency department is expected to be less.

This study has several limitations. The obvious one is retrospective design of the study. Clinical signs and symptoms that were not documented either could be absent of such clinical findings or were not evaluated. The different observers may have different interpretations of physical examination, and clinical signs that change over time may not be well recorded.

Using of final professional diagnoses as the reference standard is another limitation. The problem of different follow-up times and different clinical judgments amongst doctors also leads to misclassification. These limitations can be reduced if a prospective validation study of the diagnostic scoring system is performed, with interobserver agreement of measurements, including standardized criteria for diagnostic indicators, objective criteria for final diagnosis of each condition, and standardized follow-up time.

The result of this study should be used with caution. Patients in our setting were mainly referred from smaller hospitals in Chiang Mai. Most of them needed to be admitted to either general surgery department or obstetrics and gynecology department. Different patients' characteristics and different patient flows in other settings would affect the accuracy of the scoring system. For example, myoma uteri complications such as necrosis or torsion were rare in our settings. In other hospitals where myoma uteri complications are major causes of acute lower abdominal pain, this diagnostic score may not be suitable for such settings. Applying this scoring system to different settings, different patterns of patients flow, could probably lead to misdiagnoses in some conditions. External validation in different settings should be performed prior to adoption into clinical practice in other settings. Further impact studies of the score to assess its impacts on multidimensions of clinical practice, such as time spent in emergency department, additional diagnostic value on top of unaided junior physicians' judgments, and time and cost of diagnosis, should be conducted in the future.

## 5. Conclusion

The clinical diagnostic score can triage appendicitis, OB-GYNc, and NSAP in female patients with acute lower abdominal pain. The diagnostic score can guide emergency department physicians for proper admissions and selective managements.

## Conflict of Interests

The authors declare that there is no conflict of interests regarding the publication of this paper.

## References

[1] F. A. Bhuiya, S. R. Pitts, and L. F. McCaig, "Emergency department visits for chest pain and abdominal pain: United States, 1999–2008," *NCHS Data Brief*, no. 43, pp. 1–8, 2010.

[2] S. W. Wen and C. D. Naylor, "Diagnostic accuracy and short-term surgical outcomes in cases of suspected acute appendicitis," *Canadian Medical Association Journal*, vol. 152, no. 10, pp. 1617–1626, 1995.

[3] S. A. Seetahal, O. B. Bolorunduro, T. C. Sookdeo et al., "Negative appendectomy: a 10-year review of a nationally representative sample," *American Journal of Surgery*, vol. 201, no. 4, pp. 433–437, 2011.

[4] E. K. Paulson, M. F. Kalady, and T. N. Pappas, "Clinical practice. Suspected appendicitis," *The New England Journal of Medicine*, vol. 348, no. 3, pp. 236–242, 2003.

[5] B. C. Morse, R. H. Roettger, C. A. Kalbaugh, D. W. Blackhurst, and W. B. Hines Jr., "Abdominal CT scanning in reproductive-age women with right lower quadrant abdominal pain: does its use reduce negative appendectomy rates and healthcare costs?" *American Surgeon*, vol. 73, no. 6, pp. 580–584, 2007.

[6] K.-H. Lin, W.-S. Leung, C.-P. Wang, and W.-K. Chen, "Cost analysis of management in acute appendicitis with CT scanning under a hospital global budgeting scheme," *Emergency Medicine Journal*, vol. 25, no. 3, pp. 149–152, 2008.

[7] K. Soda, K. Nemoto, S. Yoshizawa, T. Hibiki, K. Shizuya, and F. Konishi, "Detection of pinpoint tenderness on the appendix under ultrasonography is useful to confirm acute appendicitis," *Archives of Surgery*, vol. 136, no. 10, pp. 1136–1140, 2001.

[8] W. B. Schwerk, B. Wichtrup, M. Rothmund, and J. Ruschoff, "Ultrasonography in the diagnosis of acute appendicitis: a prospective study," *Gastroenterology*, vol. 97, no. 3, pp. 630–639, 1989.

[9] H. Jahn, F. K. Mathiesen, K. Neckelmann, C. P. Hovendal, T. Bellstrom, and F. Gottrup, "Comparison of clinical judgment and diagnostic ultrasonography in the diagnosis of acute appendicitis: experience with a score-aided diagnosis," *European Journal of Surgery*, vol. 163, no. 6, pp. 433–443, 1997.

[10] P. Beattie and R. Nelson, "Clinical prediction rules: what are they and what do they tell us?" *Australian Journal of Physiotherapy*, vol. 52, no. 3, pp. 157–163, 2006.

[11] A. Alvarado, "A practical score for the early diagnosis of acute appendicitis," *Annals of Emergency Medicine*, vol. 15, no. 5, pp. 557–564, 1986.

[12] M. Y. P. Chan, C. Tan, M. T. Chiu, and Y. Y. Ng, "Alvarado score: an admission criterion in patients with right iliac fossa pain," *Surgeon*, vol. 1, no. 1, pp. 39–41, 2003.

[13] R. McKay and J. Shepherd, "The use of the clinical scoring system by Alvarado in the decision to perform computed tomography for acute appendicitis in the ED," *American Journal of Emergency Medicine*, vol. 25, no. 5, pp. 489–493, 2007.

[14] K. Jearwattanakanok, S. Yamada, W. Suntornlimsiri, W. Smuthtai, and J. Patumanond, "Clinical scoring for diagnosis of acute lower abdominal pain in female of reproductive age," *Emergency Medicine International*, vol. 2013, Article ID 730167, 6 pages, 2013.

[15] T. G. McGinn, G. H. Guyatt, P. C. Wyer, C. D. Naylor, I. G. Stiell, and W. S. Richardson, "Users' guides to the medical literature XXII: how to use articles about clinical decision rules. Evidence-Based Medicine Working Group," *Journal of the American Medical Association*, vol. 284, no. 1, pp. 79–84, 2000.

[16] T. Fahey and J. van der Lei, "Producing and using clinical prediction rules," in *The Evidence Base of Clinical Diagnosis: Theory and Methods of Diagnostic Research*, J. A. Knottnerus and F. Buntinx, Eds., pp. 213–236, Blackwell Publishing, Oxford, UK, 2nd edition, 2009.

[17] H. Sitter, S. Hoffmann, I. Hassan, and A. Zielke, "Diagnostic score in appendicitis: validation of a diagnostic score (Eskelinen score) in patients in whom acute appendicitis is suspected," *Langenbeck's Archives of Surgery*, vol. 389, no. 3, pp. 213–218, 2004.

[18] D. M. Kulik, E. M. Uleryk, and J. L. Maguire, "Does this child have appendicitis? A systematic review of clinical prediction rules for children with acute abdominal pain," *Journal of Clinical Epidemiology*, vol. 66, no. 1, pp. 95–104, 2013.

[19] S. M. M. de Castro, Ç. Ünlü, E. P. Steller, B. A. van Wagensveld, and B. C. Vrouenraets, "Evaluation of the appendicitis inflammatory response score for patients with acute appendicitis," *World Journal of Surgery*, vol. 36, no. 7, pp. 1540–1545, 2012.

[20] C. Ohmann, Q. Yang, and C. Franke, "Diagnostic scores for acute appendicitis," *European Journal of Surgery*, vol. 161, no. 4, pp. 273–281, 1995.

[21] R. Ohle, F. O'Reilly, K. K. O'Brien, T. Fahey, and B. D. Dimitrov, "The Alvarado score for predicting acute appendicitis: a systematic review," *BMC Medicine*, vol. 9, article 139, 2011.

[22] C. Ohmann, C. Franke, and Q. Yang, "Clinical benefit of a diagnostic score for appendicitis: results of a prospective interventional study. German Study Group of Acute Abdominal Pain," *Archives of Surgery*, vol. 134, no. 9, pp. 993–996, 1999.

[23] C. Huchon, P. Panel, G. Kayem et al., "Is a standardized questionnaire useful for tubal rupture screening in patients with ectopic pregnancy?" *Academic Emergency Medicine*, vol. 19, no. 1, pp. 24–30, 2012.

[24] K. Morishita, M. Gushimiyagi, M. Hashiguchi, G. H. Stein, and Y. Tokuda, "Clinical prediction rule to distinguish pelvic inflammatory disease from acute appendicitis in women of childbearing age," *American Journal of Emergency Medicine*, vol. 25, no. 2, pp. 152–157, 2007.

[25] C. Huchon, S. Staraci, and A. Fauconnier, "Adnexal torsion: a predictive score for pre-operative diagnosis," *Human Reproduction*, vol. 25, no. 9, pp. 2276–2280, 2010.

# 16

# Exploring Factors Affecting Emergency Medical Services Staffs' Decision about Transporting Medical Patients to Medical Facilities

**Abbasali Ebrahimian,[1] Hesam Seyedin,[1] Roohangiz Jamshidi-Orak,[2] and Gholamreza Masoumi[3]**

[1] *Department of Health Services Management, School of Health Management and Information Sciences, Iran University of Medical Sciences, No. 6, Rashid Yasemi Street, Vali-e-asr Avenue, Tehran 1995614111, Iran*
[2] *School of Health Management and Information Sciences, Iran University of Medical Sciences, Tehran, Iran*
[3] *Department of Emergency Medicine, School of Medicine, Iran University of Medical Sciences, Tehran, Iran*

Correspondence should be addressed to Hesam Seyedin; h.seyedin@iums.ac.ir

Academic Editor: Wen-Jone Chen

Transfer of patients in medical emergency situations is one of the most important missions of emergency medical service (EMS) staffs. So this study was performed to explore affecting factors in EMS staffs' decision during transporting of patients in medical situations to medical facilities. The participants in this qualitative study consisted of 18 EMS staffs working in prehospital care facilities in Tehran, Iran. Data were gathered through semistructured interviews. The data were analyzed using a content analysis approach. The data analysis revealed the following theme: "degree of perceived risk in EMS staffs and their patients." This theme consisted of two main categories: (1) patient's condition' and (2) the context of the EMS mission'. The patent's condition category emerged from "physical health statuses," "socioeconomic statuses," and "cultural background" subcategories. The context of the EMS mission also emerged from two subcategories of "characteristics of the mission" and EMS staffs characteristics'. EMS system managers can consider adequate technical, informational, financial, educational, and emotional supports to facilitate the decision making of their staffs. Also, development of an effective and user-friendly checklist and scoring system was recommended for quick and easy recognition of patients' needs for transportation in a prehospital situation.

## 1. Introduction

Ambulance service is at the forefront of healthcare services [1]. During the past decade, the need for ambulance service and patient transportation by emergency medical services (EMS) has increased significantly. For example, in England, this increase has been about 16% [2]. In our country, Iran, about 80–85% of all EMS missions are performed for providing prehospital care to patients with medical problems and transporting them to medical facilities [3, 4]. However, not all of these transportations are really urgent. Evidence shows that a large number of EMS missions performed in Iran, the United States of America, and Great Britain are dispensable [3–6]. Knapp et al. also noted that inappropriate and excessive use of EMS is a common problem faced by prehospital care providers [7]. EMS misuse expands EMS staffs' workload, imposes a significant financial burden on the prehospital care system [8], and increases the rate of undue hospital admissions [9]. Consequently, developing an effective control system for determining patients who really need transportation is of the utmost urgency. A basic prerequisite for developing such a system is to determine "who" really needs ambulance services, "why" he/she needs such services, and "where" he/she is located [10].

In many countries, determining patients' need for transportation is up to EMS staffs. They have the opportunity to visit, assess, and provide care to patients in prehospital settings and make decisions about their need for transportation [11, 12]. Consequently, EMS staffs have a unique status for identifying patients' real need for transportation [11]. However, research findings do not support the accuracy of all the judgments and decisions made by EMS staffs about patients' need for transportation [8, 11, 12]. For example, Mann and Guly invited two groups of emergency and family physicians to determine the need for transportation among seventeen patients hospitalized in the emergency ward. They found that the physicians of the two groups had consensus only over 20% of cases [5]. Ebrahimian and Khalesi also found that EMS workers and emergency physicians' agreement on the need of 798 medical patients for transportation was equal to 50.14% [4]. In another study, Challen and Walter found that only 65% of all 215 patients who had been transported to hospital by EMS needed hospitalization [2]. Regarding these disagreements, Fullerton et al. noted that transportation-related judgments and decisions are made mainly based on mental processes and the context of the emergency situation, rather than scientific evidence [12]. This is mainly due to the fact that EMS staffs have different levels of knowledge, expertise, and clinical judgment and decision-making abilities [4, 12]. On the other hand, there is no clear accepted definition for "medical necessity" [8]. Accordingly, deciding about the accuracy of EMS staffs' clinical judgments and decisions is increasingly difficult. Moreover, although the majority of EMS missions are performed for transporting medical patients, predictors of need among these patients for transportation are poorly known [3, 4]. Consequently, exploring EMS staffs' transportation experiences and criteria seems crucial. We conducted this study to reduce this gap. The aim of this study was to explore factors affecting EMS staffs' decision about transporting medical patients to medical facilities.

## 2. Methods

*2.1. Design.* This was a qualitative study conducted by using the qualitative content analysis approach. Content analysis is an analytic approach and a scientific method that provides new insight and better understanding about the intended phenomena [13]. This study was conducted in 2013.

*2.2. Participants.* The study population consisted of all EMS staffs working in prehospital care facilities located in the northern, eastern, western, and southern districts of Tehran, Iran. At the time of the study, there were a total of 140 EMS stations in these four districts. Sampling was performed in several rounds. During each round, we randomly selected one station from each district and then one EMS staffs from the selected station. The inclusion criteria were having the desire for participating in the study, having an at least five-year work experience, and holding college diploma in either a two-year course of Medical Emergency or a four-year Nursing course. Finally, eighteen EMS staffs were recruited to the study by using the purposive sampling technique.

*2.3. Data Collection.* We collected the study data by conducting semistructured personal interviews. Primarily, the interview questions were framed as follows.

(i) How do you identify that a medical patient needs transportation?

(ii) What do medical patients and their families expect from you?

(iii) How do medical patients and their families react to your decisions about patient transportation to medical facilities?

(iv) What are your criteria for transportation?

Moreover, we employed probing questions for acquiring detailed information about experiences shared by the study participants. Data collection was pursued until reaching data saturation. The sixteenth interview yielded no further helpful information or insights. However, to ensure data saturation, we conducted two more interviews. Accordingly, we conducted eighteen interviews in total. Interviews were scheduled according to participants' preferences. All participants were inclined toward being interviewed at their station and at the beginning of their working shift. Interviews lasted for 23–41 minutes (36 minutes in average). We recorded all the interviews by using a digital sound recorder. Immediately after each interview, we transcribed the interview content verbatim.

*2.4. Data Analysis.* Data analysis was carried out concurrently with data collection. We employed the qualitative content analysis approach [14] for data analysis. Whole interviews were considered as the unit of analysis. Accordingly, we read each interview several times to achieve a general understanding about it. Then, we started to code the meaning units, that is, words, sentences, or paragraphs, by using either participants' own expressions or our constructed codes. Simultaneously, codes were compared with each other and also with the new ones and categorized according to their differences and similarities. Categories were in turn compared and categorized into a higher-level overarching theme.

*2.5. Rigor.* The credibility of the study findings was established by using the member- and the peer-checking techniques [15]. Accordingly, we provided several participants with their own interview transcripts as well as our generated codes and asked them to determine whether our generated codes and concepts reflected their experiences or not. In case of any incongruence between the participants' shared experiences and our generated codes, we revised the codes based on their comments through negotiation. Moreover, we invited two qualitative content analysts to check the accuracy and appropriateness of our codes.

Table 1: Affecting factors of emergency medical services staffs' decision about transporting medical patients to medical facilities.

| Main theme: degree of perceived risk to staffs' selves and to patients | | |
|---|---|---|
| Categories | Subcategories | Concepts |
| Patient's condition | Physical health status | Presence of normal physiological parameters; the presence of pathologic conditions |
| | | Absence of normal physiological parameters |
| | | Presence of an obvious, serious disease |
| | Socioeconomic status | *Patient's support system* |
| | | *Patient and his family's educational status* |
| | | *Patient and his family's financial status* |
| | Cultural background | *Confidence* |
| | | *Beliefs and attitudes* |
| The context of the EMS mission | Characteristics of the mission | *Response time* |
| | | *Possibility of obtaining advice* |
| | | *Equipment* |
| | | *Special cases* |
| | EMS staffs' characteristics | *Reasoning ability* |
| | | *Physical health status* |
| | | *Perceived support* |

*2.6. Ethical Considerations.* The Institutional Review Board and the Ethics Committee of Tehran Medical University of Medical Sciences approved the study. We provided the study participants with information about the aim and the process of the study and asked them to read and sign the study informed consent form. All of the invited participants gave written informed consent for participation.

## 3. Findings

In total, eighteen male EMS staffs with an age range of 28–39 years and a mean of work experience of 6.61 years participated in the study.

The main theme of the study was the "Degree of perceived risk to staffs" selves and to patient's. In other words, the degree of the perceived risk of the emergency situation to staffs' selves and their patient determined whether a certain medical patient really needs transportation or not. This theme implied that when faced with making decision about whether to transport a patient to medical facilities or not, our participating EMS staffs considered all factors that might pose potential or real risk to them and also to their patient. This theme consisted of two main categories including "patient's condition" and "the context of the EMS mission" (Table 1). In what follows, we explain the main theme and the main categories of the study.

*3.1. Patient's Condition.* One of the most important factors affecting our participants' decision about whether to transport a patient or not was patient's condition. This category comprised three subcategories including physical health status, socioeconomic status, and cultural background.

*3.2. Physical Health Status.* Our participants mentioned that the presence of a serious disease or obvious acute signs and symptoms directly helps them decide about transporting a patient.

> *"When you are certain that your patient has developed an MI (myocardial infarction), transportation is absolutely essential" (Participant 14).*

They also noted that patient's healthy physical state as well as the absence of a serious disease or obvious acute signs and symptoms made them suspicious about a real need for transportation.

> *"When patient is conscious and has normal vital signs, you feel unsure about transportation" (Participant 10).*

> *"When you cannot find anything abnormal in patient's body and only he says that he is not feeling good, you remain doubtful about what you should do" (Participant 1).*

*3.3. Socioeconomic Status.* Patient's socioeconomic status was another factor contributing to our participants' decision about transportation. This subcategory consisted of three main concepts including patient's support system as well as patient and his family's educational and financial status.

*3.3.1. Patient's Support System.* The strength of patient's support system—including legal support, family, and neighbors support as well as insurance coverage—also affected our participants' decision about transportation. Legal support included health-related rules and regulations that in most cases safeguard patients' not care providers' rights. Moreover, to make sure of their patient's health, some families obliged our participants, either kindly or forcefully, to transport their patient to medical facilities. Patient's health insurance coverage was also an important factor contributing to families' insistence upon transportation.

> *"When patient's family ask and insist on transportation, you have no option but to transport him even if he has no serious problem" (Participant 11).*

Another aspect of family support was related to EMS staffs' judgment about family members' ability to re-call for ambulance and successfully deliver care to their patient until ambulance arrives.

> *"When you feel that patient's family members can care for him in case of developing any problem, you are more comfortable about deciding not to transport him" (Participant 16).*

*3.3.2. Patient and His Family's Educational Status.* Another subcategory of the socioeconomic status main category was patient and his family's educational status. This factor both facilitated and hindered our participants' ability to make a right decision about patient transportation. Having higher educational status as well as having health-related education facilitated patients and their families' understanding of EMS staffs' duties, encouraged them to provide staffs with accurate information about patient's condition, and helped them respect staffs' decisions.

> *"Communicating and interacting with people who have higher educational status is relatively easier" (Participant 10).*

However, in some instances, patients and family members who had higher educational status tended to hold higher expectations. Moreover, patients and family members who held health-related degrees, sometimes, meddled in EMS staffs' affairs and negatively affected their decisions. On the other hand, regarding patients and family members who had low educational status, factors such as misunderstandings and misconceptions about EMS staffs' duties, inability to establish effective communication with staffs, inability to recall patient's medical history, and indifference towards the importance of keeping patient's medical records brought about difficulties for our participants in making rational transportation-related decisions.

> *"People who hold health-related degrees tend to meddle in our affairs. Then, it is hard to arrive at a right decision" (Participant 8).*

> *"You cannot judge about patients and their family members based on their degrees. Some people who hold higher degrees have higher expectations while some of them who have low educational status barely understand you" (Participant 13).*

*3.3.3. Patient and His Family's Financial Status.* Another factor affecting our participants' decision about transportation was patient and his family's financial status. According to our participants, patients and families with better financial status sometimes hold higher expectations and show higher sensitivity to their health.

> *"Those who have better financial status have higher expectations. For example, (we are sure that) their patient has no problem. However, they call for ambulance and despite our advice, insist on transportation to hospital" (Participant 2).*

On the other hand, patients and families who had lower financial status were more willing to receive care at home. Moreover, if transportation was needed, they liked their patient to be transported to local clinics located in their own neighborhood. The reason was that they could not afford their own subsequent public transportation costs needed for referring to hospital for visitation.

> *"The families who have financial problems and do not have insurance ask us to manage their patient's problem at home" (Participant 7).*

*3.4. Cultural Background.* The third subcategory of the patient's condition main category was patient and his family's cultural background. This subcategory comprised two main concepts including confidence as well as beliefs and attitudes.

*3.4.1. Confidence.* Confidence affected our participants' transportation-related decisions in several ways. Our participants noted that patients and families who trust in EMS staffs' abilities are more cooperative, provide more accurate information, and respect EMS staffs' views and decisions. Conversely, lack of confidence could result in having reluctance to provide information about patient's past medical history and present illness.

> *"Some patients think that if they play ill, we will transport them to hospital" (Participant 12).*

> *"We also had patients who told us that in previous episodes of the same disease, they had referred to hospital and they (hospital staffs) hospitalized them" (Participant 9).*

*3.4.2. Beliefs and Attitudes.* Our participants also noted that patients and families' beliefs and attitudes significantly contribute to their tendency to abide by EMS staffs' decisions. Previous first- or second-hand experiences of transportation as well as misconceptions and superstitions about the fate of patients who are transported by ambulance significantly affect patients and families' beliefs and attitudes about the efficiency and safety of ambulance services.

> *"There was a patient who strongly insisted on transportation. He said that last year his colleague developed the same problem and ambulance didn't transport him to hospital and hence,*

*he experienced a heart attack several hours later" (Participant 9).*

*"We had a patient who was scared of getting into ambulance because his mother had died after being transported to medical facility by ambulance" (Participant 3).*

*3.5. The Context of the EMS Mission.* The second main category of the study was the context of the EMS mission. This category consisted of two subcategories including the characteristics of the mission and EMS staffs' characteristics. These subcategories with the corresponding concepts are discussed below.

*3.6. Characteristics of the Mission.* Our participants noted that although most of the EMS missions follow a similar consistent pattern, the conditions and the characteristics of each mission are unique and differ from other missions. This subcategory comprised four main concepts including response time, possibility of obtaining advice, equipment, and special conditions.

*3.6.1. Response Time.* According to our participants, response or arrival time is a major challenge of emergency care delivery. Late arrival, irrespective of its cause, presents EMS staffs with difficulties in deciding on transportation. In such circumstances, the most important factor that might have affected EMS staffs' decision was the unfavorable emotional atmosphere of the emergency situation. Accordingly, in case of late arrival, EMS staffs usually decided to transport patient to alleviate the condition and lighten the atmosphere.

*"Some emergency locations are remote. Sometimes, alleys have no sign and hence, patient's location is difficult to find. Accordingly, we arrive late. Sometimes, we arrive soon but the alley is too narrow or patient is located at the tenth floor and the elevator is out of order. When we finally arrive at the destination, both patient and family members are filled with intense anger with us. You are also both tired and angry. In such situations, can we make a right decision?" (Participant 6).*

*3.6.2. Possibility of Obtaining Advice.* Our participants noted that for deciding on transportation, EMS staffs sometimes need to obtain advice from different sources including emergency physician attending at the dispatching center, colleagues attending at the emergency situation, as well as patients and their family members. An important factor contributing to the usefulness of a piece of advice was its applicability. For example, novice physicians usually recommended EMS staff to transport patients while experienced physicians provided constructive advice.

*"Sometimes, our emergency physician is novice and has not yet experienced even an EMS mission. "Transport the patient" is the only advice given by such physician" (Participant 8).*

Our participants also highlighted that the availability of an efficient wireless communication device, the ability of EMS staffs in accurately assessing the emergency situation and effectively transferring assessment data to the attending emergency physician, and physicians' ability in providing constructive advice were the important factors contributing to the possibility of obtaining advice. Other EMS colleagues were also good sources of information. Our participants mentioned that an educated, experienced EMS staff can provide other staffs with constructive advice. Moreover, patients and family members can also provide invaluable information and excellent advice in case of being communicated effectively.

*"You may call the emergency center to consult with the attending physician. However, the physician is, sometimes, so busy that you prefer to decide about transportation by seeking help and advice from your own colleague and the patient" (Participant 4).*

*3.6.3. Equipment.* The type and the accessibility of medical equipment also were among the other factors affecting our participants' decision about transportation. They reported that inaccessibility or defectiveness of the essential equipment, such as stethoscope, sphygmomanometer, pulse oximeter, electrocardiogram machine, glucometer, and so forth, make them suspicious about assessment data, and, therefore, compel them to transport patient to medical facilities for further assessment. Conversely, availability of basic high-tech equipment helped them make more accurate decisions.

*"Since we have been equipped with portable glucometers, we have fewer difficulties in making decision about transporting diabetic patients. However, some glucometers are defective and accordingly, we cannot diagnose whether patients' weakness is related to his low blood glucose level or not. In such instances, we feel compelled to transport the patient" (Participant 9).*

*3.6.4. Special Cases.* According to our participants, some of the EMS missions are performed for providing care to special cases such as patients who hold strategic management or administrative positions, elderly people who live alone and call for ambulance at midnight, students who develop problems at school, culprits and prisoners, and foreigners. They noted that in these cases, they have to transport the patient irrespective of the severity or the seriousness of the problem.

*"For example, in case of confronting a culprit in a police station who is holding his belly, shouting that 'I'm having pain', we are left with no option but transport him even if he is shamming. Otherwise, if he develops any problem later, they will accuse us of negligence and malpractice" (Participant 5).*

*"When they call ambulance for a (foreign) tourist, we immediately transport him. Because, if we do*

> *not transport him and something wrong happens to him, our hosting country would get into trouble" (Participant 9).*

*3.7. EMS Staffs' Characteristics.* Personal characteristics of EMS staffs as well as their working environment were also key factors in transportation-related decisions. This subcategory consisted of three main concepts including reasoning ability, physical health status, and perceived support.

*3.7.1. Reasoning Ability.* EMS staffs' reasoning—developed over time through gaining knowledge and experience—also could affect their transportation-related decisions. Our participants noted that compared with obvious injuries and traumas, diagnosing medical problems is much more difficult. Accordingly, EMS staffs who have more knowledge and experience have better reasoning ability and hence reach sensible decisions more easily and more quickly.

> *"Since participating in a workshop on acute heart problems, I have become more sensitive to the manifestations of heart problems" (Participant 15).*

> *"We have had so many medical patients that now we can diagnose medical problems easily" (Participant 17).*

*3.7.2. Physical Health Status.* EMS staffs' physical condition also affected their transportation-related decisions. According to our participants, physical problems such as fatigue, sleepiness, the flu, headache, and musculoskeletal pain may negatively affect EMS staffs' concentration, resulting in poor decisions and subsequently serious consequences.

> *"My colleague was awfully tired and hence failed to diagnose a true myocardial infarction. He transferred the afflicted patient from the fourth floor to ambulance without using a stretcher. Accordingly, patient's condition deteriorated" (Participant 1).*

> *"When you are on a long 24-hour shift, you are no longer in mood for assessing and talking to patient. Instead, you transport all patients to avoid getting into trouble later on" (Participant 18).*

*3.7.3. Perceived Support.* The strength of EMS staffs' support system—including legal, organizational, professional, managerial, and financial support as well as liability insurance coverage—was also a key factor affecting our participants' decision about patient transportation. EMS technicians who did not have an effective support system made decisions that carried minimal risk.

> *"When your senior is looking for an opportunity to pick on you for your faults and on the other hand, patient's family members insist on transportation, you prefer to transport the patient. Otherwise, if anything wrong happens, you will be alone (i.e. the senior will not support you)" (Participant 11).*

## 4. Discussion

The aim of this study was to explore factors affecting EMS staffs' decision about transporting medical patients to medical facilities. Study findings revealed that the main factor affecting our participants' transportation-related decisions was the degree of the perceived risk of the emergency situation to staffs' selves and their patient. Other factors such as patient's physical condition, socioeconomic status, cultural background, characteristics of the mission, and EMS staffs' characteristics contributed to the abovementioned main factor. We discuss these factors below.

Patients' physical health status was a contributing factor affecting our participants' decision about transportation. For example, patients' vital signs are among the main criteria for decision making. Generally, vital signs are the key components of prehospital assessment checklist. Duckitt et al. noted that physiological parameters such as heart rate, systolic blood pressure, body temperature, oxygen saturation, and level of consciousness are among the most important factors determining the need for medical admission [16]. Rees and Mann also used physiological parameters such as central nervous system response, respiratory rate, heart rate, and systolic blood pressure for identifying high-risk patients in emergency department [17]. Our findings also revealed that besides the absence of normal physiological parameters, the presence of pathologic conditions also played an important role in deciding on transportation. For example, if our participants noticed a life-threatening condition (such as an acute myocardial infarction), they immediately decided to transport the patient irrespective of other parameters and conditions. The important fact here is that the signs and the symptoms of pathologic conditions are not necessarily obvious and hence EMS staffs require a great amount of knowledge and expertise for diagnosing them. Consequently, EMS staffs need education to be empowered enough for easily and correctly diagnosing medical problems. Nonetheless, Frost and Wise noted that even if the underlying disease has not yet been diagnosed, life-threatening conditions—such as coma, convulsion, restlessness and confusion, tachycardia, bradycardia, decreased blood pressure, coldness, cyanosis, tachypnea, bradypnea, and anuria—are easily identifiable [18].

Patients' socioeconomic status and cultural background were the other factors affecting our participants' decision about transportation. Other studies have also shown that socioeconomic status is a determinant of health [19–21] and lack of resources and facilities makes patients and families vulnerable [22]. However, these parameters are not routinely used for making standard clinical judgments. These findings indicate that prehospital decision making is not performed solely based on clinical judgment criteria.

We also found that the characteristics of EMS mission—including response time, possibility of obtaining advice, equipment, and special conditions—also affected our participants' decision about transportation. The response time (the time between patient's call for ambulance and the arrival of ambulance) is a determining factor in decreasing the risk of life-threatening complications and improving survival

[23, 24]. In large cities like Tehran, the response time is below the international standards—14.98 [25] versus less than eight minutes [26]. Possibility of obtaining advice also contributed to our participants' decision about transportation. In different complicated situations, our participants tended to get advice from different sources such as the attending emergency physician, other EMS staffs, as well as patients and their family members. If our participants could obtain constructive advice, they could make better decisions about transportation. Otherwise, they felt doubt over the best decision and, in most cases, finally decided to transport the patient irrespective of the real need for transportation. McCaughan et al. also found that in awkward situations, nurses usually preferred to get advice from physicians and their own colleagues [27]. Defectiveness or inaccessibility of medical equipment were another factor affecting our participants' decision about transportation. We found that equipment malfunction required our participants to quickly decide on transportation. Assar-roudi also reported that shortage of medical equipment interferes with efficient emergency care delivery [28]. Moreover, the study findings revealed that in special cases, EMS staffs needed to take into account different political or security considerations when deciding on transportation. This finding indicates that EMS staffs are under uncontrollable external pressures that negatively affect their decisions and professional practice.

Another factor affecting our participants' decision about transportation was their own characteristics—including their reasoning ability, physical health status, and perceived support. We found that our participating staffs integrated their knowledge and expertise to better understand patients' conditions and hence make more sensible decisions. Integration of knowledge and expertise—which is sometimes referred to as intuition—helps clinicians make important clinical decisions [29, 30]. EMS staffs' physical condition also affected their decisions about transportation. Poor physical health negatively affected their concentration as well as their relationship with patients and family members. West et al. reported that care providers' physical disorders led to problems in establishing relationship with their clients and providing care to them [31]. Ozyurt et al. also noted that fatigue negatively affects workers' professional commitment and performance as well as their practical effectiveness [32].

The level of perceived socioeconomic and organizational support also affected our participants' decisions about transportation. When they perceived stronger support, they could make decisions that were more sensible. According to Taylor, there are different types of support available to individuals—appraisal support, financial support, informational support, and emotional support [33]. Rosenfeld et al. noted that weak social support creates distrust and uncertainty, which in turn might result in rule violation [34]. Accordingly, inadequate support perceived by EMS staffs may result in the violation of transportation rules. We found that EMS staffs who perceived weak support tended to transport all medical patients, irrespective of their real need for transportation. However, in case of lack of support, there is also a potential risk of refraining from transporting patients who really need transportation.

## 5. Conclusion

Study findings suggest that many factors—with different degrees of importance—contribute to EMS staffs' decision about patients' need for transportation. The multiplicity of these factors implies the tremendous responsibility of EMS staffs in accurately diagnosing medical problems. They need to analyze these factors in a short period of time and finally reach a right decision about transportation. Consequently, EMS staffs should be recruited from well-educated highly-experienced healthcare professionals. Moreover, EMS system managers can help facilitate their staffs' decision making and lighten their workload through providing them with adequate technical, informational, financial, educational, and emotional support. The study findings also provide EMS staffs with considerable support against criticism about EMS staffs' judgments and decisions being non-evidence-based.

Given the diversity and the multiplicity of factors that affect EMS staffs' decision about patient transportation, the development of effective, user-friendly checklists and scoring systems for quickly and easily identifying medical patients' need for transportation is recommended. Moreover, as other factors may contribute to EMS patient transportation decision, replicating this study in other contexts and settings is also recommended.

## 6. Limitations of the Study

We strived to create a comfortable and supportive environment during the interviews. Nonetheless, some of the participants might have taken into account different personal and organizational considerations when sharing their experiences.

## Conflict of Interests

The authors declare that there is no conflict of interests regarding the publishing of this paper.

## Acknowledgment

This study was a part of a Ph.D. thesis supported financially by Iran University of Medical Sciences (Grant no. IUMS/SHMIS_2013.4.7/7).

## References

[1] "Providing Leadership for the Provision of Ambulance Services," The Council of Ambulance Authorities Inc., May 2008.

[2] K. Challen and D. Walter, "Physiological scoring: an aid to emergency medical services transport decisions?" *Prehospital and Disaster Medicine*, vol. 25, no. 4, pp. 320–323, 2010.

[3] A. A. Ebrahimian, H. R. Shabanikiya, and N. Khalesi, "The role of physiological scores for decision making in internal pre-hospital emergency situations," *HealthMed*, vol. 6, no. 11, pp. 3612–3615, 2012.

[4] A. A. Ebrahimian, N. Khalesi, G. Mohamadi, M. Tordeh, and M. Naghipour, "Transportation management in pre-hospital

emergency whit physiological early warning scores," *Journal of Health Administration*, vol. 15, no. 49, 2012 (Persian).

[5] C. Mann and H. Guly, "Is the emergency (999) service being misused? Retrospective analysis," *British Medical Journal*, vol. 316, no. 7129, pp. 437–438, 1998.

[6] M. Kamper, B. D. Mahoney, S. Nelson, and J. Peterson, "Feasibility of paramedic treatment and referral of minor illnesses and injuries," *Prehospital Emergency Care*, vol. 5, no. 4, pp. 371–378, 2001.

[7] B. J. Knapp, B. L. Kerns, I. Riley, and J. Powers, "EMS-initiated refusal of transport: the current state of affairs," *The Journal of Emergency Medicine*, vol. 36, no. 2, pp. 157–161, 2009.

[8] L. H. Brown, M. W. Hubble, D. C. Cone et al., "Paramedic determinations of medical necessity: a meta-analysis," *Prehospital Emergency Care*, vol. 13, no. 4, pp. 516–527, 2009.

[9] J. Nicholl, "Case-mix adjustment in non-randomised observational evaluations: the constant risk fallacy," *Journal of Epidemiology & Community Health*, vol. 61, no. 11, pp. 1010–1013, 2007.

[10] J. Y. S. Ting and A. M. Z. Chang, "Focus on EMS transport: path analysis modeling indicates free transport increases ambulance use for minor indications," *Prehospital Emergency Care*, vol. 10, no. 4, pp. 476–481, 2006.

[11] S. A. Mulholland, B. J. Gabbe, and P. Cameron, "Is paramedic judgement useful in prehospital trauma triage?" *Injury*, vol. 36, no. 11, pp. 1298–1305, 2005.

[12] J. N. Fullerton, C. L. Price, N. E. Silvey, S. J. Brace, and G. D. Perkins, "Is the Modified Early Warning Score (MEWS) superior to clinician judgement in detecting critical illness in the pre-hospital environment?" *Resuscitation*, vol. 83, no. 5, pp. 557–562, 2012.

[13] K. H. Krippendorff, *Content Analysis: An Introductory to Its Methodology*, Sage, Thousand Oaks, Calif, USA, 2nd edition, 2004.

[14] U. H. Graneheim and B. Lundman, "Qualitative content analysis in nursing research: concepts, procedures and measures to achieve trustworthiness," *Nurse Education Today*, vol. 24, no. 2, pp. 105–112, 2004.

[15] P. H. Mayring, "Qualitative content analysis," *Forum: Qualitative Social Research*, vol. 1, no. 2, pp. 1–10, 2000.

[16] R. W. Duckitt, R. Buxton-Thomas, J. Walker et al., "Worthing physiological scoring system: derivation and validation of a physiological early-warning system for medical admissions. An observational, population-based single-centre study," *British Journal of Anaesthesia*, vol. 98, no. 6, pp. 769–774, 2007.

[17] J. E. Rees and C. Mann, "Use of the patient at risk scores in the emergency department: a preliminary study," *Emergency Medicine Journal*, vol. 21, no. 6, pp. 698–699, 2004.

[18] P. J. Frost and M. P. Wise, "Early management of acutely ill ward patients," *British Medical Journal*, vol. 345, Article ID e5677, pp. 1–8, 2012.

[19] N. Jerliu, E. Toçi, G. Burazeri, N. Ramadani, and H. Brand, "Socioeconomic conditions of elderly people in Kosovo: a crosssectional study," *BMC Public Health*, vol. 12, article 512, 2012.

[20] G. N. Pereira, G. A. N. Bastos, G. F. Del Duca, and Â. J. G. Bós, "Socioeconomic and demographic indicators associated with functional disability in the elderly," *Cadernos de Saúde Pública*, vol. 28, no. 11, pp. 2035–2042, 2012.

[21] J. J. Siracuse, D. D. Odell, S. P. Gondek et al., "Health care and socioeconomic impact of falls in the elderly," *The American Journal of Surgery*, vol. 203, no. 3, pp. 335–338, 2012.

[22] J. Sutton and K. Tierney, *Disaster Preparedness: Concept, Guidance and Research*, Natural Hazards Center, Institute of Behavioral Science, University of Colorado Boulder, 2006.

[23] K. Peleg and J. S. Pliskin, "A geographic information system simulation model of EMS: reducing ambulance response time," *The American Journal of Emergency Medicine*, vol. 22, no. 3, pp. 164–170, 2004.

[24] J. P. Pell, J. M. Sirel, A. K. Marsden, I. Ford, and S. M. Cobbe, "Effect of reducing ambulance response times on deaths from out of hospital cardiac arrest: cohort study," *British Medical Journal*, vol. 322, no. 7299, pp. 1385–1388, 2001.

[25] M. J. Moradian et al., "Response time to emergency cases inShiraz," *Journal of Rescue and Relief*, vol. 5, no. 2, pp. 30–39, 2013 (Persian).

[26] R. Skinner, "Improving ambulance estimated time of arrival (ETA) at hospital emergency department," *Health GIS Guy*, vol. 6, pp. 78–79, 2008.

[27] D. McCaughan, C. Thompson, N. Cullum, T. Sheldon, and P. Raynor, "Nurse practitioner and practice nurses' use of research information in clinical decision making: findings from an exploratory study," *Family Practice*, vol. 22, no. 5, pp. 490–497, 2005.

[28] A. Assar-roudi, "The causes of late arrival of pre-hospital emergency from the point of view of clinical emergency personnel of the 115 of Mashhad in 2006," *Dena Journal*, vol. 3, no. 3, pp. 1–15, 2009 (Persian).

[29] H. H. I. McCutcheon and J. Pincombe, "Intuition: an important tool in the practice of nursing," *Journal of Advanced Nursing*, vol. 35, no. 3, pp. 342–348, 2001.

[30] M. E. Burman, M. B. Stepans, N. Jansa, and S. Steiner, "How do NPs make clinical decisions?" *Nurse Practitioner*, vol. 27, no. 5, pp. 57–64, 2002.

[31] C. P. West, M. M. Huschka, P. J. Novotny et al., "Association of perceived medical errors with resident distress and empathy: a prospective longitudinal study," *The Journal of the American Medical Association*, vol. 296, no. 9, pp. 1071–1078, 2006.

[32] A. Ozyurt, O. Hayran, and H. Sur, "Predictors of burnout and job satisfaction among Turkish physicians," *QJM*, vol. 99, no. 3, pp. 161–169, 2006.

[33] S. E. Taylor, *Health Psychology*, McGraw-Hill, 4th edition, 1999.

[34] R. Rosenfeld, S. F. Messner, and E. P. Baumer, "Social capital and homicide," *Social Forces*, vol. 80, no. 1, pp. 283–310, 2001.

# 17

# Medical History of Elderly Patients in the Emergency Setting: Not an Easy Point-of-Care Diagnostic Marker

**Tobias Lindner, Anna Slagman, Arthur Senkin, Martin Möckel, and Julia Searle**

*Division of Emergency Medicine, Charité-Universitätsmedizin Berlin, Campus Virchow Klinikum (CVK), Augustenburger Platz 1, 13353 Berlin, Germany*

Correspondence should be addressed to Tobias Lindner; tobias.lindner@charite.de

Academic Editor: Chak W. Kam

*Background.* Medical histories are a crucially important diagnostic tool. Elderly patients represent a large and increasing group of emergency patients. Due to cognitive deficits, taking a reliable medical history in this patient group can be difficult. We sought to evaluate the medical history-taking in emergency patients above 75 years of age with respect to duration and completeness. *Methods.* Anonymous data of consecutive patients were recorded. Times for the defined basic medical history-taking were documented, as were the availability of other sources and times to assess these. *Results.* Data of 104 patients were included in the analysis. In a quarter of patients (25%, $n = 26$) no complete basic medical history could be obtained. In the group of patients where complete data could be gathered, only 16 patients were able to provide all necessary information on their own. Including other sources like relatives or GPs prolonged the time until complete medical history from 7.3 minutes (patient only) to 26.4 (+relatives) and 56.3 (+GP) minutes. *Conclusions.* Medical histories are important diagnostic tools in the emergency setting and are prolonged in the elderly, especially if additional documentation and third parties need to be involved. New technologies like emergency medical cards might help to improve the availability of important patient data but implementation of these technologies is costly and faces data protection issues.

## 1. Introduction

Life-threatening emergencies in the preclinical and clinical setting often require a symptom-based approach, especially if information on the patient's medical history is unreliable or lacking. Information on preexisting diseases, medication, allergies, and incompatibilities is crucially important for a suitable diagnostic and therapeutic strategy. Unfortunately, due to either the specific emergency setting and/or due to patient-related factors like impaired vigilance, cognitive deficiencies, and psychological stress, evaluating a medical history can be difficult or even impossible [1]. Even for patients who are electively transferred for hospitalization by their general practitioner, information on the medical history can be very sparse, because the transfer process is not standardized. Likewise, information accompanying patients who are transferred from nursing homes or the outpatient sector is of very varying quality [2–4]. Often, the treating physician in the emergency department is reliant on medication packaging, medication lists of unknown date, or loose papers which are found amongst the patient's belongings.

A lack of knowledge regarding concomitant diseases including organ failure, medication [4–6], or allergies can cause unsafe, inadequate, delayed, or prolonged treatment [7]. For example, recent adjustment of a patient's medication might explain his/her symptoms, prevent potentially harmful measures [8], and enable a simple and cost-effective treatment strategy. Likewise, information on concomitant diseases, the availability of recent laboratory results, and the knowledge of, for example, an allergy to contrast media can help to speed up emergency management processes, avoid unnecessarily duplicated diagnostic testing, and improve risk stratification.

Assessment of a patient's medical history potentially takes up a considerable amount of time in the acute setting, where time is often sparse. Particularly in elderly (and often multimorbid) patients with cognitive deficiencies, taking a medical history can be time consuming and information is potentially unreliable.

We sought to investigate the physician-related time effort of assessing a standard medical history in patients with an age above 75 years presenting to the trauma unit in the emergency department of a tertiary care hospital. Secondary objectives were to evaluate how often a complete medical history can be obtained in these patients, to which extent information can be provided by the patient themselves, and what other measures were necessary to retrieve relevant information.

## 2. Patients and Methods

We performed a prospective cohort study in the trauma unit of our emergency department at Campus Virchow Klinikum of the Charité Berlin, Germany. The unit cares for around 50.000 cases of predominantly traumatologic and orthopedic origin. The study complies with the Declaration of Helsinki and was approved by the ethics committee of our institution (Ethikkommission Charité Berlin EA1/367/13). All data were attained by medical students doing their internship in the emergency department during routine patient management and were documented anonymously into a case report form.

From August 2013 to January 2014, data on men and women ≥75 years of age who presented to the trauma unit were reported by 5 medical students in 5 periods of 2 weeks each. For convenience reasons data were recorded if patients presented on workdays between 9 a.m. and 4 p.m. Students were asked to constantly check the central screen in the emergency department on which patients appear after triage and the administrative procedure in order to be seen by a physician. Among other things, details on the monitor contain the exact age of the patients, so that students could identify the group ≥75 years and immediately enroll them. Patients with life-threatening emergencies or in severe pain were excluded (assessment by physician on-call).

Documentation of the basic medical history included current medication, known diseases, allergies, and name and address of the general practitioner. Additionally, the students documented whether and to which extend these data could be obtained from the patient. Questions were open without suggestion of possible answers. The time needed for obtaining the available information was also recorded. In patients who could provide no or incomplete information, written medical documentation provided by the patient, especially medication lists, and an assessment of when these had been created or updated were sought.

If any written documentation was available, the time it took to look through and gather the necessary information from these documents was recorded.

In cases of doubt regarding the information provided by the patient or his/her written documents, other sources were sought, for example, relatives or the patient's GP. Again, the time it took to contact these sources and to retrieve the necessary information was recorded. The time needed to be invested by a physician was recorded only if it led to successful retrieval of the medical history.

All documentation was carried out on a prepared one-sided examination sheet. This sheet was blinded and also exact age and gender were not documented with respect to data protection issues and avoidance of the possibility of reidentification.

*Statistics.* Data were analyzed using SPSS software (IBM SPSS Statistics, Version 19). Nominal variables are shown as absolute and relative frequencies; categorical variables are shown as median with interquartile ranges (IQR), as well as minimum and maximum values.

## 3. Results

We recorded data on a total of 104 patients with an age of 75 years or above. The majority of patients came to the ED from their home ($n = 72$; 69.2%) or were brought in from a nursing home ($n = 24$; 23.1%). Two patients (1.9%) were brought in from a public place (street), another two were brought in from a GP (1.9%), and one was brought in from a rehabilitation clinic. In three cases (2.9%) documentation of the patients origin was left blank.

*3.1. Availability of Basic Medical History Information.* We differentiated between two groups, with regard to the availability of a complete basic medical information (defined as complete information about current medication, preknown diseases, allergies, and general practitioner).

*3.1.1. Group 1: No Complete Basic Medical Data Achievable.* A total of 25% ($n = 26$) of the patients included had to be treated without the knowledge of their complete basic medical history (current medication, preknown diseases, allergies, and GP) (Figure 1), although 12 of these patients (46.2%) were carrying medical reports with them.

*Current Medication.* 25 patients (24%) in this group could not give appropriate answer to a current medication actively by themselves. 11 medical reports contained a list of medications (one set of data concerning eventual existence of list of medications missing), but only five of these lists were recognizably not older than 3 months, so that these five patients at least could ensure sufficient evidence about the drugs they currently take, leaving 20 patients (19.2%) without adequate information on this item (Figure 1).

*Preknown Diseases.* 19 patients (18.3%) could not give appropriate answer to their preexisting illnesses actively by themselves. Medical reports of eight of these patients contained a list of preknown diseases (one set of data concerning eventual notification of preknown diseases in medical record missing), leaving 11 patients (10.6%) without adequate information on this item (Figure 1).

*Allergies.* Ten patients (9.6%) could not provide safe information on eventually existing allergies actively on their own. Only in one medical record of these patients an allergy status was retrieved to help out, leaving nine patients (8.7%) without adequate information on this item (Figure 1).

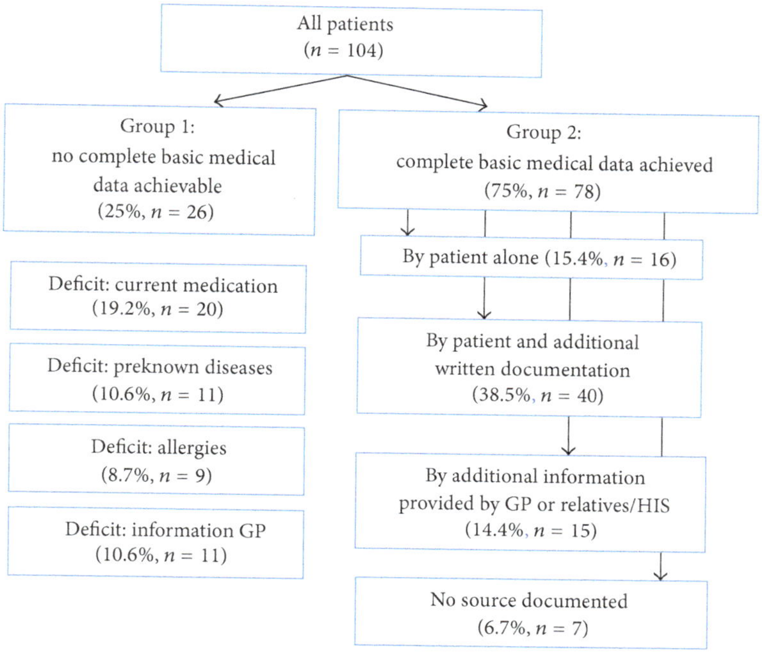


FIGURE 1: Distribution of patients included (Groups 1 and 2) (total number and % of all patients included): Group 1: no complete basic medical data achieved: single item deficit. Group 2: complete basic medical data achieved: by what means.

*General Practitioner.* 15 patients (14.4%) could not give sufficient information on their GP themselves that enabled medical staff to contact those. In four medical records of this patient group this information was achievable (one set of data concerning information on GP in medical record missing), leaving 11 patients (10.6%) without adequate information on this item (Figure 1).

*3.1.2. Group 2: Complete Basic Medical Data Achieved.* In 75% ($n = 78$) of all patients complete basic medical data as defined was achievable (Figure 1).

However, only 15.4% of all patients ($n = 16$) were able to provide the necessary information completely on their own without any support of documents or other sources.

In 38.5% ($n = 40$) complete data was obtained through the information given by the patient himself combined with written documentation the patient had brought with him to hospital. In 14.4% ($n = 15$) data had to be completed by a third party (GP or relatives) or the hospital information system (Figure 1).

*3.1.3. Time Resources for Taking the Complete Medical History.* In patients where a complete medical history could be established no matter how ($n = 78$), this took a median time of 12 minutes (interquartile range (IQR) 8/16.25; minimum 3 min., maximum 240 min.). The active physician's engagement time was 6 (5/10) minutes in patients who could provide a full medical history and was prolonged to around 11 (8/15) minutes if medical documents needed to be looked at. In cases where the GP needed to be contacted, establishing the medical history took a median time of 20 (15/81) minutes with a wide range (minimum 15 minutes, maximum 240 minutes) (Table 1).

TABLE 1: Sources of information and time until successfully completed basic medical history ($n = 78$).

| Source(s) of information | Relative frequency in % | Duration [min.] Median (IQR) Minimum–maximum |
|---|---|---|
| Self-reported medical history only | 15.4 ($n = 16$) | 6 (5/10) 3–15 |
| Self-reported medical history plus medical documentation | 38.5 ($n = 40$) | 11 (8/15) 4–26 |
| Third-party medical history (GP) | 8.7 ($n = 9$) | 20 (15/81) 15–240 |
| Third-party medical history (relatives) | 4.8 ($n = 5$) | 19 (14/43) 10–62 |
| Data from hospital information system | 0.1 ($n = 1$) | 16 |
| *No source documented* | 6.7 ($n = 7$) | 14 (12/19) 11–25 |

IQR: interquartile range.

## 4. Discussion

Our data show how difficult and time consuming it is to establish a reliable and complete medical history in emergency patients above 75 years of age.

A quarter of the patients in our study had to be managed without complete information about current medication, preknown diseases, possible allergies, or a contact's information of their GP. In particular, the availability of up-to-date medication charts seems to be problematic as almost every fifth patient had to be treated without adequate information on this item. Only 15% were able to provide all the information without the help of other sources. In most cases a successful completion of medical history was achieved by combination of talking to the patient and reading the documents he brought with him. As was to be expected, the physician's engagement time was shortest for patients who could provide all data of their medical history themselves. In cases where the GP had to be contacted, completion of the medical history was prolonged to 20 minutes (median) with a maximum time of 240 minutes, although this included waiting times for return calls, faxes, and so forth, during which time the physician is not actively bound. According to the German Medical Council, establishing a patient's medical history is a nondelegable responsibility of the treating physician [9]. If the process of taking the medical history is being improved to make it more reliable (and thereby safer) and faster, emergency departments gain valuable physician resources needed to diagnose and treat the patient's acute condition.

*4.1. Elderly Patients in the Emergency Department.* Due to the demographic changes in western developed countries, emergency departments face an increasing number of elderly patients. A systematic review from Canada published in 2002 analyzed 11 international studies and found the ED attendance rate of elderly patients to be between 12 and 21%. The authors found a consistent overrepresentation rate in this age group as compared to the respective general population. Two of the included studies with a longitudinal design showed a constant increase of elderly patients within the previous decade [10]. From 2006 to 2011, ED visit rates in the US were consistently highest for patients aged 85 years and above (around 90 per 100.000 inhabitants) [11]. In our institution in 2013, a total of 2931 patients with an age ≥75 years were treated in the trauma unit of the emergency department, which equals 7.5% of all patients presenting to this unit. When extrapolating our data to these total numbers, 733 patients above the age of 75 years would have been cared for without knowledge of their basic medical history. With the information the patients were able to provide themselves alone, 1172 might have received medication without the cognition of possible allergies and 1465 might have received nonappropriate medication considering their preexisting diseases and possible pharmacological interactions.

Tambyln et al. recently published a study on the information gap between community-based pharmacy records and medication records in the ED of patients admitted to hospital [4]. They included 613 patients in two Canadian hospitals and found that the ED records did not list 41.5% of the medication documented in the community records. They concluded that there is a big need for health technologies that allow information transfer of current medication between hospital and community especially for elderly and multimorbid patients.

Morphet et al. recently published a retrospective study analyzing data of 408 resident transfers from aged care facilities to emergency departments in Australia in terms of transfer documentation [3]. Median age of transferred patients was 86 years. The authors defined seven essential sets of data for their quality control of information transfer to an ED. Amongst others, they also examined "past medical history," "medication chart," "allergy status," and "GP contact details." In 2007, Australian authorities had introduced the "transfer-to-hospital" envelope, which should contain patient's key clinical information for admission to an ED but also discharge information from hospital back into the outpatient system. Information on "past medical history" was present in 63%, on "medication" in 65%, on "allergies" in 56%, and on "GP details" in 69% of the 408 cases. In comparison to our data, this "envelope" seemed to improve information transfer but still is insufficient and it might be unreliable regarding updates and actuality.

*4.2. Possible Solutions.* To meet the requirements of emergency medicine to be safe and effective, new technologies for process optimization in emergency and acute care have been asked for in this issue and also in recent publications [2, 3, 5, 12, 13].

A possible solution to improve the currently unreliable and time consuming process of history-taking in the elderly could be offered by medical emergency cards that can provide updated and relevant patient information. A pilot survey by Olola et al. [14] in Utah evaluated the perceived usefulness of an emergency card and a continuity-of-care report in users. In the online survey amongst the 101 users (75,3% female, median age 56 years), 68% reported the card to be helpful, especially the emergency card. Users clearly prioritized up-to-date information emergency situations over information for routine visits. The same group evaluated what medical professionals (from outpatient clinics) thought about the usefulness of their card/report [15]. In accordance with the patients, 94% found the emergency medical card to be of help in medical decision making at the point of care, whereas only 74% were persuaded by the usefulness of the continuity-of-care report. However, with respect to decreasing time effort and increasing overall knowledge both documents were voted 100% helpful; regarding the influence on the process of decision making the agreement rate was 94% for both. The authors put emphasis on the fact that the stored information has to be accessible for and modifiable by the user, who should have a control function over his file.

In Germany, an electronic health card was introduced in 2009, but so far information attainable through this card is restricted to only basic data (name, date of birth, address, etc.). In a next step, it is planned to include an emergency data set, which should increase patient safety during emergency treatment and help to gain a more effective use of physician resources. However, there have been a lot of setbacks in the technical development of this card and there is still ongoing political discussion especially with regard to data protection issues. The World Medical Card (Bergen, Norway) (http://www.wmc-card.com/) is an already readily available product that covers all these aspects and stores patient-centered and patient-controlled medical and paramedical information for emergencies but also for routine visits. Knowing his own medical risk profile the user can individually weigh up the risk of disclosing relevant information for emergency situations against the risk that despite all efforts of data protection his data might become visible for persons he does not want to share this information with. It also serves as an organ donator card. Information transfer is ensured by a haptic card, on web (with an additional data storage for reports, X-rays, patient's provision, etc.) and on mobile devices. This emergency card was primarily introduced to assure information transfer for international travels. For communicating medical data it deploys international ATC-codes for medication and ICD.-10 codes for diseases as developed by the World Health Organization (WHO).

From a procedural point of view, however, even more extensive systems which also allow feed of approved data from a closed and patient-centered system like the World Medical Card directly into the hospital information system are favorable. This function in addition to its impact on medical history duration could potentially increase the time-saving aspect by avoiding noncurative activities like manually transcribing long lists of medication and concomitant diseases from a piece of paper into the hospital information system.

## 5. Limitations

Data were recorded anonymously and thus no data on age and gender are available. Patients were included if their age was above 75 years.

The quality of the medical history reported by the patients was not validated. Thus, the proportion of incomplete (or wrong) information might have been even higher.

We did not record any diagnoses or further treatment and we therefore have no data on disease severity. We also did not record whether an incomplete or prolonged medical history led to any delays in diagnostics or treatment. In our study, in 11.5% of patients basic data were only available through the patient's GP. We only included patients during working hours, where it should have potentially been easy to contact the patient's GP. It is to be expected that there are more cases with incomplete medical history outside these hours. Last, we did not record the time invested in the cases in which no basic medical history was achieved in the end. The medical histories in this study were taken and documented by medical students in their last year (PJ students/interns). Taking a medical history may be faster when this is done by an experienced physician.

## 6. Conclusion

Medical histories are important diagnostic tools in the emergency setting and are prolonged in the elderly, especially if additional documentation and third parties need to be involved. New technologies like emergency medical cards might help to improve the availability of important patient data but a general implementation of these technologies is costly and faces data protection issues.

Given the potentially high impact on the safety of emergency care in elderly patients, who present a large and increasing patient group in emergency departments, all efforts should be made to make these technologies available.

## Conflict of Interests

Tobias Lindner is a member of the Medical Advisory Board and a consultant of the World Medical Card. Anna Slagman, Arthur Senkin, Martin Möckel, and Julia Searle declare no conflict of interests.

## References

[1] D. A. Redelmeier, M. J. Schull, J. E. Hux, J. V. Tu, and L. E. Ferris, "Problems for clinical judgement: 1. Eliciting an insightful history of present illness," *Canadian Medical Association Journal*, vol. 164, no. 5, pp. 647–651, 2001.

[2] D. Griffiths, J. Morphet, K. Innes, K. Crawford, and A. Williams, "Communication between residential aged care facilities and the emergency department: a review of the literature," *International Journal of Nursing Studies*, vol. 51, no. 11, pp. 1517–1523, 2014.

[3] J. Morphet, D. L. Griffiths, K. Innes, K. Crawford, S. Crow, and A. Williams, "Shortfalls in residents' transfer documentation: challenges for emergency department staff," *Australasian Emergency Nursing Journal*, vol. 17, no. 3, pp. 98–105, 2014.

[4] R. Tamblyn, L. Poissant, A. Huang et al., "Estimating the information gap between emergency department records of community medication compared to on-line access to the community-based pharmacy records," *Journal of the American Medical Informatics Association*, vol. 21, no. 3, pp. 391–398, 2014.

[5] S. Caglar, P. L. Henneman, F. S. Blank, H. A. Smithline, and E. A. Henneman, "Emergency department medication lists are not accurate," *The Journal of Emergency Medicine*, vol. 40, no. 6, pp. 613–616, 2011.

[6] V. C. Tam, S. R. Knowles, P. L. Cornish, N. Fine, R. Marchesano, and E. E. Etchells, "Frequency, type and clinical importance of medication history errors at admission to hospital: a systematic review," *Canadian Medical Association Journal*, vol. 173, no. 5, pp. 510–515, 2005.

[7] A. Stiell, A. J. Forster, I. G. Stiell, and C. van Walraven, "Prevalence of information gaps in the emergency department and the effect on patient outcomes," *Canadian Medical Association Journal*, vol. 169, no. 10, Article ID 14609971, pp. 1023–1028, 2003.

[8] I. Akwagyriam, L. I. Goodyer, L. Harding, S. Khakoo, and H. Millington, "Drug history taking and the identification of drug related problems in an accident and emergency department," *Emergency Medicine Journal*, vol. 13, no. 3, pp. 166–168, 1996.

[9] Bundesvereinigung BuK, "Persönliche Leistungserbringung—Möglichkeiten und Grenzen der Delegation ärztlicher Tätigkeiten 2008," 2008, http://www.bundesaerztekammer.de/downloads/Empfehlungen_Persoenliche_Leistungserbringung.pdf.

[10] F. Aminzadeh and W. B. Dalziel, "Older adults in the emergency department: a systematic review of patterns of use, adverse outcomes, and effectiveness of interventions," *Annals of Emergency Medicine*, vol. 39, no. 3, pp. 238–247, 2002.

[11] H. G. Skinner, J. Blanchard, and A. Elixhauser, "Trends in emergency department visits, 2006–2011," Statistical Brief 179, Healthcare Cost and Utilization Project (HCUP) Statistical Briefs, Rockville, Md, USA, 2006.

[12] K. W. Fung, M. Kayaalp, F. Callaghan, and C. J. McDonald, "Comparison of electronic pharmacy prescription records with manually collected medication histories in an emergency department," *Annals of Emergency Medicine*, vol. 62, no. 3, pp. 205–211, 2013.

[13] S. Arora, A. D. Goldberg, and M. Menchine, "Patient impression and satisfaction of a self-administered, automated medical history-taking device in the emergency department," *The Western Journal of Emergency Medicine*, vol. 15, no. 1, pp. 35–40, 2014.

[14] C. H. O. Olola, S. Narus, M. Poynton et al., "Patient-perceived usefulness of an emergency medical card and a continuity-of-care report in enhancing the quality of care," *International Journal for Quality in Health Care*, vol. 23, no. 1, pp. 60–67, 2011.

[15] C. H. O. Olola, S. Narus, J. Nebeker et al., "The perception of medical professionals and medical students on the usefulness of an emergency medical card and a continuity of care report in enhancing continuity of care," *International Journal of Medical Informatics*, vol. 80, no. 6, pp. 412–420, 2011.

# 18

# Direct-Acting Oral Anticoagulants: Practical Considerations for Emergency Medicine Physicians

**W. Frank Peacock,[1] Zubaid Rafique,[1] and Adam J. Singer[2]**

[1]*Section of Emergency Medicine, Baylor College of Medicine, Ben Taub General Hospital, 1504 Taub Loop, Houston, TX 77030, USA*
[2]*Department of Emergency Medicine, Stony Brook School of Medicine, University Medical Center L4, 100 Nicolls Road, Stony Brook, NY 11794-8350, USA*

Correspondence should be addressed to W. Frank Peacock; frankpeacock@gmail.com

Academic Editor: Chak W. Kam

Nonvalvular atrial fibrillation- (NVAF-) related stroke and venous thromboembolism (VTE) are cardiovascular diseases associated with significant morbidity and economic burden. The historical standard treatment of VTE has been the administration of parenteral heparinoid until oral warfarin therapy attains a therapeutic international normalized ratio. Warfarin has been the most common medication for stroke prevention in NVAF. Warfarin use is complicated by a narrow therapeutic window, unpredictable dose response, numerous food and drug interactions, and requirements for frequent monitoring. To overcome these disadvantages, direct-acting oral anticoagulants (DOACs)—dabigatran, rivaroxaban, apixaban, and edoxaban—have been developed for the prevention of stroke or systemic embolic events (SEE) in patients with NVAF and for the treatment of VTE. Advantages of DOACs include predictable pharmacokinetics, few drug-drug interactions, and low monitoring requirements. In clinical studies, DOACs are noninferior to warfarin for the prevention of NVAF-related stroke and the treatment and prevention of VTE as well as postoperative knee and hip surgery VTE prophylaxis, with decreased bleeding risks. This review addresses the practical considerations for the emergency physician in DOAC use, including dosing recommendations, laboratory monitoring, anticoagulation reversal, and cost-effectiveness. The challenges of DOACs, such as the lack of specific laboratory measurements and antidotes, are also discussed.

## 1. Introduction

Stroke is associated with nonvalvular atrial fibrillation (NVAF), occurring in a yearly average of 5% of untreated NVAF patients and equaling approximately 700,000 cases per year [1]. Venous thromboembolism (VTE), including deep-vein thrombosis (DVT) and pulmonary embolism (PE), occurs at a rate of 117 people per 100,000 person-years annually, with increased incidence in select patient populations [2, 3]. Both NVAF-related stroke and VTE are causes of significant economic burden. In the United States, the healthcare costs associated with VTE exceed $1.5 billion per year, and the direct cost to treat the first year of AF-related strokes is $2.6 billion (2003 US dollars) [1, 4, 5].

The historical standard of care for VTE treatment is initiated by the administration of a parenteral anticoagulant for 5 to 10 days, followed by overlapping treatment with the vitamin K antagonist (VKA) warfarin [6]. The parenteral anticoagulant options for VTE treatment include intravenous unfractionated heparin, subcutaneous low-molecular-weight heparin (LMWH) (e.g., enoxaparin), or fondaparinux [6]. Intravenous administration requires vascular access, and subcutaneous injections may lead to increased patient discomfort and injection hematoma [7]. Patients receiving heparin are at risk for heparin-induced thrombocytopenia, although this risk is lower for LMWH than for unfractionated heparin [8, 9]. Despite the convenience of oral administration, the use of warfarin is complicated by delayed onset of action, narrow target therapeutic range, unpredictable dose responses, and numerous food and drug interactions [10, 11]. Patients taking warfarin also require frequent monitoring, as variable levels of anticoagulation increase the risk for both recurrent thromboembolism and bleeding [10, 11]. In a study of 395 patients receiving warfarin in a US Veterans Affairs facility, the estimated annual total cost of preventable warfarin-related adverse events (AEs) was $270,000 [12].

Dabigatran (Pradaxa®; Boehringer Ingelheim Pharmaceuticals, Inc., Ridgefield, CT), rivaroxaban (Xarelto®; Janssen Pharmaceuticals, Inc., Titusville, NJ), apixaban (Eliquis®; Bristol-Myers Squibb Co., Princeton, NJ), and edoxaban (Savaysa® (United States) and Lixiana® (European Union and Japan); Daiichi Sankyo, Parsippany, NJ) are direct-acting oral anticoagulants (DOACs) that have been approved in many regions of the world for the prevention of stroke or systemic embolic events (SEE) in patients with NVAF and for the treatment of VTE [13–18]. Direct-acting oral anticoagulants act by inhibiting a single component in the coagulation cascade: either factor Xa (rivaroxaban, apixaban, and edoxaban) or thrombin (dabigatran) [13–16]. Compared with warfarin, the advantages of DOACs include much faster onset of action, simpler dosing, reduced monitoring requirements, reduced food and drug interactions, and a decreased risk of bleeding [13–16]. The properties of DOACs are summarized in Table 1.

## 2. Summary of Efficacy and Safety of DOACs in Phase 3 Clinical Trials

In the pivotal phase 3 clinical trials in patients with NVAF, the 4 DOACs were at least as effective as warfarin in reducing the risk of stroke or SEE (see Supplementary Table 1 in Supplementary Material available online at http://dx.doi.org/10.1155/2016/1781684). In addition, DOACs were associated with similar or decreased rates of major bleeding, and patients experienced decreased rates of intracranial bleeding compared with warfarin [19–22]. A meta-analysis of these trials confirmed that DOACs were associated with reduced risk of stroke or SEE as well as decreased rates of all-cause mortality and intracranial hemorrhage (ICH) compared with warfarin [23]. However, nonfatal gastrointestinal (GI) bleeding events were increased with the use of DOACs relative to warfarin [23]. While the exact reasons for decreased ICH remain unclear, hypotheses include that DOACs target a single component (rather than multiple components) in the coagulation cascade and have no direct effect on factor VIIa, a vitamin K-dependent coagulation factor whose receptor (tissue factor) is expressed in high levels in the blood vessels of the brain [24–26]. The increased GI bleeding associated with DOACs may be attributed to the lower absorption of DOACs across the GI mucosa relative to that of warfarin [27]. With incomplete DOAC absorption, the active anticoagulant in the GI tract lumen may aggravate bleeding from vulnerable lesions [27]. Table 2 summarizes the bleeding outcomes of DOACs from phase 3 clinical trials for the prevention of stroke and SEE in patients with NVAF.

In the pivotal phase 3 clinical trials in patients with VTE, DOACs were noninferior for the treatment of acute symptomatic VTE and were associated with significantly decreased bleeding risks compared with standard therapy (LMWH or unfractionated heparin followed by treatment with an overlapping VKA (warfarin or acenocoumarol); see Supplemental Table 2) [29–33]. Table 3 summarizes the bleeding outcomes of DOACs from phase 3 clinical trials for the treatment and secondary prevention of VTE.

## 3. DOACs for the Treatment of DVT or PE

Pulmonary embolism is a potentially life-threatening condition that, in the US, has historically resulted in hospitalization in a vast majority of cases. This compares unfavorably with DVT, as 1 cost-effectiveness study has shown that approximately 40% of DVT patients are treated entirely in an outpatient fashion [39]. Among patients with DVT, the need for hospitalization is determined by the presence of any of the following criteria: massive DVT, high risk for anticoagulant-related bleeding, uncontrolled pain, signs of limb ischemia, or another comorbidity that warrants in-hospital care [40]. Before the approvals of DOACs, most DVT patients received initial therapy with an LMWH (e.g., enoxaparin) as a lead-in combined with warfarin as primary treatment; this allowed for the opportunity to educate patients on heparin administration and make arrangements for follow-up visits for warfarin monitoring.

Like other oral anticoagulants, DOACs can increase the risk for bleeding [41]. Therefore, bleeding risk assessment is important for the determination of anticoagulant regimens. Limited evidence suggests that several DOACs and warfarin may have similar bleeding risk factors [42]. In general, clinical factors that may increase a patient's warfarin-associated bleeding risk include advanced age; hypertension; malignancy; bleeding history; certain concomitant medications; and comorbidities such as heart failure, diabetes, and renal or hepatic diseases [43]. Furthermore, most bleeding risk factors, except for concomitant medications, are also risk factors for adverse VTE outcomes. This requires physicians to carefully balance the risks for an adverse VTE event, such as VTE recurrence [44], chronic thromboembolic pulmonary hypertension [45], and death [44], against the risk of bleeding when using anticoagulants. Notably, DOACs increase the risk for GI bleeding (which is rarely fatal) but decrease the risk for ICH (which is commonly fatal) compared with warfarin. Thus, a challenge of using DOACs is to manage their bleeding risk profile, which differs from that of warfarin, to minimize the risk of stroke or an adverse VTE event [46]. Given the complexity of assessing bleeding potential, tools have been developed to quantify the bleeding risk for an individual taking oral anticoagulants [43]. For example, the HAS-BLED scoring tool evaluates common bleeding risk factors such as hypertension, abnormal renal/liver function, stroke, and bleeding history [47].

For the treatment of DVT or PE, DOAC dose regimens vary between the individual agents and may be influenced by patient characteristics. For example, dabigatran and edoxaban require heparinoid lead-in, while apixaban and rivaroxaban start with higher initial doses that are subsequently lowered to a maintenance dose [13–16]. It should be noted that initiation of rivaroxaban or apixaban is not recommended as an alternative to unfractionated heparin in patients with PE who present with hemodynamic instability or who may receive thrombolysis or pulmonary embolectomy [13, 15].

Table 1: Properties of DOACs [13–16, 28].

| | Dabigatran | Rivaroxaban | Apixaban | Edoxaban |
|---|---|---|---|---|
| Class | Oral thrombin inhibitor | Oral factor Xa inhibitor | Oral factor Xa inhibitor | Oral factor Xa inhibitor |
| FDA-approved indication | Reduction of stroke and SEE risk for patients with NVAF; treatment of DVT and PE following 5–10 days of parenteral anticoagulant; and reduction of recurrence risk for DVT and PE | Reduction of stroke and SEE risk for patients with NVAF; treatment of DVT and PE and reduction of recurrence risk for DVT and PE; prophylaxis of DVT in patients undergoing knee or hip replacement surgery | Reduction of stroke and SEE risk for patients with NVAF; treatment of DVT and PE and reduction of recurrence risk for DVT and PE; prophylaxis of DVT in patients undergoing knee or hip replacement surgery | Reduction of stroke and SEE risk for patients with NVAF and treatment of DVT and PE following 5–10 days of parenteral anticoagulant[a] |
| Time to $C_{max}$ (h) | 1-2 | 2–4 | 3-4 | 1-2 |
| Half-life (h) | 12–17 | 5–13 | 12 | 10–14 |
| Renal elimination | 80% of absorbed dose | 66% of oral dose | 27% of absorbed dose | 50% of absorbed dose |
| Transporters[b] | P-gp | P-gp/BCRP | P-gp/BCRP | P-gp |
| Cytochrome P450 metabolism | No | Yes | Yes | Minimal |
| Bioavailability (%) | 3–7 | ≥80[c] | 50[d] | 62 |
| Potential drug interactions | Potent P-gp inhibitors and P-gp/CYP3A4 dual inducer rifampin | Potent dual CYP3A4 and P-gp inhibitors or inducers | Potent dual CYP3A4 and P-gp inhibitors or inducers | Potent P-gp inhibitors and P-gp/CYP3A4 dual inducer rifampin |

[a]Edoxaban should not be used in NVAF patients with creatinine clearance >95 mL/min [16].
[b]DOACs are substrates of these transporters.
[c]For 10 mg dose. For 20 mg dose in the fasted state, it is 66%.
[d]For doses up to 10 mg.
BCRP, breast cancer resistance protein; $C_{max}$, maximum observed plasma concentration; CYP3A4, cytochrome P450 3A4 enzyme; DOACs, direct-acting oral anticoagulants; DVT, deep-vein thrombosis; NVAF, nonvalvular atrial fibrillation; P-gp, P-glycoprotein; PE, pulmonary embolism; SEE, systemic embolic event; VTE, venous thromboembolism.

Further, most DOACs either require dose adjustment or are not recommended for patients with renal insufficiency [13–16]. Finally, while DOACs have fewer drug-drug interactions than warfarin, they do carry some concomitant drug restrictions. All DOACs are substrates of P-glycoprotein (P-gp), a cell membrane efflux transport protein that is known to pump drugs out of cells [48] and are metabolized by cytochrome P450 3A4 (CYP3A4), a family of oxidases that metabolizes drugs, to varying degrees, with dabigatran and edoxaban having the lowest metabolic dependence on CYP3A4 [49]. Thus, concomitant use of P-gp or CYP3A4 modulators may alter DOAC exposure [13–16]. P-gp or CYP3A4 inducers decrease DOAC exposure and thereby increase the risk of VTE, while P-gp or CYP3A4 inhibitors generally increase DOAC exposure and may lead to increased bleeding risk. However, the effect of drug-drug interactions on DOAC exposure varies across the DOACs. A detailed list of DOAC dosing for treatment and secondary prevention of VTE is available in Table 4.

Patients who have undergone anticoagulation for the prevention or treatment of VTE are at an increased risk for VTE recurrence after the discontinuation of anticoagulants [50]. However, the risk of VTE recurrence upon anticoagulant cessation is not significantly higher than the initial risk of developing a VTE (should the patient not be anticoagulated), indicating no rebound effect for anticoagulant treatment. Data from phase 3 clinical trials indicate that patients treated with DOACs and standard therapy (heparin/VKA) have similar VTE recurrence risks as shown in Supplementary Table 2.

## 4. Assessing the Anticoagulant Effect of DOACs at the Time of Bleeding

Laboratory measurement of DOACs, though not required for regular use, may be necessary in circumstances of bleeding management or perioperative monitoring. While US Food and Drug Administration- (FDA-) approved measurements for rivaroxaban, apixaban, and edoxaban are unavailable, the anticoagulant activity of dabigatran can be detected using activated partial thromboplastin time (aPTT) [13–16, 51]. However, limitations still exist in the use of aPTT

Table 2: Summary of bleeding outcomes of DOACs from phase 3 clinical trials for the prevention of stroke and SEE in patients with NVAF [19–22].

| | Major bleeding | | Intracranial bleeding | | Gastrointestinal bleeding | |
|---|---|---|---|---|---|---|
| | *N* (%) | HR (95% CI) *P* value | *N* (%) | HR (95% CI) *P* value | *N* (%) | HR (95% CI) *P* value |
| RE-LY | | | | | | |
| Dabigatran 150 mg BID | 375 | 0.93 (0.81–1.07) | 36 | 0.40 (0.27–0.60) | 182 | 1.50 (1.19–1.89) |
| (*n* = 6076) | (3.11) | 0.31 | (0.30) | <0.001 | (1.51) | <0.001 |
| Dabigatran 110 mg BID | 322 | 0.80 (0.69–0.93) | 27 | 0.31 (0.20–0.47) | 133 | 1.10 (0.86–1.41) |
| (*n* = 6015) | (2.71) | 0.003 | (0.23) | <0.001 | (1.12) | 0.43 |
| Warfarin | 397 | | 87 | | 120 | |
| (*n* = 6022) | (3.36) | | (0.74) | | (1.02) | |
| ROCKET AF | | | | | | |
| Rivaroxaban 20 mg QD[a] | 395 | 1.04 (0.90–1.20) | 55 | 0.67 (0.47–0.93) | 224 | NR |
| (*n* = 7111) | (5.60) | 0.58 | (0.80) | 0.02 | (3.15) | |
| Warfarin | 386 | | 84 | | 154 | |
| (*n* = 7125) | (5.40) | | (1.20) | | (2.16) | |
| ARISTOTLE | | | | | | |
| Apixaban 5 mg BID[b] | 327 | 0.69 (0.60–0.80) | 52 | 0.42 (0.30–0.58) | 105 | 0.89 (0.70–1.15) |
| (*n* = 9088) | (2.13) | <0.001 | (0.33) | <0.001 | (0.76) | 0.37 |
| Warfarin | 462 | | 122 | | 119 | |
| (*n* = 9052) | (3.09) | | (0.80) | | (0.86) | |
| ENGAGE AF-TIMI 48 | | | | | | |
| Edoxaban 60 mg QD | 418 | 0.80 (0.71–0.91) | 61 | 0.47 (0.34–0.63) | 232 | 1.23 (1.02–1.50) |
| (*n* = 7012) | (2.75) | <0.001 | (0.39) | <0.001 | (1.51) | 0.03 |
| Edoxaban 30 mg QD | 254 | 0.47 (0.41–0.55) | 41 | 0.30 (0.21–0.43) | 129 | 0.67 (0.53–0.83) |
| (*n* = 7002) | (1.61) | <0.001 | (0.26) | <0.001 | (0.82) | <0.001 |
| Warfarin | 524 | | 132 | | 190 | |
| (*n* = 7012) | (3.43) | | (0.85) | | (1.23) | |

[a] 15 mg QD in patients with creatinine clearance 30–49 mL/min.
[b] 2.5 mg BID in patients meeting 2 or more of the following criteria: age ≥80 years, body weight ≤60 kg, or serum creatinine ≥15 mg/L.
ARISTOTLE, apixaban for reduction in stroke and other thromboembolic events in atrial fibrillation; BID, twice daily; CI, confidence interval; DOACs, direct-acting oral anticoagulants; ENGAGE AF-TIMI 48, effective anticoagulation with factor Xa next generation in atrial fibrillation-thrombolysis in myocardial infarction 48; HR, hazard ratio; NR, not reported; QD, once daily; NVAF, nonvalvular atrial fibrillation; RE-LY, randomized evaluation of long-term anticoagulation therapy; ROCKET AF, rivaroxaban once daily oral direct factor Xa inhibition compared with vitamin K antagonism for prevention of stroke and embolism trial in atrial fibrillation; SEE, systemic embolic event.

for dabigatran monitoring, including the lack of a defined therapeutic range [52, 53], low sensitivity to different plasma concentrations [52–54], and inapplicability in patients with lupus anticoagulant or intrinsic clotting factor deficiency that may prolong aPTT [55]. The ecarin clotting time (ECT) assay responds to dabigatran in a dose-dependent fashion and therefore can be used to quantify dabigatran concentrations [56, 57]. However, this approach is unavailable in real time for most hospital labs [58, 59]. Another method for dabigatran quantification is the thrombin time (TT) test, which can detect dabigatran with exquisite sensitivity. While the traditional TT cannot be used for quantification purposes because of the lack of standardization, commercially available assay kits based on calibrated dilute TT (dTT) can provide results linearly correlated with dabigatran plasma concentrations spanning the therapeutic range and, therefore, represent a rapid method for measuring dabigatran plasma levels [60].

Although rivaroxaban and apixaban affect both aPTT and PT, some studies suggest that PT, but not aPTT, may represent a relatively sensitive assessment for the activity of these 2 DOACs [52, 59, 61]. However, the utility of absolute PT for estimating anticoagulant activity varies greatly based on the specific assay used and timing relative to the last dose. Edoxaban may be measured by both aPTT and PT, but there is considerable variability among different reagents for each of these assays [62]. Thrombin generation-endogenous thrombin potential (ETP) has been put forth as a reliable measure of the anticoagulant effect of DOACs in multiple studies [63–66]. While commercial assay kits are available for thrombin generation-ETP, using this method for DOAC measurement requires standardization and primarily occurs in research laboratories rather than clinical practice. The chromogenic antifactor Xa assay may be used for quantitative assessment of oral FXa inhibitors. Although this method

TABLE 3: Summary of bleeding outcomes of DOACs from phase 3 clinical trials for the treatment and secondary prevention of VTE [29–33].

| | Major bleeding | | Clinically relevant bleeding | |
|---|---|---|---|---|
| | *N* (%) | HR (95% CI) *P* value | *N*(%) | HR (95% CI) *P* value |
| RECOVER I/II | | | | |
| Dabigatran 150 mg BID[a] | 37 | 0.73 (0.48–1.11) | 136 | 0.62 (0.50–0.76) |
| (*n* = 2553) | (1.4) | NR | (5.3) | NR |
| Heparin/VKA | 51 | | 217 | |
| (*n* = 2554) | (2.0) | | (8.5) | |
| EINSTEIN-DVT | | | | |
| Rivaroxaban[b] | 14 | 0.65 (0.33–1.30) | 139 | 0.97 (0.76–1.22) |
| (*n* = 1718) | (0.8) | 0.21 | (8.1) | 0.77 |
| Heparin/VKA | 20 | | 138 | |
| (*n* = 1711) | (1.2) | | (8.1) | |
| EINSTEIN-PE | | | | |
| Rivaroxaban[b] | 26 | 0.49 (0.31–0.79) | 249 | 0.90 (0.76–1.07) |
| (*n* = 2412) | (1.1) | 0.003 | (10.3) | 0.23 |
| Heparin/VKA | 52 | | 274 | |
| (*n* = 2405) | (2.2) | | (11.4) | |
| AMPLIFY | | | | |
| Apixaban[c] | 15 | 0.31 (0.17–0.55) | 115 | 0.44 (0.36–0.55) |
| (*n* = 2676) | (0.6) | <0.001 | (4.3) | <0.001 |
| Heparin/VKA | 49 | | 261 | |
| (*n* = 2689) | (1.8) | | (9.7) | |
| Hokusai-VTE | | | | |
| Edoxaban 60 mg QD[a,d] | 56 | 0.84 (0.59–1.21) | 349 | 0.81 (0.71–0.94) |
| (*n* = 4118) | (1.4) | 0.35 | (8.5) | 0.004 |
| Heparin/VKA | 66 | | 423 | |
| (*n* = 4122) | (1.6) | | (10.3) | |

[a]With a parenteral anticoagulation lead-in.
[b]15 mg BID for 3 weeks followed by 20 mg QD.
[c]10 mg BID for the first 7 days followed by 5 mg BID for 6 months.
[d]30 mg QD in patients with creatinine clearance 30–50 mL/min or body weight ≤60 kg or receiving concomitant potent P-glycoprotein inhibitors.
AMPLIFY, apixaban for the initial management of pulmonary embolism and deep-vein thrombosis as first-line therapy; BID, twice daily; CI, confidence interval; DOACs, direct-acting oral anticoagulants; DVT, deep-vein thrombosis; HR, hazard ratio; NR, not reported; PE, pulmonary embolism; QD, once daily; VKA, vitamin K antagonist; VTE, venous thromboembolism.

requires standardization, the availability of commercial assay kits along with DOAC-specific calibrators has enabled reliable DOAC quantification using antifactor Xa assay [52, 57, 60, 67–70].

Clinical guidance regarding bleeding management based on DOAC laboratory measurement is limited, but the recently published guidelines from the International Society on Thrombosis and Haemostasis (ISTH) have provided some insights [71]. Qualitative measurement of DOACs can help determine their contribution to bleeding or the timing for an unplanned procedure [71]. For example, as aPTT and TT are sensitive tests for dabigatran, a normal aPTT or TT result may exclude the actual effect of dabigatran in a patient who has received this agent [71]. In addition, quantification of DOAC levels contributes to the decision as to whether a reversal agent should be administered. Except for patients who experience life-threatening bleeding or require emergency surgery for life-threatening conditions, factors that influence the need for a reversal agent include the time of the last DOAC dose, creatinine clearance (CrCl), and the DOAC plasma concentration obtained from laboratory tests. In patients with serious bleeding, a drug concentration over 50 ng/mL may warrant antidote administration, while in patients requiring an urgent procedure associated with a high risk of bleeding, antidote use should be considered at a DOAC concentration exceeding 30 ng/mL [71]. Although pharmacokinetic studies have provided reference plasma concentration ranges for DOACs, the clinical significance of an out-of-range measurement remains unclear [60]. Also, patients' DOAC plasma concentrations and anticoagulant effect may vary over time [60]. Therefore, clinicians should interpret DOAC laboratory measurement results with caution and should not overreact at laboratory measurement results slightly beyond the reference range [60].

## 5. Management of Bleeding

*5.1. General Approaches for Managing Oral Anticoagulant-Related Bleeding.* Bleeding remains a serious risk for all patients receiving anticoagulants. Therefore, bleeding management is an important consideration in anticoagulation therapies. General approaches for managing DOAC- and warfarin-related bleeding are similar and include applying mechanical pressure or performing endoscopic/surgical procedures at the bleeding site, as well as using supportive measures [72]. Bleeding related to antithrombotic therapy can also be controlled by hemostatic agents or anticoagulant antidotes; however, these agents may differ between DOACs and warfarin.

*5.2. Management of Warfarin-Related Bleeding.* For managing bleeding in patients receiving warfarin, guidelines published by the American College of Chest Physicians (ACCP) recommend the use of vitamin K, fresh frozen plasma (FFP), prothrombin complex concentrate (PCC), or recombinant activated factor VIIa (rVIIa), depending on the urgency of the situation [10]. Because vitamin K is slow acting, concomitant administration of FFP or PCC may be necessary to speed the reversal process [73, 74]. However, the use of FFP is associated with significant limitations, including thaw time, the need for ABO blood type matching, potential pathogen transmission, and insufficient reversal due to varying levels of coagulation factors [75–77]. More importantly, FFP must be given in large volumes for patients with greatly elevated international normalized ratios (INRs), which may lead to the development of transfusion-associated circulatory overload (TACO), a

TABLE 4: DOAC dosing for treatment and secondary prevention of VTE in the US [13–16].

| Patient population | Dabigatran | Rivaroxaban | Apixaban | Edoxaban |
|---|---|---|---|---|
| General population | 150 mg twice daily after 5–10 days of initial parenteral therapy if CrCl >30 mL/min | 15 mg[a] twice daily for 21 days and then 20 mg[a] once daily | 10 mg twice daily for 7 days and then 5 mg twice daily | 60 mg once daily following 5–10 days of initial parenteral anticoagulant therapy |
| Renal impairment | No recommendations if CrCl ≤30 mL/min or on dialysis | Avoid if CrCl <30 mL/min | No dose change | Reduce dose to 30 mg once daily if CrCl is 15–50 mL/min |
| Elderly | No dose change[b] | No dose change[b] | No dose change | No dose change |
| Low body weight | NR | No dose change | NR | Reduce dose to 30 mg once daily if weight ≤60 kg |
| Concomitant P-gp inhibitor | Avoid if CrCl <50 mL/min | Avoid if P-gp inhibitor is also a strong CYP3A4 inhibitor | Reduce to 5.0 or 2.5 mg (for 10.0 and 5.0 mg doses, resp.) if P-gp inhibitor is also a strong CYP3A4 inhibitor; avoid if already taking 2.5-mg dose | Reduce dose to 30 mg once daily |
| Concomitant P-gp inducer | Avoid (e.g., rifampin) | Avoid if P-gp inducer is also a strong CYP3A4 inducer | Avoid if P-gp inducer is also a strong CYP3A4 inducer | Avoid concomitant use with rifampin |

[a]Should be taken with food.
[b]Risk of stroke and bleeding increases with age but risk/benefit is favorable.
CrCl, creatinine clearance; CYP3A4, cytochrome P450 3A4 enzyme; DOAC, direct-acting oral anticoagulant; NR, not reported; P-gp, P-glycoprotein; VTE, venous thromboembolism.

type of noncardiogenic lung edema [78]. FFP may also induce transfusion-related acute lung injury (TRALI), another type of lung edema resulting from immunologic reactions to the transfusion components, although this occurs at a much lower rate than TACO [77, 78]. In contrast, PCC is easy to use and can be administered more quickly, with significantly decreased risks of pathogen transmission, TACO, and TRALI [74, 77, 79, 80]. For these reasons, PCC is recommended over FFP for the reversal of anticoagulation in clinical practice in patients with life-threatening bleeding. Although not specifically included in the guidelines, Kcentra® (CSL Behring LLC, King of Prussia, PA), a 4-factor PCC (clotting factors II, VII, IX, and X) (4F-PCC) that also contains protein S, protein C, and antithrombin, is approved by the FDA specifically for warfarin reversal in cases of acute major bleeding or in need of urgent surgery [81, 82]. In a pivotal phase 3 clinical trial, Kcentra was noninferior in achieving effective hemostasis and superior in reducing INR compared with FFP; the safety profile is similar between Kcentra and FFP [82].

*5.3. Management of DOAC-Related Bleeding.* Reversal agents for DOACs are very limited, and there are no reversal agents currently approved by the FDA specifically to reverse the anticoagulant effects of rivaroxaban, apixaban, or edoxaban. This poses a potential challenge to bleeding management or perioperative interruption, especially for emergency surgeries in patients receiving DOACs. However, DOACs may be associated with better outcomes after major bleeding than warfarin. A study comparing outcomes of major bleeding between patients receiving dabigatran and warfarin revealed that dabigatran-treated patients had a lower 30-day mortality rate, significantly shorter stays in the intensive care unit, and reduced need for plasma transfusions after major bleeding than those treated with warfarin, although the dabigatran-treated patients in the study were older, had lower creatinine clearance, and more frequently used aspirin or nonsteroidal anti-inflammatory agents [83]. In the pivotal clinical trials, rivaroxaban and apixaban were associated with lower rates of vitamin K-related medication uses and FFP transfusions after major bleeding than warfarin; patients receiving rivaroxaban who experienced major bleeding also had fewer PCC administrations and shorter hospitalization [84, 85]. A meta-analysis including studies of all 4 DOACs has also reported lower risks of death after major bleeding for DOACs than for warfarin [86]. In addition, DOACs are fast acting with relatively short half-lives, which may translate to a short periprocedural interruption in anticoagulation [13–16]. Practice guidelines suggest that heparin bridging for periprocedural DOAC interruption may not be required, as is the case for warfarin [87]. Circumventing the need for bridging not only improves convenience but also decreases the risk for major bleeding, especially in patients who undergo major procedures [88]. However, definitive guidance regarding periprocedural DOAC interruption is lacking because of limited clinical evidence and the rapid progression of this research field [89, 90]. In general, surgical procedures should be delayed for at least 24 hours after the discontinuation of DOACs, as indicated by current practice guidelines [87]. The effect of renal function, age, drug affected half-life, concomitant medications, and timing of the last dosage should be considered. The DOAC package inserts and some clinical guidelines recommend that DOACs should be withheld 1 to 2 days before surgical procedures depending on the individual agents and the risk levels of the procedures [13–16, 87]. In the case of an emergency procedure, the risk of bleeding should be weighed against the urgency of intervention [13–16]. After the procedure, DOACs can generally be resumed as soon as adequate hemostasis has been established, and the anticoagulation effect will take place quickly, typically in 1 to 2 hours after restarting the medications [13–16].

Although specific reversal agents for most DOACs are currently lacking, several nonspecific reversal approaches may be applicable to the reversal of DOACs in case of emergency or serious bleeding. Dabigatran, which is 35% protein-bound, may be removed by dialysis as recommended by the prescribing information in the package insert [14, 51]. However, dialysis is ineffective in removing rivaroxaban, apixaban, or edoxaban, which exist in higher protein-bound forms [57, 91–93]. Some evidence suggests that activated charcoal may reduce absorption of dabigatran, rivaroxaban, and apixaban if administered 1 to 2 hours after ingestion [13, 15, 52, 53, 94].

Except for vitamin K, most hemostatic agents used for managing warfarin-related bleeding are applicable to the reversal of DOACs [34, 63, 66, 95–98]. In several human volunteer studies, 4F-PCC has demonstrated effectiveness in reversing the anticoagulant effect of rivaroxaban, apixaban, and edoxaban, as determined by measurements of prothrombin time (PT) or thrombin generation-ETP [63, 66, 95, 97]. The reversal of edoxaban by 4F-PCC has also been established by punch biopsy, an invasive method that may be more representative of clinical bleeding situations than measurements of coagulation parameters [66]. However, 4F-PCC had no effect on dabigatran-induced changes in aPTT, ETP lag time, thrombin clotting time, or ECT [63]. Factor VIII Inhibitor Bypassing Activity (a commercial anti-inhibitor coagulant complex) and an active recombinant form of factor VII have also been tested for feasibility as DOAC reversal agents and have reversed DOAC-induced changes in some coagulation parameters [96–99].

In addition to PCC, tranexamic acid—a synthetic analog of the amino acid lysine, which inhibits fibrinolysis—may be used as an adjuvant therapy to manage bleeding in patients receiving dabigatran [100, 101]. However, this agent is not expected to reverse the anticoagulant activity of edoxaban [16]. Although direct reversal of rivaroxaban by tranexamic acid has not been reported, 1 clinical study suggests that this agent may reduce postoperative blood loss in patients who undergo total hip replacement and receive rivaroxaban for thromboprophylaxis [102]. The effect of tranexamic acid in patients receiving apixaban has not been reported.

The only FDA-approved DOAC-specific reversal agent is Praxbind® (idarucizumab, Boehringer Ingelheim Pharmaceuticals, Inc., Ridgefield, CT), which is indicated to reverse the anticoagulant effects of dabigatran in situations of emergency surgery/urgent procedures or life-threatening/uncontrolled bleeding [35]. Praxbind is a monoclonal antibody fragment that binds dabigatran with an affinity that is 350 times higher than thrombin [103]. Thus, this agent is expected to bind free and thrombin-bound dabigatran and neutralize its activity [103]. In a recent clinical study, idarucizumab reversed the anticoagulant effect of dabigatran to a near complete extent in patients who experienced serious bleeding or required an urgent procedure [103].

Several DOAC-specific antidotes are under development and have shown promise in preliminary studies. PER977 (Perosphere, Inc., Danbury, CT) [104, 105], a small synthetic molecule with binding activity to all 4 DOACs, reduces the whole-blood clotting time prolonged by edoxaban [106]. Further, andexanet alfa (PRT064445, Portola Pharmaceuticals, Inc., South San Francisco, CA), a recombinant catalytically inactive FXa decoy molecule, may provide a rapid and sustained reversal of DOACs as measured by anti-Xa activity in subjects taking apixaban and rivaroxaban [105, 107–110]. Ongoing clinical studies are evaluating the effect of andexanet alfa on edoxaban [105]. Bleeding management in patients receiving warfarin or DOACs is illustrated in Figure 1.

Thromboembolic complications are the primary concern when anticoagulant reversal agents are used. Infusion of PCC may lead to the development of thrombotic stroke, DVT, and myocardial infarction [111, 112], although a patient's underlying thrombotic risk factors may also contribute to these AEs [111]. Thrombotic events such as DVT, PE, myocardial infarction, and ischemic stroke have also been reported in patients receiving idarucizumab [103]. The safety of PER977 and andexanet alfa is still under evaluation in several ongoing clinical studies [105]. No evidence has shown that the use of reversal agents reduces patient mortality.

## 6. Implications for Care

*6.1. DOAC Cost-Effectiveness.* The costs of DOACs average from $300 to $600 per month depending on the specific DOAC type and the dosing regimens [113]. However, there are also high costs associated with NVAF-related stroke and VTE. The estimated 1-time cost of ischemic stroke in AF is $15,497 with moderate-to-severe sequelae and $9,562 with minor sequelae. Furthermore, the continuing monthly costs of AF-related ischemic stroke with moderate-to-severe sequelae and minor sequelae are $5,605 and $2,528, respectively (costs adjusted from 2008 US dollars to 2011 US dollars) [113]. The costs for a single event of DVT and PE are $7,712 and $9,566, respectively, accounting for the expense of both immediate and follow-up treatment for VTE [4, 114].

Cost-effectiveness analyses of DOACs versus warfarin have been performed [115, 116]. For stroke prevention in NVAF, the annual total cost reduction associated with the use of dabigatran, rivaroxaban, apixaban, and edoxaban relative to warfarin is $204, $140, $495, and $340 per patient, respectively [115]. This overall reduction is primarily attributed to the decreased incidence and incremental costs associated with major bleeding [115]. In a hypothetical insured population of 1 million people, including both NVAF

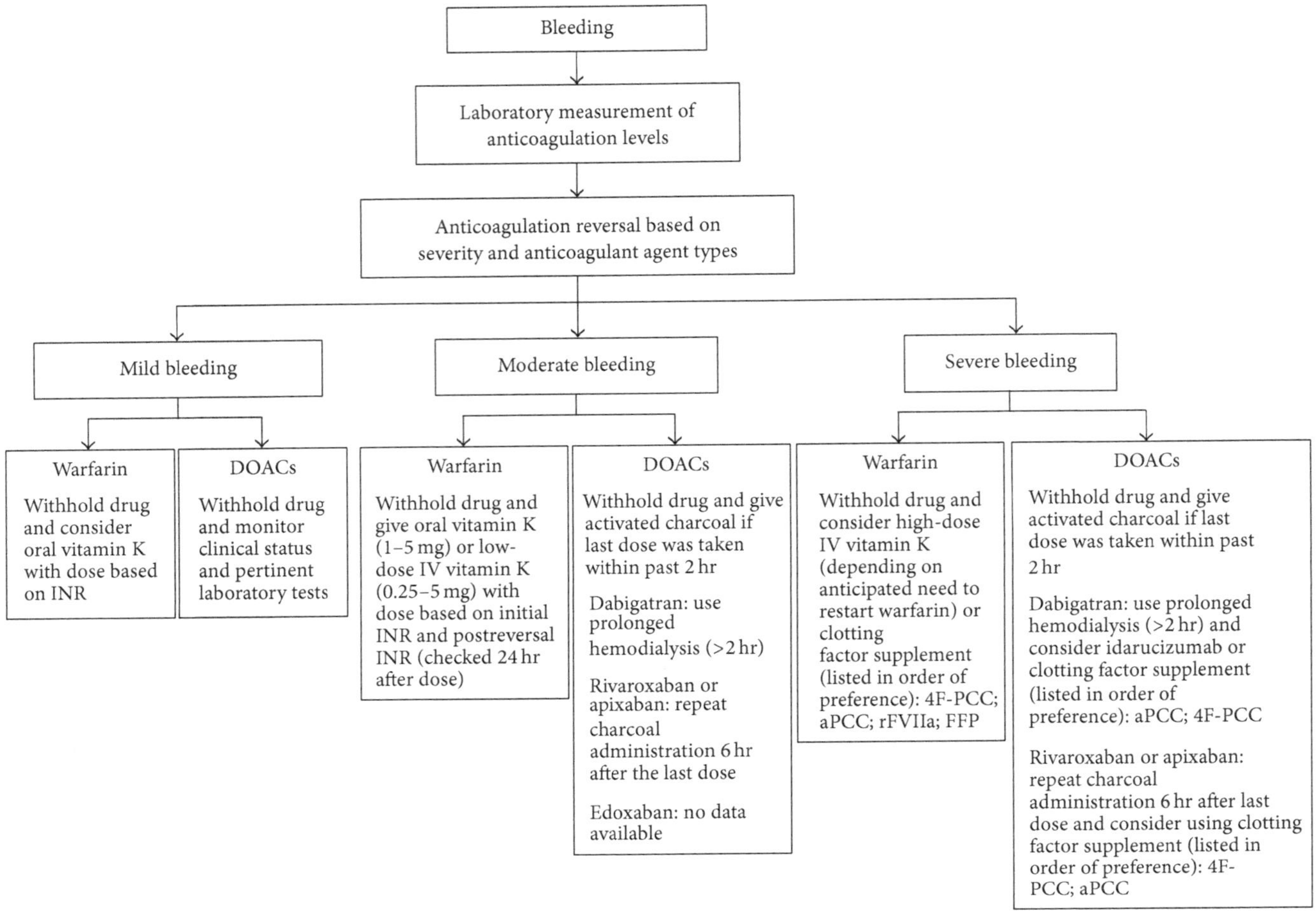


FIGURE 1: Bleeding management in patients receiving warfarin or DOACs [10, 34–38]. 4F-PCC, 4-factor prothrombin complex concentrate; aPCC, activated prothrombin complex concentrate; DOACs, direct-acting oral anticoagulants; FFP, fresh frozen plasma; INR, international normalized ratio; IV, intravenous; rFVIIa, recombinant activated factor VII.

and VTE patients, the medical cost reductions resulting from DOACs relative to warfarin are estimated to be \$3.0, \$2.1, \$7.3, and \$5.0 million for NVAF patients treated with dabigatran, rivaroxaban, apixaban, and edoxaban, respectively; \$0.7, \$2.2, \$4.1, and \$1.6 million for patients with acute VTE treated with dabigatran, rivaroxaban, apixaban, and edoxaban, respectively; and \$3.7, \$4.2, \$11.5, and \$6.6 million for the whole population treated with dabigatran, rivaroxaban, apixaban, and edoxaban, respectively [115]. The medical cost reductions associated with DOAC use are projected to steadily increase [115]. On the other hand, cost-effectiveness analyses are predominantly based on data from the phase 3 clinical trials and may not represent the use of DOACs in a real-world setting [115]. With the increasing adoption of DOACs, data derived from routine clinical practice will bring additional insights into the cost considerations for choice of oral anticoagulant use [117].

*6.2. Outpatient Management of VTE Using DOACs.* The use of DOACs facilitates the transition of VTE management from hospitals or emergency departments to a patient's home. The ACCP guidelines recommend initial home treatment for patients with lower limb DVT and early discharge for patients with low-risk PE if the patient's home circumstances are adequate [6]. The required circumstances include well-maintained living conditions, strong support from family or friends, phone access, and the ability to quickly return to the hospital if deterioration occurs [6]. Home care is associated with the benefits of comfort, convenience, and significant cost savings [6]. Outpatient management of VTE is also supported by clinical evidence. A study comparing home versus in-hospital initial treatment of outpatients with acute DVT revealed that home treatment was associated with a lower rate of major bleeding or death than in-hospital treatment [118], although this conclusion may be confounded by the fact that the home-treated patients in this study were younger and had fewer comorbidities than the hospital-treated ones [118]. Additionally, a US and European open-label, randomized noninferiority trial indicated that for selected low-risk patients with PE, outpatient treatment could be as effective and safe as inpatient treatment [119]. A recently published study conducted in 2 US emergency departments has established the effectiveness of DOACs in VTE outpatient treatment. In this study, patients with low-risk DVT or PE were discharged immediately after diagnosis, received home treatment with rivaroxaban, and demonstrated a low rate of VTE recurrence and bleeding [120].

Patients with VTE suffer from impaired quality of life (QOL) [121]. A study conducted in patients with newly diagnosed VTE or AF discovered that patients' QOL was significantly improved at 3 months after the initiation of VKA therapy [122]. While the study did not address whether the initial low QOL was due to the disease diagnosis or the start of VKA treatment, the investigators speculated that the improvement in QOL may result from "the patient's acceptance of the diagnosis as well as the benefits of treatment" [122]. The impact of DOACs on patients' QOL is not yet well studied. Limited evidence suggests that dabigatran and warfarin have similar impacts on QOL, which was unexpected by the study investigators because of "the known complexities of warfarin treatment" [123]. As DOACs are easy to use, with fewer food and drug interactions and reduced monitoring requirements compared with warfarin, they are expected to improve patients' QOL. Additional research is necessary to provide a better understanding of the impact of DOACs on patients' QOL.

## 7. Conclusions

Four DOACs are available for the prevention of stroke in patients with NVAF and for the treatment of VTE. Compared with the traditional oral anticoagulant warfarin, advantages of the DOACs include faster onset of action, fewer food and drug interactions, and lower requirements for monitoring. Clinical studies have demonstrated that DOACs are at least as effective as warfarin for the prevention of NVAF-related stroke, the treatment of acute VTE, and the prevention of recurrent VTE and are associated with similar or decreased risks of bleeding. Despite these advantages, several important factors should be taken into consideration regarding the appropriate use of DOACs in clinical practice. Different DOACs vary in dose regimens, and dose adjustments are necessary in patients with low body weight, renal impairment, or concomitant medications. Bleeding is a concern for all anticoagulants, and the lack of specific laboratory measurements and reversal agents poses additional challenges to its management in patients using DOACs. If bleeding occurs, knowledge of nonspecific measurements and reversal approaches may mitigate AEs associated with DOACs. Overall, DOACs represent effective, safe, and likely cost-effective alternatives to warfarin. Appropriate use of DOACs will maximize their benefits and improve the prevention of NVAF-related stroke and the treatment of VTE.

## Competing Interests

Dr. W. Frank Peacock has received research grants from Abbott, Alere, Banyan, Cardiorentis, Janssen, Portola, Roche, the Medicines Company, and ZS Pharma. He serves as a consultant for Prevencio, Singulex, Janssen, Portola, Roche, the Medicines Company, Comprehensive Research Associates, and Emergencies in Medicine. Dr. Adam J. Singer is a member of the speaker's bureau for Janssen and the advisory board for Daiichi Sankyo. He has received research grants from Boehringer Ingelheim. Dr. Zubaid Rafique is a principal investigator at ZS Pharma.

## Acknowledgments

Writing and editorial support was provided by Liqing Xiao, Ph.D., and Terri Schochet, Ph.D., of AlphaBioCom, LLC, and funded by Daiichi Sankyo.

## References

[1] J. J. Caro, "An economic model of stroke in atrial fibrillation: the cost of suboptimal oral anticoagulation," *American Journal of Managed Care*, vol. 10, no. 14, pp. S451–S461, 2004.

[2] J. A. Heit, T. M. Petterson, S. A. Farmer, K. R. Bailey, and L. J. Melton III, "Trends in the incidence of deep vein thrombosis and pulmonary embolism: a 35-year population-based study," *ASH Annual Meeting Abstracts*, vol. 108, p. 1488, 2006.

[3] M. D. Silverstein, J. A. Heit, D. N. Mohr, T. M. Petterson, W. M. O'Fallon, and L. J. Melton III, "Trends in the incidence of deep vein thrombosis and pulmonary embolism: a 25-year population-based study," *Archives of Internal Medicine*, vol. 158, no. 6, pp. 585–593, 1998.

[4] P. P. Dobesh, "Economic burden of venous thromboembolism in hospitalized patients," *Pharmacotherapy*, vol. 29, no. 8, pp. 943–953, 2009.

[5] C. J. Mercaldi, M. Ciarametaro, B. Hahn et al., "Cost efficiency of anticoagulation with warfarin to prevent stroke in medicare beneficiaries with nonvalvular atrial fibrillation," *Stroke*, vol. 42, no. 1, pp. 112–118, 2011.

[6] C. Kearon, E. A. Akl, A. J. Comerota et al., "Antithrombotic therapy for VTE disease: antithrombotic therapy and prevention of thrombosis, 9th ed: American College of Chest Physicians evidence-based clinical practice guidelines," *Chest*, vol. 141, no. 2, pp. e419S–e494S, 2012.

[7] C. Stellbrink, U. Nixdorff, T. Hofmann et al., "Safety and efficacy of enoxaparin compared with unfractionated heparin and oral anticoagulants for prevention of thromboembolic complications in cardioversion of nonvalvular atrial fibrillation: the Anticoagulation in Cardioversion using Enoxaparin (ACE) trial," *Circulation*, vol. 109, no. 8, pp. 997–1003, 2004.

[8] S. V. Rao and E. M. Ohman, "Anticoagulant therapy for percutaneous coronary intervention," *Circulation: Cardiovascular Interventions*, vol. 3, no. 1, pp. 80–88, 2010.

[9] N. Martel, J. Lee, and P. S. Wells, "Risk for heparin-induced thrombocytopenia with unfractionated and low-molecular-weight heparin thromboprophylaxis: a meta-analysis," *Blood*, vol. 106, no. 8, pp. 2710–2715, 2005.

[10] W. Ageno, A. S. Gallus, A. Wittkowsky, M. Crowther, E. M. Hylek, and G. Palareti, "Oral anticoagulant therapy: antithrombotic therapy and prevention of thrombosis, 9th ed: American College of Chest Physicians evidence-based clinical practice guidelines," *Chest*, vol. 141, no. 2, pp. e44S–e88S, 2012.

[11] J. Ansell, J. Hirsh, E. Hylek et al., "Pharmacology and management of the vitamin K antagonists: American College of Chest Physicians Evidence-Based Clinical Practice Guidelines (8th Edition)," *Chest*, vol. 133, pp. 160S–198S, 2008.

[12] L. Hamby, W. B. Weeks, and C. Malikowski, "Complications of warfarin therapy: causes, costs, and the role of the anticoagulation clinic," *Effective Clinical Practice*, vol. 3, no. 4, pp. 179–184, 2000.

[13] *ELIQUIS®*, Bristol-Myers Squibb Company, Princeton, NJ, USA; Pfizer Inc., New York, NY, USA, 2015, http://packageinserts.bms.com/pi/pi_eliquis.pdf.

[14] PRADAXA®, Boehringer Ingelheim Pharmaceuticals Inc, Ridgefield, Conn, USA, 2015, http://docs.boehringer-ingelheim.com/Prescribing%20Information/PIs/Pradaxa/Pradaxa.pdf.

[15] *XARELTO®*, Janssen Pharmaceuticals, Titusville, NJ, USA, 2015, https://www.xarelto-us.com/shared/product/xarelto/prescribing-information.pdf.

[16] SAVAYSA™, Daiichi Sankyo Inc, Parsippany, NJ, USA, 2015, http://www.accessdata.fda.gov/drugsatfda_docs/label/2015/206316lbl.pdf.

[17] *Lixiana®*, Daiichi Sankyo Europe GmbH, Munich, Germany, 2015, https://www.medicines.org.uk/emc/PIL.30504.latest.pdf.

[18] Daiichi Sankyo, *Daiichi Sankyo Launches LIXIANA(R) (edoxaban), a Direct Oral Factor Xa Inhibitor, in Japan for the Prevention of Venous Thromboembolism after Major Orthopedic Surgery*, Daiichi Sankyo, Tokyo, Japan, 2011, http://www.daiichisankyo.com/media_investors/media_relations/press_releases/detail/005784.html.

[19] S. J. Connolly, M. D. Ezekowitz, S. Yusuf et al., "Dabigatran versus warfarin in patients with atrial fibrillation," *The New England Journal of Medicine*, vol. 361, pp. 1139–1151, 2009.

[20] R. P. Giugliano, C. T. Ruff, E. Braunwald et al., "Edoxaban versus warfarin in patients with atrial fibrillation," *The New England Journal of Medicine*, vol. 369, no. 22, pp. 2093–2104, 2013.

[21] C. B. Granger, J. H. Alexander, J. J. McMurray et al., "Apixaban versus warfarin in patients with atrial fibrillation," *The New England Journal of Medicine*, vol. 365, pp. 981–992, 2011.

[22] M. R. Patel, K. W. Mahaffey, J. Garg et al., "Rivaroxaban versus warfarin in nonvalvular atrial fibrillation," *The New England Journal of Medicine*, vol. 365, no. 10, pp. 883–891, 2011.

[23] C. T. Ruff, R. P. Giugliano, E. Braunwald et al., "Comparison of the efficacy and safety of new oral anticoagulants with warfarin in patients with atrial fibrillation: a meta-analysis of randomised trials," *The Lancet*, vol. 383, no. 9921, pp. 955–962, 2014.

[24] S. Chatterjee, P. Sardar, G. Biondi-Zoccai, and D. J. Kumbhani, "New oral anticoagulants and the risk of intracranial hemorrhage: traditional and Bayesian meta-analysis and mixed treatment comparison of randomized trials of new oral anticoagulants in atrial fibrillation," *JAMA Neurology*, vol. 70, no. 12, pp. 1486–1490, 2013.

[25] N. Mackman, "The role of tissue factor and factor VIIa in hemostasis," *Anesthesia and Analgesia*, vol. 108, no. 5, pp. 1447–1452, 2009.

[26] J. Hirsh, V. Fuster, J. Ansell, and J. L. Halperin, "American Heart Association/American College of Cardiology Foundation guide to warfarin therapy," *Circulation*, vol. 107, no. 12, pp. 1692–1711, 2003.

[27] J. Desai, J. M. Kolb, J. I. Weitz, and J. Aisenberg, "Gastrointestinal bleeding with the new oral anticoagulants—defining the issues and the management strategies," *Thrombosis and Haemostasis*, vol. 110, no. 2, pp. 205–212, 2013.

[28] M. S. Bathala, H. Masumoto, T. Oguma, L. He, C. Lowrie, and J. Mendell, "Pharmacokinetics, biotransformation, and mass balance of edoxaban, a selective, direct factor Xa inhibitor, in humans," *Drug Metabolism and Disposition*, vol. 40, no. 12, pp. 2250–2255, 2012.

[29] G. Agnelli, H. R. Buller, A. Cohen et al., "Oral apixaban for the treatment of acute venous thromboembolism," *The New England Journal of Medicine*, vol. 369, no. 9, pp. 799–808, 2013.

[30] R. Bauersachs, S. D. Berkowitz, B. Brenner et al., "Oral rivaroxaban for symptomatic venous thromboembolism," *The New England Journal of Medicine*, vol. 363, pp. 2499–2510, 2010.

[31] H. R. Buller, H. Decousus, M. A. Grosso et al., "Edoxaban versus warfarin for the treatment of symptomatic venous thromboembolism," *The New England Journal of Medicine*, vol. 369, pp. 1406–1415, 2013.

[32] H. R. Buller, M. H. Prins, A. W. Lensin et al., "Oral rivaroxaban for the treatment of symptomatic pulmonary embolism," *The New England Journal of Medicine*, vol. 366, pp. 1287–1297, 2012.

[33] S. Schulman, A. K. Kakkar, S. Z. Goldhaber et al., "Treatment of acute venous thromboembolism with dabigatran or warfarin and pooled analysis," *Circulation*, vol. 129, no. 7, pp. 764–772, 2014.

[34] E. A. Nutescu, W. E. Dager, J. S. Kalus, J. J. Lewin, and M. D. Cipolle, "Management of bleeding and reversal strategies for oral anticoagulants: clinical practice considerations," *American Journal of Health-System Pharmacy*, vol. 70, no. 21, pp. 1914–1929, 2013.

[35] *PRAXBIND®*, Boehringer Ingelheim Pharmaceuticals, Ridgefield, Conn, USA, 2015, http://www.accessdata.fda.gov/drugsatfda_docs/label/2015/761025lbl.pdf.

[36] Thrombosis Canda, *New/Noval Oral Anticoagulants (NOACs): Management of Bleeding*, Thrombosis Canda, 2015, http://thrombosiscanada.ca/wp-content/uploads/2016/02/22_NOACs-Management-Bleeding_2016Jan12-FINAL.pdf.

[37] *Bleeding—Management in Patients Taking Oral Anticoagulants*, Wirral University Teaching Hospital (NHS), 2016, http://www.wuth.nhs.uk/media/984539/Bleeding-Management-in-patients-taking-oral-anticoagulants-4-July-13.pdf.

[38] D. M. Siegal, D. A. Garcia, and M. A. Crowther, "How I treat target-specific oral anticoagulant-associated bleeding," *Blood*, vol. 123, no. 8, pp. 1152–1158, 2014.

[39] A. C. Spyropoulos, "Reimbursement strategies in an outpatient-based disease management program for the treatment of deep venous thrombosis in an integrated health care system," *Managed Care*, vol. 8, supplement 1, pp. 14–20, 1999, http://www.managedcaremag.com/sites/default/files/supplements/9912_dvt_suppl/9912.dvt.pdf.

[40] J. D. Douketis, "Treatment of deep vein thrombosis: what factors determine appropriate treatment?" *Canadian Family Physician*, vol. 51, pp. 217–223, 2005.

[41] J. I. Weitz and C. V. Pollack Jr., "Practical management of bleeding in patients receiving non-vitamin K antagonist oral anticoagulants," *Thrombosis and Haemostasis*, vol. 114, no. 6, pp. 1113–1126, 2015.

[42] S. G. Goodman, D. M. Wojdyla, J. P. Piccini et al., "Factors associated with major bleeding events: insights from the ROCKET AF trial (rivaroxaban once-daily oral direct factor Xa inhibition compared with vitamin K antagonism for prevention of stroke and embolism trial in atrial fibrillation)," *Journal of the American College of Cardiology*, vol. 63, no. 9, pp. 891–900, 2014.

[43] M. Shoeb and M. C. Fang, "Assessing bleeding risk in patients taking anticoagulants," *Journal of Thrombosis and Thrombolysis*, vol. 35, no. 3, pp. 312–319, 2013.

[44] J. A. Heit, "Venous thromboembolism: disease burden, outcomes and risk factors," *Journal of Thrombosis and Haemostasis*, vol. 3, no. 8, pp. 1611–1617, 2005.

[45] V. Pengo, A. W. Lensing, M. H. Prins et al., "Incidence of chronic thromboembolic pulmonary hypertension after pulmonary embolism," *The New England Journal of Medicine*, vol. 350, no. 22, pp. 2257–2264, 2004.

[46] S. S. Adam, J. R. McDuffie, T. L. Ortel, and J. W. Williams Jr., "Comparative effectiveness of warfarin and new oral anticoagulants for the management of atrial fibrillation and venous thromboembolism: a systematic review," *Annals of Internal Medicine*, vol. 157, no. 11, pp. 796–807, 2012.

[47] R. Pisters, D. A. Lane, R. Nieuwlaat, C. B. de Vos, H. J. Crijns, and G. Y. Lip, "A novel user-friendly score (HAS-BLED) to assess 1-year risk of major bleeding in patients with atrial fibrillation: the Euro Heart Survey," *Chest*, vol. 138, no. 5, pp. 1093–1100, 2010.

[48] S. G. Aller, J. Yu, A. Ward et al., "Structure of P-glycoprotein reveals a molecular basis for poly-specific drug binding," *Science*, vol. 323, no. 5922, pp. 1718–1722, 2009.

[49] L. C. Quattrochi and P. S. Guzelian, "CYP3A regulation: from pharmacology to nuclear receptors," *Drug Metabolism and Disposition*, vol. 29, no. 5, pp. 615–622, 2001.

[50] C. Kearon, S. R. Kahn, G. Agnelli, S. Goldhaber, G. E. Raskob, and A. J. Comerota, "Antithrombotic therapy for venous thromboembolic disease: American College of Chest Physicians Evidence-Based Clinical Practice Guidelines (8th Edition)," *Chest*, vol. 133, no. 6, pp. 454S–545S, 2008.

[51] K. Babilonia and T. Trujillo, "The role of prothrombin complex concentrates in reversal of target specific anticoagulants," *Thrombosis Journal*, vol. 12, article 8, 2014.

[52] E. Gehrie and C. Tormey, "Novel oral anticoagulants: efficacy, laboratory measurement, and approaches to emergent reversal," *Archives of Pathology and Laboratory Medicine*, vol. 139, no. 5, pp. 687–692, 2015.

[53] A. M. Winkler and C. A. Tormey, "Pathology consultation on monitoring direct thrombin inhibitors and overcoming their effects in bleeding patients," *The American Journal of Clinical Pathology*, vol. 140, no. 5, pp. 610–622, 2013.

[54] J. Curvers, D. van de Kerkhof, A. K. Stroobants, E.-J. van den Dool, and V. Scharnhorst, "Measuring direct thrombin inhibitors with routine and dedicated coagulation assays: which assay is helpful?" *American Journal of Clinical Pathology*, vol. 138, no. 4, pp. 551–558, 2012.

[55] D. D. Castellone and E. M. Van Cott, "Laboratory monitoring of new anticoagulants," *American Journal of Hematology*, vol. 85, no. 3, pp. 185–187, 2010.

[56] R. C. Gosselin, D. M. Dwyre, and W. E. Dager, "Measuring dabigatran concentrations using a chromogenic ecarin clotting time assay," *Annals of Pharmacotherapy*, vol. 47, no. 12, pp. 1635–1640, 2013.

[57] W. Mueck, S. Schwers, and J. Stampfuss, "Rivaroxaban and other novel oral anticoagulants: pharmacokinetics in healthy subjects, specific patient populations and relevance of coagulation monitoring," *Thrombosis Journal*, vol. 11, article 10, 2013.

[58] M. A. Miyares and K. Davis, "Newer oral anticoagulants: a review of laboratory monitoring options and reversal agents in the hemorrhagic patient," *American Journal of Health-System Pharmacy*, vol. 69, no. 17, pp. 1473–1484, 2012.

[59] T. Baglin, "The role of the laboratory in treatment with new oral anticoagulants," *Journal of Thrombosis and Haemostasis*, vol. 11, supplement 1, pp. 122–128, 2013.

[60] D. Garcia, Y. C. Barrett, E. Ramacciotti, and J. I. Weitz, "Laboratory assessment of the anticoagulant effects of the next generation of oral anticoagulants," *Journal of Thrombosis and Haemostasis*, vol. 11, no. 2, pp. 245–252, 2013.

[61] J. Douxfils, F. Mullier, C. Loosen, C. Chatelain, B. Chatelain, and J.-M. Dogné, "Assessment of the impact of rivaroxaban on coagulation assays: laboratory recommendations for the monitoring of rivaroxaban and review of the literature," *Thrombosis Research*, vol. 130, no. 6, pp. 956–966, 2012.

[62] Y. Morishima and C. Kamisato, "Laboratory measurements of the oral direct factor Xa inhibitor edoxaban: comparison of prothrombin time, activated partial thromboplastin time, and thrombin generation assay," *American Journal of Clinical Pathology*, vol. 143, no. 2, pp. 241–247, 2015.

[63] E. S. Eerenberg, P. W. Kamphuisen, M. K. Sijpkens, J. C. Meijers, H. R. Buller, and M. Levi, "Reversal of rivaroxaban and dabigatran by prothrombin complex concentrate: a randomized, placebo-controlled, crossover study in healthy subjects," *Circulation*, vol. 124, no. 14, pp. 1573–1579, 2011.

[64] R. Herrmann, J. Thom, A. Wood, M. Phillips, S. Muhammad, and R. Baker, "Thrombin generation using the calibrated automated thrombinoscope to assess reversibility of dabigatran and rivaroxaban," *Thrombosis and Haemostasis*, vol. 111, no. 5, pp. 989–995, 2014.

[65] A. Tripodi, L. Padovan, C. Veena, E. Scalambrino, S. Testa, and F. Peyvandi, "How the direct oral anticoagulant apixaban affects thrombin generation parameters," *Thrombosis Research*, vol. 135, no. 6, pp. 1186–1190, 2015.

[66] H. Zahir, K. S. Brown, A. G. Vandell et al., "Edoxaban effects on bleeding following punch biopsy and reversal by a 4-factor prothrombin complex concentrate," *Circulation*, vol. 131, no. 1, pp. 82–90, 2015.

[67] L. M. Asmis, L. Alberio, A. Angelillo-Scherrer et al., "Rivaroxaban: quantification by anti-FXa assay and influence on coagulation tests: a study in 9 swiss laboratories," *Thrombosis Research*, vol. 129, no. 4, pp. 492–498, 2012.

[68] Y. C. Barrett, Z. Wang, C. Frost, and A. Shenker, "Clinical laboratory measurement of direct factor Xa inhibitors: anti-Xa assay is preferable to prothrombin time assay," *Thrombosis and Haemostasis*, vol. 104, no. 6, pp. 1263–1271, 2010.

[69] A. Cuker and H. Husseinzadeh, "Laboratory measurement of the anticoagulant activity of edoxaban: a systematic review," *Journal of Thrombosis and Thrombolysis*, vol. 39, no. 3, pp. 288–294, 2015.

[70] D. M. Adcock and R. Gosselin, "Direct oral anticoagulants (DOACs) in the laboratory: 2015 review," *Thrombosis Research*, vol. 136, no. 1, pp. 7–12, 2015.

[71] J. H. Levy, W. Ageno, N. C. Chan, M. Crowther, P. Verhamme, and J. I. Weitz, "When and how to use antidotes for the reversal of direct oral anticoagulants: guidance from the SSC of the ISTH," *Journal of Thrombosis and Haemostasis*, vol. 14, no. 3, pp. 623–627, 2016.

[72] M. Makris, J. J. Van Veen, C. R. Tait, A. D. Mumford, and M. Laffan, "Guideline on the management of bleeding in patients on antithrombotic agents," *British Journal of Haematology*, vol. 160, no. 1, pp. 35–46, 2013.

[73] D. A. Garcia and M. A. Crowther, "Reversal of warfarin: case-based practice recommendations," *Circulation*, vol. 125, no. 23, pp. 2944–2947, 2012.

[74] R. I. Baker, P. B. Coughlin, A. S. Gallus, P. L. Harper, H. H. Salem, and E. M. Wood, "Warfarin reversal: consensus guidelines, on behalf of the Australasian Society of Thrombosis and Haemostasis," *The Medical Journal of Australia*, vol. 181, no. 9, pp. 492–497, 2004.

[75] M. Makris and H. G. Watson, "The management of coumarin-induced over-anticoagulation Annotation," *British Journal of Haematology*, vol. 114, no. 2, pp. 271–280, 2001.

[76] D. F. O'Shaughnessy, C. Atterbury, P. Bolton Maggs et al., "Guidelines for the use of fresh-frozen plasma, cryoprecipitate and cryosupernatant," *British Journal of Haematology*, vol. 126, no. 1, pp. 11–28, 2004.

[77] M. Zareh, A. Davis, and S. Henderson, "Reversal of warfarin-induced hemorrhage in the emergency department," *Western Journal of Emergency Medicine*, vol. 12, no. 4, pp. 386–392, 2011.

[78] S. Pandey and G. N. Vyas, "Adverse effects of plasma transfusion," *Transfusion*, vol. 52, supplement 1, pp. 65S–79S, 2012.

[79] M. Makris, M. Greaves, W. S. Phillips, S. Kitchen, F. R. Rosendaal, and F. E. Preston, "Emergency oral anticoagulant reversal: the relative efficacy of infusions of fresh frozen plasma and clotting factor concentrate on correction of the coagulopathy," *Thrombosis and Haemostasis*, vol. 77, no. 3, pp. 477–480, 1997.

[80] S. Schulman and N. R. Bijsterveld, "Anticoagulants and their reversal," *Transfusion Medicine Reviews*, vol. 21, no. 1, pp. 37–48, 2007.

[81] KCENTRA™, CSL Behring, King of Prussia, Pa, USA, 2013, http://www.fda.gov/ucm/groups/fdagov-public/@fdagov-bio-gen/documents/document/ucm350239.pdf.

[82] R. Sarode, T. J. Milling, M. A. Refaai et al., "Efficacy and safety of a 4-factor prothrombin complex concentrate in patients on vitamin K antagonists presenting with major bleeding: a randomized, plasma-controlled, phase iiib study," *Circulation*, vol. 128, no. 11, pp. 1234–1243, 2013.

[83] A. Majeed, H.-G. Hwang, S. J. Connolly et al., "Management and outcomes of major bleeding during treatment with dabigatran or warfarin," *Circulation*, vol. 128, no. 21, pp. 2325–2332, 2013.

[84] C. Held, E. M. Hylek, J. H. Alexander et al., "Clinical outcomes and management associated with major bleeding in patients with atrial fibrillation treated with apixaban or warfarin: insights from the ARISTOTLE trial," *European Heart Journal*, vol. 36, no. 20, pp. 1264–1272, 2015.

[85] J. P. Piccini, J. Garg, M. R. Patel et al., "Management of major bleeding events in patients treated with rivaroxaban vs. warfarin: results from the ROCKET AF trial," *European Heart Journal*, vol. 35, no. 28, pp. 1873–1880, 2014.

[86] J. Skaistis and T. Tagami, "Risk of fatal bleeding in episodes of major bleeding with new oral anticoagulants and vitamin k antagonists: a systematic review and meta-analysis," *PLoS ONE*, vol. 10, no. 9, Article ID e0137444, 2015.

[87] C. T. January, L. S. Wann, J. S. Alpert et al., "2014 AHA/ACC/HRS guideline for the management of patients with atrial fibrillation: a report of the American College of Cardiology/American Heart Association Task Force on Practice Guidelines and the Heart Rhythm Society," *Journal of the American College of Cardiology*, vol. 64, no. 21, pp. e1–e76, 2014.

[88] D. Faraoni, J. H. Levy, P. Albaladejo, and C. Samama, "Updates in the perioperative and emergency management of non-vitamin K antagonist oral anticoagulants," *Critical Care*, vol. 19, article 203, 2015.

[89] G. Breuer, D. R. Weiss, and J. Ringwald, "'New' direct oral anticoagulants in the perioperative setting," *Current Opinion in Anaesthesiology*, vol. 27, no. 4, pp. 409–419, 2014.

[90] R. Ferrandis, J. Castillo, J. de Andrés et al., "The perioperative management of new direct oral anticoagulants: a question without answers," *Thrombosis and Haemostasis*, vol. 110, no. 3, pp. 515–522, 2013.

[91] W. I. Gonsalves, R. K. Pruthi, and M. M. Patnaik, "The new oral anticoagulants in clinical practice," *Mayo Clinic Proceedings*, vol. 88, no. 5, pp. 495–511, 2013.

[92] K. Ogata, J. Mendell-Harary, M. Tachibana et al., "Clinical safety, tolerability, pharmacokinetics, and pharmacodynamics of the novel factor Xa inhibitor edoxaban in healthy volunteers," *Journal of Clinical Pharmacology*, vol. 50, no. 7, pp. 743–753, 2010.

[93] D. A. Parasrampuria, T. Marbury, N. Matsushima et al., "Pharmacokinetics, safety, and tolerability of edoxaban in end-stage renal disease subjects undergoing haemodialysis," *Thrombosis and Haemostasis*, vol. 113, no. 4, pp. 719–727, 2015.

[94] J. van Ryn, J. Stangier, S. Haertter et al., "Dabigatran etexilate—a novel, reversible, oral direct thrombin inhibitor: interpretation of coagulation assays and reversal of anticoagulant activity," *Thrombosis and Haemostasis*, vol. 103, no. 6, pp. 1116–1127, 2010.

[95] M. Levi, K. T. Moore, C. F. Castillejos et al., "Comparison of three-factor and four-factor prothrombin complex concentrates regarding reversal of the anticoagulant effects of rivaroxaban in healthy volunteers," *Journal of Thrombosis and Haemostasis*, vol. 12, no. 9, pp. 1428–1436, 2014.

[96] R. Marlu, E. Hodaj, A. Paris, P. Albaladejo, J. L. Crackowski, and G. Pernod, "Effect of non-specific reversal agents on anticoagulant activity of dabigatran and rivaroxaban: a randomised crossover ex vivo study in healthy volunteers," *Thrombosis and Haemostasis*, vol. 108, no. 2, pp. 217–224, 2012.

[97] G. Escolar, V. Fernandez-Gallego, E. Arellano-Rodrigo et al., "Reversal of apixaban induced alterations in hemostasis by different coagulation factor concentrates: significance of studies in vitro with circulating human blood," *PLoS ONE*, vol. 8, no. 11, Article ID e78696, 2013.

[98] T. Fukuda, Y. Honda, C. Kamisato, Y. Morishima, and T. Shibano, "Reversal of anticoagulant effects of edoxaban, an oral, direct factor Xa inhibitor, with haemostatic agents," *Thrombosis and Haemostasis*, vol. 107, no. 2, pp. 253–259, 2012.

[99] FEIBA, Baxter Healthcare Corporation, Westlake Village, Calif, USA, 2013, http://www.fda.gov/downloads/BiologicsBloodVaccines/BloodBloodProducts/ApprovedProducts/LicensedProductsBLAs/FractionatedPlasmaProducts/UCM221749.pdf.

[100] R. Alikhan, R. Rayment, D. Keeling et al., "The acute management of haemorrhage, surgery and overdose in patients receiving dabigatran," *Emergency Medicine Journal*, vol. 31, no. 2, pp. 163–168, 2014.

[101] H. Shakur, I. Roberts, R. Bautista et al., "Effects of tranexamic acid on death, vascular occlusive events, and blood transfusion in trauma patients with significant haemorrhage (CRASH-2): a randomised, placebo-controlled trial," *The Lancet*, vol. 376, no. 9734, pp. 23–32, 2010.

[102] A. Clavé, F. Fazilleau, D. Dumser, and J. Lacroix, "Efficacy of tranexamic acid on blood loss after primary cementless total hip replacement with rivaroxaban thromboprophylaxis: a case-control study in 70 patients," *Orthopaedics and Traumatology: Surgery and Research*, vol. 98, no. 5, pp. 484–490, 2012.

[103] C. V. Pollack Jr., P. A. Reilly, J. Eikelboom et al., "Idarucizumab for dabigatran reversal," *The New England Journal of Medicine*, vol. 373, pp. 511–520, 2015.

[104] S. Hollenbach, G. Lu, F. DeGuzman et al., "Abstract 14657: andexanet-alfa and PER977 (Arapazine) correct blood loss in a rabbit liver laceration model—only andexanet reverses markers of fXa-mediated anticoagulation," *Circulation*, vol. 130, abstract A14657, 2014.

[105] A. Gómez-Outes, M. L. Suárez-Gea, R. Lecumberri, A. I. Terleira-Fernández, and E. Vargas-Castrillón, "Specific antidotes in development for reversal of novel anticoagulants: a review," *Recent Patents on Cardiovascular Drug Discovery*, vol. 9, no. 1, pp. 2–10, 2014.

[106] J. E. Ansell, S. H. Bakhru, B. E. Laulicht et al., "Use of PER977 to reverse the anticoagulant effect of edoxaban," *The New England Journal of Medicine*, vol. 371, no. 22, pp. 2141–2142, 2014.

[107] G. Lu, F. R. DeGuzman, S. J. Hollenbach et al., "A specific antidote for reversal of anticoagulation by direct and indirect inhibitors of coagulation factor Xa," *Nature Medicine*, vol. 19, no. 4, pp. 446–451, 2013.

[108] D. M. Siegal and A. Cuker, "Reversal of target-specific oral anticoagulants," *Drug Discovery Today*, vol. 19, no. 9, pp. 1465–1470, 2014.

[109] A. M. Gold, M. Crowther, G. Levy et al., "ANNEXA™-R: a phase 3 randomized, double-blind, placebo-controlled trial, demonstrating reversal of rivaroxaban-induced anticoagulation in older subjects by andexanet alfa (PRT064445), a universal antidote for factor Xa (fXa) inhibitors," *Journal of the American College of Cardiology*, vol. 65, no. 10, article A23, 2015.

[110] M. Crowther, G. G. Levy, G. Lu et al., "ANNEXA™-A: a phase 3 randomized, double-blind, placebo-controlled trial, demonstrating reversal of apixaban-induced anticoagulation in older subjects by andexanet alfa (PRT064445), a universal antidote for factor Xa (fXa) inhibitors," in *Proceedings of the American Heart Association Scientific Sessions "Clinical Science: Special Reports"*, Chicago, Ill, USA, November 2014.

[111] M. Franchini and G. Lippi, "Prothrombin complex concentrates: an update," *Blood Transfusion*, vol. 8, no. 3, pp. 149–154, 2010.

[112] A.-C. Martin, B. Le Bonniec, A.-M. Fischer et al., "Evaluation of recombinant activated factor VII, prothrombin complex concentrate, and fibrinogen concentrate to reverse apixaban in a rabbit model of bleeding and thrombosis," *International Journal of Cardiology*, vol. 168, no. 4, pp. 4228–4233, 2013.

[113] J. Biskupiak, S. R. Ghate, T. Jiao, and D. Brixner, "Cost implications of formulary decisions on oral anticoagulants in nonvalvular atrial fibrillation," *Journal of Managed Care Pharmacy*, vol. 19, no. 9, pp. 789–798, 2013.

[114] M. F. Bullano, V. Willey, O. Hauch, G. Wygant, A. C. Spyropoulos, and L. Hoffman, "Longitudinal evaluation of health plan cost per venous thromboembolism or bleed event in patients with a prior venous thromboembolism event during hospitalization," *Journal of Managed Care Pharmacy*, vol. 11, no. 8, pp. 663–673, 2005.

[115] A. Amin, A. Bruno, J. Trocio, J. Lin, and M. Lingohr-Smith, "Comparison of differences in medical costs when new oral anticoagulants are used for the treatment of patients with non-valvular atrial fibrillation and venous thromboembolism vs warfarin or placebo in the US," *Journal of Medical Economics*, vol. 18, no. 6, pp. 399–409, 2015.

[116] S. M. Singh and H. C. Wijeysundera, "Cost-effectiveness of novel oral anticoagulants for stroke prevention in non-valvular atrial fibrillation," *Current Cardiology Reports*, vol. 17, article 61, 2015.

[117] A. Maan, E. K. Heist, J. N. Ruskin, and M. Mansour, "Practical issues in the management of novel oral anticoagulants-cardioversion and ablation," *Journal of Thoracic Disease*, vol. 7, no. 2, pp. 115–131, 2015.

[118] F. Lozano, J. Trujillo-Santos, M. Barrón et al., "Home versus in-hospital treatment of outpatients with acute deep venous thrombosis of the lower limbs," *Journal of Vascular Surgery*, vol. 59, no. 5, pp. 1362.e1–1367.e1, 2014.

[119] D. Aujesky, P.-M. Roy, F. Verschuren et al., "Outpatient versus inpatient treatment for patients with acute pulmonary embolism: an international, open-label, randomised, non-inferiority trial," *The Lancet*, vol. 378, no. 9785, pp. 41–48, 2011.

[120] D. M. Beam, Z. P. Kahler, and J. A. Kline, "Immediate discharge and home treatment with rivaroxaban of low-risk venous thromboembolism diagnosed in two U.S. emergency departments: a one-year preplanned analysis," *Academic Emergency Medicine*, vol. 22, no. 7, pp. 788–795, 2015.

[121] I. M. van Korlaar, C. Y. Vossen, F. R. Rosendaal et al., "The impact of venous thrombosis on quality of life," *Thrombosis Research*, vol. 114, no. 1, pp. 11–18, 2004.

[122] C. L. Marvig, T. I. Verhoef, A. de Boer et al., "Quality of life in patients with venous thromboembolism and atrial fibrillation treated with coumarin anticoagulants," *Thrombosis Research*, vol. 136, no. 1, pp. 69–75, 2015.

[123] B. U. Monz, S. J. Connolly, M. Korhonen, H. Noack, and J. Pooley, "Assessing the impact of dabigatran and warfarin on health-related quality of life: results from an RE-LY sub-study," *International Journal of Cardiology*, vol. 168, no. 3, pp. 2540–2547, 2013.

# 19

# E-Bike Injuries: Experience from an Urban Emergency Department—A Retrospective Study from Switzerland

**Sylvana Papoutsi, Luca Martinolli, Christian Tasso Braun, and Aristomenis K. Exadaktylos**

*Department of Emergency Medicine, University Hospital and University of Bern, Freiburgstraße 16c, 3010 Bern, Switzerland*

Correspondence should be addressed to Sylvana Papoutsi; dr.papoutsi@gmail.com

Academic Editor: Chak W. Kam

*Background.* Between 2005 and 2012, annual sales of E-bikes in Switzerland increased from 1,792 to 52,941. This continuous and rapid transition from human-powered bicycles to an electric bicycle technology may indicate the increasing demand for low-cost transportation technology in combination with a healthy lifestyle. *Material and Methods.* In the present study, from April 2012 to September 2013, we retrospectively analysed E-bike accidents treated in the Emergency Department of our hospital by focusing on the following parameters: age, gender, time, period, and cause of the accident, as well as injury and outcome. *Results.* Patients were predominantly male. The mean age of injured E-cyclists was 47.5 years. The main causes of injury were self-accident. Most injuries were to the head/neck. The mean ISS was 8.48. The outcome showed that 9 patients were treated as outpatients, 9 were inpatients, and 5 patients were kept in the Intensive Care Unit (ICU). Only six patients underwent surgery (S). *Discussion.* This is the first attempt to evaluate E-bike injuries in Switzerland in an acute hospital setting. Since there is increasing popular preference for E-bikes as means of transportation and injuries to the head or neck are prevalent among E-cyclists, the hazard should not to be underestimated.

## 1. Introduction

Electric bikes or E-bikes are a category of modern vehicles that includes two-wheel bikes propelled by human pedalling, supplemented by electrical power from a storage battery (bicycle-style). The main technical components include a hub motor and lead-acid (VRLA) battery regulated by a controlled valve. Bicycle-style E-bikes typically have 36 V batteries and 180–250 W motors. E-bikes are regulated not to exceed 20 km/h on electric power alone; however, many E-bikes can travel at speeds in excess of that limit and some are advertised as being able to reach 40 km/h and more [1].

Approximately 29 million E-bikes were produced in 2010, representing a 24.7% increase over 2009 [2]. By 2011, 120 million E-bikes had been registered in China [3], which might account for 90% of the global market [2]. Furthermore, a worldwide increase in demand is expected; it is estimated that 466 million E-bikes will have hit the road by 2016 [4].

These vehicles have also become a popular transportation mode for the Swiss [5], as they provide a long-term, less expensive, and convenient form of private mobility and are thus an attractive alternative to public transport, private cars, motorbikes, or normal cycling. Due to their low energy consumption and almost zero emissions [6], these vehicles are promoted by local governments [7]. They are safer than motorcycles, more comfortable and cheaper than the bus, and cheaper than the car. Longer distances can be travelled than with normal bikes [8]. Thus, from the user's perspective, E-bikes offer many advantages over regular bikes and walking.

As was mentioned before, E-bikes are gaining an increasing share of two-wheel transportation. Swiss statistics have shown that in 2005 there were a total of 1,792 E-bikes. The latest statistics from the Swiss Institute for Bicycles (SFZ) indicate that E-bike sales in Switzerland have "sky rocketed," with 52,941 annual E-bike sales and an annual rate of increase of 15.2% (Table 1) [5].

TABLE 1: Overview of Switzerland's bicycle market [5].

| Year | Total bike sales | E-bike sales | Proportion % |
|---|---|---|---|
| 2005 | 280,840 | 1,792 | +0.6% |
| 2006 | 299,286 | 3,181 | +1.1% |
| 2007 | 314,161 | 5,825 | +1.9% |
| 2008 | 314,784 | 11,631 | +3.7% |
| 2009 | 349,903 | 23,886 | +6.8% |
| 2010 | 351,003 | 39,247 | +11.2% |
| 2011 | 351,808 | 49,615 | +14.1% |
| 2012 | 348,643 | 52,941 | +15.2% |

Notwithstanding the huge increase in the number of E-cyclists, the literature on E-bikes injuries is relatively limited. We have now performed the first retrospective study of E-bike injuries at a European level I trauma centre.

## 2. Material and Methods

Our University Department of Emergency Medicine, the only Level I centre in the canton of Bern, serves about 1,8 million people and treats more than 35,000 cases per year, caring for patients older than 16 years. Our retrospective 18-month observational study, from April 2012 to September 2013, comprised adult patients (≥16 years old) admitted to our Emergency Department (ED) in relation to an accident that had occurred with an E-bike. All patients presenting to the ED with an E-bike accident during the study period were included in our study. Patients were identified using the appropriate search string in the patient demographic field of our computerised patient database. Since this medical database allows instantaneous recall of past diagnostic reports, consultations, X-rays, and other relevant medical documents, the authors retrospectively analysed the E-bike injured patients, including gender, age (<40 or ≥40 years old), time (morning 05:01 am–13:30 pm, afternoon 13:31 pm–17:30 pm, evening 17:31 pm–21:00 pm, and night 21:01 pm–05:00 am), season (spring, summer, autumn, and winter), and cause of accident: being caught in a tram rail (occurred after being caught in a tram rail), vehicle collision (occurred after collision with a vehicle), and self-accident (occurred due to alcohol intoxication, due to high speed, or without a known reason), as well as severity of injury, medical diagnosis, and, finally, the outcome (treated as home/outpatient, kept in hospital, or as inpatient, kept in the Intensive Care Unit and mortality). Each diagnosis was classified according to the Abbreviated Injury Scale (AIS) handbook 2008 [9] and the Injury Severity Score (ISS) was calculated for each patient [10].

## 3. Results

During the 18-month study period, from April 2012 until September 2013, a total of twenty-three ($n = 23$) E-bike accidents were reported to our ED. Seventy percent ($n = 16$) of the injured were male and 30% ($n = 7$) female. A total of 18 (78.3%) of the injured E-cyclists were above the age of 40. The median age was 47.5 years. The detailed characteristics of each patient are shown in Table 2.

Additionally, 43.5% ($n = 10$) of accidents took place during the morning, 26.1% ($n = 6$) during the afternoon, 17.4% ($n = 4$) during the evening, and only 13.0% ($n = 3$) during the night. The most common season was summer, with 39.1% ($n = 9$) of accidents, followed by spring and autumn, each with 26.1% ($n = 6$), as well as winter with 8.7% ($n = 2$). Approximately 60.9% ($n = 14$) of injured E-cyclists were involved in a self-accident of known/unknown cause: these were related to a high speed ($n = 4$; 17.4%), to alcohol intoxication ($n = 2$; 8.7%), or no known reason ($n = 8$; 34.8%). Furthermore, 5 (21.7%) E-cyclists were injured after being caught in a tram rail and 4 (17.4%) due to a collision with a vehicle.

The head/neck was the most common body region injured (27.4%). Injuries to the upper extremities (22.6%) and face (19.3%) were almost as common. Injuries to the chest (11.3%), abdomen (9.7%), lower extremities (6.4%), and external skin (3.2%) were less frequent (Figure 1). The types and locations of the injuries are summarised in Table 3. In particular, the most common injuries to the head/neck were mild brain injury (14.9%) and subarachnoid haemorrhage (7.4%); to the face, contused lacerated wounds (10.4%) and fractures (4.5%); to the upper extremities, clavicle fractures (11.9%) and contusive trauma (8.9%); to the chest, rib fractures (6.0%); to the low extremities, contusive trauma (4.5%); to the abdomen, contusive trauma (3.0%); to the external skin, (4.5%) slight excoriation (without contusive trauma). The most frequent types of injuries were fractures (32.6%)—especially fractures to the clavicle (38.1%)—contusive trauma (20.9%), and mild brain injuries (14.9%) (Figure 2).

The ISS scores were between 2 and 29, with an average value of 8.48. Of the 14 (60.8%) hospitalised patients, only 6 (42.8%) underwent surgery.

Only 9 patients (39.1%) were sent home or for outpatient treatment, but 14 patients (60.81%) were treated in hospital. In the latter group, 9 patients (39.1%) were treated in general wards (3 patients in the Oral/Maxillofacial Unit, 3 in the Neurosurgery Unit, 2 in the Orthopaedics/Traumatology Unit, and 1 in the Dermatology Unit) and the remaining 5 patients (21.7%) were kept in ICU. No E-cyclist died.

## 4. Discussion

The current retrospective 18-month descriptive study aims to make a preliminary evaluation of E-bike injuries, in the Emergency Department (ED) of an acute Level I Trauma Centre in Switzerland. To the best of our knowledge, this is one of the first studies that systematically analyses the accidents related to this means of transport at a European hospital.

Our results showed that E-bike users are predominantly male; this finding is in full concordance with the current international literature [11–15]. Among accident victims, 78.3% are ≥40 years old, with a median age of 47.5. Our finding with regard to the median age is in good agreement with a recent report (SINUS-Report 2013) from The Swiss

Table 2: E-cyclists' characteristics.

| Patients (n) | Sex | Age | Time | Period | Cause of accident | Region of injury | ISS | Outcome |
|---|---|---|---|---|---|---|---|---|
| 1 | M | 38 | Evening | Summer | Being caught in a tram rail | Head/neck, face, upper extremities, external | 6 | Home |
| 2 | M | 63 | Night | Spring | Self-accident (alcohol intoxication) | Head/neck, face, upper extremities, abdomen | 12 | Hospital |
| 3 | F | 41 | Evening | Spring | Self-accident (unknown reason) | Upper extremities, chest, abdomen, external | 3 | Home |
| 4 | M | 51 | Afternoon | Summer | Being caught in a tram rail | Head/neck, face, upper extremities | 3 | Home |
| 5 | M | 54 | Afternoon | Spring | Self-accident (unknown reason) | Head/neck, face, chest | 17 | Hospital |
| 6 | M | 45 | Afternoon | Spring | Collision with vehicle | Face, upper extremities, chest, lower extremities | 6 | Hospital |
| 7 | F | 27 | Afternoon | Summer | Self-accident (high speed) | Head/neck, face, upper extremities, abdomen | 6 | Hospital/S* |
| 8 | F | 41 | Morning | Autumn | Self-accident (high speed) | Lower extremities | 4 | Home |
| 9 | F | 57 | Afternoon | Autumn | Self-accident (unknown reason) | Head/neck, face, upper extremities | 9 | Hospital |
| 10 | F | 43 | Morning | Autumn | Self-accident (unknown reason) | Head/neck, chest | 10 | ICU** |
| 11 | M | 42 | Morning | Summer | Collision with vehicle | Upper extremities, chest, lower extremities | 3 | Home |
| 12 | M | 76 | Afternoon | Autumn | Collision with vehicle | Head/neck, chest, upper extremities, abdomen | 29 | ICU/S |
| 13 | M | 59 | Night | Autumn | Self-accident (unknown reason) | Head/neck, face | 17 | ICU/S |
| 14 | M | 48 | Morning | Autumn | Being caught in a tram rail | Face, chest | 5 | Home |
| 15 | F | 64 | Morning | Winter | Self-accident (unknown reason) | Head/neck, face | 4 | Hospital |
| 16 | F | 35 | Morning | Winter | Self-accident (unknown reason) | Head/neck, face, upper extremities | 6 | Hospital/S |
| 17 | M | 62 | Morning | Spring | Collision with vehicle | Upper extremities, lower extremities | 13 | Hospital/S |
| 18 | M | 40 | Evening | Spring | Self-accident (high speed) | Head/neck, face, upper extremities | 5 | Home |
| 19 | M | 61 | Morning | Summer | Self-accident (high speed) | Head/neck | 9 | ICU |
| 20 | M | 21 | Morning | Summer | Self-accident (unknown reason) | Head/neck | 1 | Home |
| 21 | M | 41 | Morning | Summer | Being caught in a tram rail | Head/neck, upper extremities, abdomen | 6 | Hospital/S |
| 22 | M | 46 | Evening | Summer | Being caught in a tram rail | Head/neck, upper extremities | 8 | Home |
| 23 | M | 37 | Night | Summer | Self-accident (alcohol intoxication) | Head/neck, abdomen | 13 | ICU |

*Surgery; **Intensive Care Unit.

Table 3: Number and type of injuries for each body region.

| | | | | |
|---|---|---|---|---|
| Head/Neck | MBI* $n = 10$ (14.9%) | SAH** $n = 5$ (7.4%) | Fractures $n = 4$ (6.0%) | CLW*** $n = 3$ (4.5%) |
| Face | CLW $n = 7$ (10.4%) | Fractures $n = 3$ (4.5%) | Contusive trauma $n = 1$ (1.5%) | Teeth fracture $n = 1$ (1.5%) |
| Upper extremities | Clavicle fractures $n = 8$ (11.9%) | | Contusive trauma $n = 6$ (8.9%) | |
| Chest | Rib fracture $n = 4$ (6.0%) | | Contusive trauma $n = 2$ (3.0%) | Pneumothorax $n = 1$ (1.5%) |
| Abdomen | Contusive trauma $n = 2$ (3.0%) | | Free intra-abdominal fluid $n = 1$ (1.5%) | |
| Lower extremities | Fractures $n = 2$ (3.0%) | Contusive trauma $n = 3$ (4.5%) | | CLW $n = 1$ (1.5%) |
| External skin | Excoriation $n = 3$ (4.5%) | | | |

*MBI: mild brain injury; **SAH: subarachnoid haemorrhage; ***CLW: contused lacerated wounds.

Council for Accident Prevention [16]. Du et al., in a Chinese study of 323 E-bike injuries, reported an average age of 43.8 years [15]. However, some of their patients were children. More and more elderly adults in Switzerland choose E-bikes for transportation, perhaps because this takes less time and is less exhausting than riding a conventional bike. In Australia, another study reported that using an E-bike rather than a conventional bike increased the likelihood of preferring an active method of transport, and was significantly quicker, with less perceived effort [17].

The present study also showed that most E-bike accidents occurred during the morning, followed by evening and afternoon, as well as in the summer months. Du et al. also analysed the time of the day and concluded that most accidents occurred during the night (18:00 pm–23:59 pm). Our findings are consistent with peak travel to and from work; they may indicate the use of E-bikes as a means of transportation to and from work.

Furthermore, we noticed that most E-bike injuries were caused by self-accident and a significant percentage of accidents were attributed to being caught in a tram rail. It is worth mentioning that we analysed the tram rails as a cause of accident as these were very frequent among our patients. In the study of Du et al., it was reported that 48.6% of injuries involved collisions with motor vehicles. In contrast, we found that only 17.4% of accidents were caused by collision with vehicles. This may be related to the traffic density in the two countries.

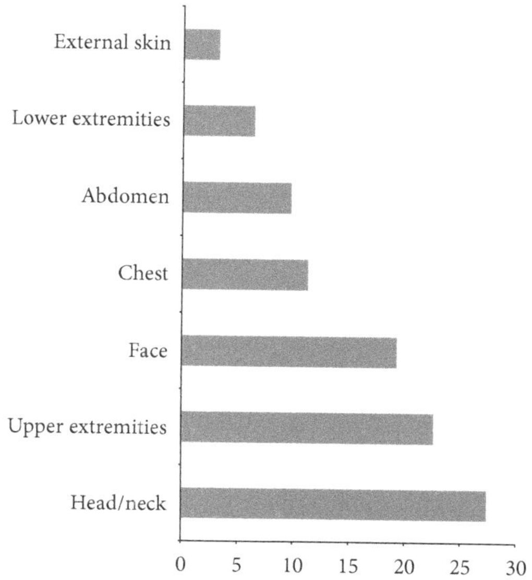


FIGURE 1: Percentage of injured regions among E-cyclists (%).

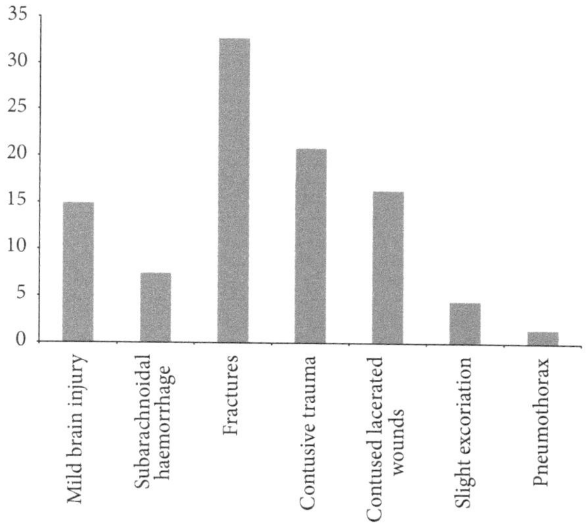


FIGURE 2: Type of injuries in E-cyclists in percentage (%).

Another Chinese study found that E-bike related casualties had increased in recent years, notwithstanding the decreases in the total number of road traffic collisions and deaths [18]. In Switzerland, the proportion of E-bikes in cycling traffic is rising steadily. In 2010, only 1.5% of cyclists rode E-bikes, with increases to 2.3% in 2011 and 3.8% in 2012 (Swiss Council for Accident Prevention). Unfortunately, no detailed data for E-bike injuries are available for Switzerland for these years.

The injuries to the head/neck region included a high proportion of mild brain injury. In the whole body, the most common injuries were fractures and contusions, followed by contused lacerated wounds and superficial excoriations (Figure 2). Du et al. made similar findings with respect to the head/neck region; however, the most common injuries they found were fractures of the limbs, whereas in our study, they were clavicle fractures. Moreover, the second most commonly injured body region in our study was the upper extremities (Figure 1). This is in contrast to Du et al., who recorded 46.4% of injuries in the head/neck and 20.7% in the trunk. These may relate to the failure of more E-cyclists to wear helmets in China. Indeed, the rate of helmet wearing among Swiss E-cyclists is currently 75.0% (Swiss Council for the Accident Prevention) in Switzerland [16] and only 9.0% in China [15]. Considering that the impacts and hazards are likely to be similar in the two countries, the evidence and the effectiveness of helmets in reducing bicyclist [19] and motorcyclist [20] head injuries clearly support helmet use for E-cyclists.

It is remarkable that we found no hospital mortality and our ISS score was relatively low. Unfortunately, no ISS scores on E-bike injuries have been published in comparable studies. Only eight E-bike deaths were reported in 2012 (Swiss Federal Roads Authority), which was six more than in the previous year [16]. However, Du et al. failed to find any hospital fatality in the course of their 6-month study in China. In another study carried out in Hangzhou, with its population of circa 7,800,000, Feng et al. recorded 397 E-bike related deaths between 2004 and 2008 [18].

In their retrospective study on motorcycle and bicycle accidents, Wagner et al. concluded that these accidents cause major injuries in older patients with more severe ISS. They concluded that fewer older bicyclists used helmets and that they suffered more sustained or severe head injuries, with greater functional decline [21]. An Australian study to evaluate the factors influencing the outcome of 208 motorcycle crash victims showed that losing control due to intoxication, collision with another vehicle, or travelling above the speed limit was associated with the worst patient outcome; travelling in excess of 50 kph increased the risk of intracranial injury [22]. Our patient group was too small to allow similar conclusions.

*Limitations*. Our findings have to be considered with some caution, as the study was conducted retrospectively. As the information in our medical history database is presented in a narrative comment, there is no guarantee that the number of E-cyclists was fully reported. Furthermore, our study was limited to adults (≥16 years old), as children are treated at a separate Emergency Department in our hospital. Since the weather conditions during each accident were not reported, as a first approximation, we analysed our data by season. It has been demonstrated that helmets protect riders of two-wheel vehicles and so correlate negatively with admission to an ICU [23, 24]. Unfortunately, our register data did not document helmet use.

## 5. Conclusions

E-bikes are a new mode of transport; prices are coming down and purchases will probably continue to rise. Injuries to the head and neck are common. Further studies are needed to compare accidents suffered by E-cyclists with those suffered by bicyclists and motor cyclists.

## Conflict of Interests

The authors declare that there is no conflict of interests regarding the publication of this paper.

## References

[1] J. Weinert, C. Ma, and C. Cherry, "The transition to electric bikes in China: history and key reasons for rapid growth," *Transportation*, vol. 34, no. 3, pp. 301–318, 2007.

[2] Research in China, "Industry report of electric bicycles in China, 2010-2011," Tech. Rep., 2011.

[3] L. Yao and C. Wu, "Traffic safety of e-bike riders in China: safety attitudes, risk perception and aberrant riding behaviors," *Transportation Research Record. Journal of the Transportation Research Board & Transportation Research Board*, vol. 2314, pp. 49–56, 2013.

[4] D. Hurst and C. Wheelock, *Electric Two-Wheel Vehicles (Electric Bicycles, Mopeds, Scooters and Motorcycles): Market Analysis and Forecasts*, Boulder Pike Research, Boulder, Colo, USA, 2010.

[5] Statistiken über den Velomarkt Schweiz. Velosuisse, http://www.velosuisse.ch/de/statistik_aktuell.html.

[6] "The electric bicycle race. MPR," July/August 2010.

[7] Mit E-Bike-Pilotstation die Nachfrage überprüfen, http://www.bernerzeitung.ch/region/thun/Mit-EBikePilotstation-die-Nachfrage-ueberpruefen/story/18104412.

[8] C. Cherry and R. Cervero, "Use characteristics and mode choice behavior of electric bike users in China," *Transport Policy*, vol. 14, no. 3, pp. 247–257, 2007.

[9] T. A. Gennarelli and E. Wodzin, "Abbreviated Injury Scale update 2008," *Association for the Advancement of Automotive Medicine*, vol. 1, no. 1, 2008.

[10] "Injury severity score 2012," http://www.trauma.org/archive/scores/iss.html.

[11] W. Du, J. Yang, B. Powis et al., "Understanding on-road practices of electric bike riders: an observational study in a developed city of China," *Accident Analysis and Prevention*, vol. 59, pp. 319–326, 2013.

[12] Y. Zhang and C. Wu, "The effects of sunshields on red light running behaviour of cyclists and electric bike riders," *Accident Analysis and Prevention*, vol. 52, pp. 210–218, 2013.

[13] C. Wu, L. Yao, and K. Zhang, "The red-light running behavior of electric bike riders and cyclists at urban intersections in China: an observational study," *Accident Analysis and Prevention*, vol. 49, pp. 186–192, 2012.

[14] L. Yao and C. Wu, "Traffic safety of E-Bike riders in China: safety attitudes, risk perception, and aberrant riding behaviours," in *Proceedings of the Annual Meeting of the Transportation Research Board (TRB '11)*, November 2011.

[15] W. Du, J. Yang, B. Powis et al., "Epidemiological profile of hospitalised injuries among electric bicycle riders admitted to a rural hospital in Suzhou: a cross-sectional study," *Injury Prevention*, vol. 20, pp. 128–133, 2014.

[16] "Unfälle mit E-Bikes häufig selbstverschuldet," http://www.news.ch/Unfaelle+mit+E+Bikes+haeufig+selbstverschuldet/603601/detail.htm.

[17] M. Ralfe and J. Williams, "Comparing electric bicycle and conventional bicycle use-implications for increasing daily activity," *Journal of Science and Medicine in Sport*, vol. 10, no. 1, 2008.

[18] Z. Feng, R. P. Raghuwanshi, Z. Xu, D. Huang, C. Zhang, and T. Jin, "Electric-bicycle-related injury: a rising traffic injury burden in china," *Injury Prevention*, vol. 16, no. 6, pp. 417–419, 2010.

[19] D. C. Thompson, F. P. Rivara, and R. Thompson, "Helmets for preventing head and facial injuries in bicyclists," *Cochrane Database of Systematic Reviews*, no. 2, Article ID CD001855, 2000.

[20] B. C. Liu, R. Ivers, R. Norton, S. Boufous, S. Blows, and S. K. Lo, "Helmets for preventing injury in motorcycle riders," *Cochrane Database of Systematic Reviews*, no. 1, Article ID CD004333, 2008.

[21] J. Wagner, A. Rai, F. Ituarte, A. Tillou, H. Cryer, and J. R. Hiatt, "Two-wheel vehicular trauma: an age-based analysis," *The American Surgeon*, vol. 78, no. 10, pp. 1066–1070, 2012.

[22] G. Cunningham, D. Chenik, and R. Zellweger, "Factors influencing motorcycle crash victim outcomes: a prospective study," *ANZ Journal of Surgery*, vol. 82, pp. 551–554, 2012.

[23] A. Philip, W. Fangman, J. Liao, M. Lilienthal, and K. Choi, "Helmets prevent motorcycle injuries with significant economic benefits," *Traffic Injury Prevention*, vol. 14, pp. 496–500, 2013.

[24] L. Ganti, A. Bodhit, Y. Daneshvar et al., "Impact of helmet use in traumatic brain injuries associated with recreational vehicles," *Advances in Preventive Medicine*, vol. 2013, Article ID 450195, 6 pages, 2013.

# 20

# Does the Integration of Personalized Ultrasound Change Patient Management in Critical Care Medicine? Observational Trials

**Raoul Breitkreutz,[1,2] Marco Campo dell' Orto,[2,3] Christian Hamm,[3] Colleen Cuca,[4] Peter M. Zechner,[5] Tanja Stenger,[6,7] Felix Walcher,[8] and Florian H. Seeger[9]**

[1] *Emergency Department, Hospital of the City of Frankfurt (Höchst), Gotenstraße 6-8, 65929 Frankfurt am Main, Germany*
[2] *Emergency Ultrasound Regional Network and the Frankfurt Institute of Emergency Medicine and Simulation Training, Johann Wolfgang Goethe University Hospital, Marienburgstraße 5-7, 60528 Frankfurt am Main, Germany*
[3] *Department of Cardiology, Kerckhoff Klinik Bad Nauheim, Benekestraße 2-8, 61231 Bad Nauheim, Germany*
[4] *Deptartment of Anaesthesiology and Intensive Care, Hospital zum Heiligen Geist, Lange Straße, 60311 Frankfurt, Germany*
[5] *Landeskrankenhaus Graz West, Abteilung für Innere Medizin, Göttinger Straße 22, 8020 Graz, Austria*
[6] *Städtisches Klinikum Neunkirchen, Brunnenstraße 20, 66538 Neunkirchen/Saar, Germany*
[7] *Brainfactory, 66288 Bildstock, Germany*
[8] *Trauma Surgery, Johann Wolfgang Goethe University Hospital, Theodor Stern Kai 7, 60590 Frankfurt am Main, Germany*
[9] *Department of Cardiology, Johann Wolfgang Goethe University Hospital, Theodor Stern Kai 7, 60590 Frankfurt am Main, Germany*

Correspondence should be addressed to Raoul Breitkreutz; raoul.breitkreutz@gmail.com

Academic Editor: Tobias Lindner

*Objective.* To test the influence of personalized ultrasound (PersUS) on patient management in critical care. *Design of the Study.* Prospective, observational, and critical care setting. Four substudies compared PersUS and mobile ultrasound, work distribution, and diagnostic and procedural quality. *Patients and Interventions.* 640 patient ultrasound exams including 548 focused diagnostic exams and 92 interventional procedures. *Main Outcome Measures.* Number of studies, physician's judgement of feasibility, time of usage per patient, and referrals to echo lab. *Results.* Randomized availability of PersUS increased its application in ICU work shifts more than twofold from 33 to 68 exams mainly for detection and therapy of effusions. Diagnostic and procedural quality was rated as excellent/very good in PersUS-guided puncture in 95% of cases. Integrating PersUS within an initial physical examination of 48 randomized cases in an emergency department, PersUS extended the examination time by 100 seconds. Interestingly, PersUS integration into 53 randomized regular ward rounds of 1007 patients significantly reduced average contact time per patient by 103 seconds from 8.9 to 7.2 minutes. Moreover, it lowered the patient referral rate to an echo lab from 20% to 2% within the study population. *Conclusions.* We propose the development of novel ultrasound-based clinical pathways by integration of PersUS.

## 1. Introduction

Point-of-care ultrasound has become more popular in the environment of acute and critical care medicine [1, 2]. Various recommendations on its use mainly address clinical indications related to acute or severe dyspnoea, hypotension and shock, trauma, and abdominal pain [1–4]. The technical concept of a "personal ultrasound imager" and an "ultrasonic stethoscope" is more than 30 years old [5]. There is a strong interest in the integration of ultrasound into clinical pathways and many context-based protocols are available. A novel technology was born when the initial idea of a personalized ultrasound device (PersUS) used like a physician's generic stethoscope was realized [5, 6], a paradigm shift that now supports real point-of-care clinical pathway concepts. In 1978 it was suggested that bringing the echo lab to the patient would be a major step forward [5]. Previously, ultrasound labs contained stationary ultrasound systems, while mobile and hand-carried ultrasound was kept at facilities like emergency departments or intensive care units, making the technology available for multiple users. In fact, "personalized" refers to the size and quick application of the PersUS, like a mobile phone or stethoscope, allowing greater flexibility in its usage. There is an ongoing debate as to whether miniaturization of ultrasound machines can improve patient care. The potential personalized usage opens up the field of ultrasound in acute and critical care medicine for a large group of new users [3]. However, only rarely have concepts or strategies for clinical integrations been tested for the critical care environment and little has been established in the way of clinical integration and workflow [7]. Our aim, therefore, was the analysis of the feasibility of clinical integration, frequency of use, decision making, and time consumption of PersUS implementation in the daily routine.

## 2. Methods

*2.1. Study Design.* Ethical approval was obtained from the Institutional Ethics Committee for Human Studies, University Hospital, Frankfurt am Main, Germany (application number 2/11, 13.1.2011). A prospective observational study with data-controlled acquisition was performed.

*2.2. Study Setting and Substudies 1–4.* Patients were enrolled between July 2010 and September 2011. Personalized ultrasound (PersUS) was performed in four centres of the coauthors and in each case using the Vscan (GE Healthcare, Wauwatosa, WI, USA). After an opening and booting time of 25 seconds, the device allows ultrasound exams with a phased array sector probe (1.7–3.8 Mhz) in B-Mode with harmonic imaging and color-coded flow mapping (color Doppler) on a 3.5-inch screen. Support was provided through the "Vscan gateway" (GE Healthcare, Wauwatosa, WI, USA) for all participating examiners. Physicians were trained in focused ultrasound exams in critical care medicine for general applications of the thorax and abdomen and documented each exam with a notation on the patient chart and/or images or clips for later review within the study protocols. Two investigators were staff attending cardiologists and three investigators were staff attending anaesthesiologists or intensivists. Junior staff with expert knowledge in emergency ultrasound performed substudies 3 and 4. Images or clips were deleted after review by the respective attending or study control centre to ensure anonymity. Alternatively, the study protocol allowed a mobile ultrasound device (MobUS) to be used. By chance this was always a Vivid-i (GE Healthcare, Wauwatosa, WI, USA) with each collaboration partner. To examine a great number of patients with a broad spectrum of diseases, this trial was subdivided into four distinct substudies.

*2.2.1. Substudy 1.* Our hypothesis was an availability-based increase in the use of PersUS. We tested this hypothesis in two independent intensive care units with two ultrasound-capable physicians (one cardiologist-intensivist and one anesthesiologist-intensivist), respectively. The practitioners had access to the PersUS device—carried on person—on either odd or even days, which was determined randomly.

*2.2.2. Substudy 2.* Four critical care physicians studied PersUS for planning an execution of ultrasound-guided needle punctures, such as pleural, pericardial, abdominal, or urinary bladder punctures for evacuation of fluid or inserting catheters (pleurocath, pigtail, or suprapubic). Linear analogue self-assessment was used to obtain semiquantitative data of the physician's impression of (i) diagnostic quality and (ii) visual support in ultrasound-guided intervention. Any relative value above 90% was graded as "excellent" and between 80 and 90% as "good" or between 70 and 80% as "satisfactory."

*2.2.3. Substudy 3.* We measured the mean duration of a physical examination with PersUS integration according to the decision of a single emergency physician who used PersUS after randomisation by coin toss. Our null hypothesis was that PersUS exam integration does not significantly prolong the examination time. Indications were acute dyspnoea, thorax pain, hypotension, or abdominal pain. The time between examinations begining and end (handshake following exam) was measured by a generic stopwatch. Any influence on patient management due to PersUS was noted. Of note, PersUS was used during the first patient contact and integrated into the examination. All patients needing ultrasound, for example, to exclude pericardial effusion, received the US with the MobUS device as usual.

*2.2.4. Substudy 4.* In a cardiological and nephrological specialty care unit a PersUS device was randomized between two wards by switching its presence or absence on alternating calendar days. One senior cardiologist alone was informed as the study coordinator of this substudy and allowed to make the PersUS available or remove it from the respective ward. The ward rounds teams, consisting of one or two staff physicians and one attending physician, were blinded to the study aims and differed from day to day. They were instructed to use PersUS whenever it was available and deemed necessary and to note the times and indications of use. Time between beginning and end of ward rounds was measured as well as the number of patients seen and the type and length per ultrasound exam. Most of the examinations during the ward rounds were focused on LV-function as well as effusions. More subtle examinations such as diastolic function of valve regurgitations were sent to the echo lab. The quality of the exam was graded on a Likert scale regarding diagnostic quality as judged by the examiner. All data was then sorted into Group A (control group without PersUS) or Group B (examination with PersUS). Exam time per patient per ward round was calculated. Our null hypothesis was that the exam time per patient would not change significantly by using PersUS on ward rounds.

*2.3. Study Entry Criteria.* Patient inclusion was based on the decision of the participating treating physician. After informed consent, patient-related data and procedure details were logged either on a data acquisition sheet or into a paperless database. If patients were unable to give their informed consent (sedation, dementia) relatives were informed. All

Table 1: Types of indications for application of a mobile ultrasound device (MobUS) in comparison to a randomized availability of a personalized ultrasound device (PersUS). $N = 101$ patients were examined (33 exams with MobUS, 68 with PersUS) with a total of 167 indications and ultrasound studies.

| Category number | Kind of indication | $N$ (% of total) MobUS studies | Time (min) Mean ± SD | $N$ (% of total) PersUS studies | Time (min) Mean ± SD | Percentage change (%) |
|---|---|---|---|---|---|---|
| 1 | Cardiac function (visual LVEF, eyeballing) | 15 (9) | 4.8 ± 1.1 | 36 (22) | 4.4 ± 1.0 | 114 |
| 2 | Focused cardiac anatomy and valve assessment | 14 (9) | 4.7 ± 1.1 | 27 (17) | 4.5 ± 1.0 | 93 |
| 3 | Dyspnoea, suspected pleural effusions | 7 (4) | 14.1 ± 9.9 | 24 (14) | 9.2 ± 4.8 | 243 |
| 4 | Pericardial effusion | 4 (2) | 4.8 ± 2.2 | 14 (9) | 4.4 ± 0.9 | 250 |
| 5 | Abdomen/ascites | 3 (2) | 21.7 ± 7.6 | 8 (4) | 9.9 ± 5.5 | 166 |
| 6 | Ultrasound-guided punctures | 2 (1) | 20 ± 0 | 5 (3) | 12.0 ± 4.5 | 150 |
| 7 | Miscellaneous (a) | 1 (1) | 10 ± 0 | 2 (1) | 4.5 ± 0.7 | 100 |
| 8 | Resuscitation | 3 (2) | 4.0 ± 1.0 | 1 (1) | 4.0 ± 0 | n.a. |
| | Total (167, 100%) | 49 (29) | 8.2 ± 7.0 | 118 (71) | 6.5 ± 3.9 | 141 |

(a) Including groin aneurysm spurium and cubital vein detection for puncture.
n.a.: not applicable. All times as estimated by the examiner from beginning (hands-on) to end (hands-off) of the examination procedure. Descriptive data presentation only. Percentage change was calculated as (the number of PersUS studies minus the number of MobUS studies) divided by the number of MobUS studies.

interventions were applied only after a generic routine MobUS confirmed the initial findings. Indication was formally only supported by MobUS findings and no additional interventions were performed based on PersUS findings alone. Participating physicians were briefed on the implementation of PersUS. Patients below 18 years of age were excluded from the study. Bias could not be controlled otherwise.

*2.4. Data Analysis.* Physicians interpreted all ultrasound exams at the time of the scan and completed the data acquisition protocols upon exam conclusion. Unless stated otherwise, continuous data is shown as mean ± standard deviation. Box plots show median (bold line), mean (dashed line), 25th and 75th quartiles, whiskers, and all outliers. The Mann-Whitney $U$ test was used for descriptive data analysis for comparison between the two groups in substudies 1, 3, and 4. Study size was planned with a fixed number of patients. Power analysis was not applicable for there were no data to precisely predefine our variables. There were no missing data to be excluded.

## 3. Results

*3.1. Substudy 1: Clinical Integration of PersUS in Intensive Care.* Of 31 work shifts (16 without and 15 with PersUS) there were a total of 101 patient exams with 167 ultrasound indications (Table 1). Major indications were diagnostic and related to cardiac anatomy and function as well as pleural effusion (Table 1).

When only a MobUS was available, 33 patients received a focused ultrasound exam. In contrast, the availability of the PersUS markedly increased the number of patients receiving an ultrasound exam up to 68 (relative change: 106%; Figure 1(a), Table 1) and allowed interventions such as pleural puncture to be applied at an earlier point in time. Mean PersUS operation time per patient was 6.5 ± 3.9 minutes, 1.7 minutes faster than MobUS (Table 1). There was hardly any difference in cardiac evaluations; however, for thoracic and other ultrasound examinations there was a remarkable reduction of hands-on/hands-off time per patient (Table 1). During a 3-shift intensive care system, PersUS was most likely to be requested by the physician directly after the morning ward rounds, followed by afternoon or night shift ward rounds (Figure 1(b)).

*3.2. Substudy 2: Evaluation of Image Quality and Interventional Support.* Four attending physicians in critical care evaluated diagnostic and image quality of the PersUS exam and its image quality as well as feasibility in interventional procedures (Figure 2(a)). For pleural effusions, which were the most common diagnoses within the study, PersUS was rated "excellent" (Figure 2(a)(B)). PersUS use demonstrating pericardial effusion and urinary bladder status (Figure 2(a)((A), (C))) as well as during PersUS-guided procedural intervention was rated "good," except in the case of urinary bladder puncture (Figure 2(a)). Numbers for ascites punctures (2) were judged similarly. After PersUS-guided intervention was complete, physician requests for device use in later punctures increased substantially (Figure 2(b)).

*3.3. Substudy 3: Time Requirements of PersUS.* Within nineteen work shifts in an ED, 48 patients with leading symptoms acute dyspnoea ($n = 21$; 44%), abdominal pain (15; 31%), thorax pain (11; 23%), and hypotension/shock (1; 2%) were randomized to be examined on admission either without (Group A; 26 patient admissions, 14 female and 12 male, aged 59 ± 22 years) or with the assistance of PersUS (Group B; 22 patient admissions, 9 female and 13 male, 62 ± 21 years). The duration of this "quick check" initial physical exam in Group A was 59 ± 3 seconds (mean ± SD, 95% CI of mean; 6.8; Figure 3(a)). Integration of PersUS into an initial physical exam directly upon patient admission in the ED allowed the quantification of possible excess time

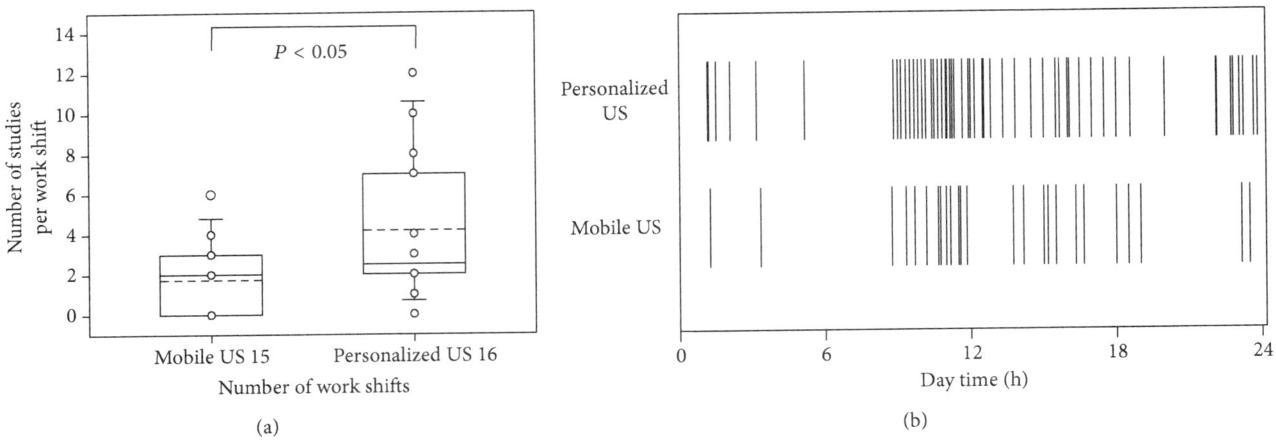


FIGURE 1: Increased personalized ultrasound use in critical care medicine (substudy 1). Randomized comparison of personalized versus mobile ultrasound. (a) number of exams per work shift; (b) distribution pattern over three work shifts. These results indicate the increase in request of the frequency for ultrasound exams during ward rounds (8 a.m., 1 p.m., 8 p.m.) or shortly thereafter, which can be better implemented with personalized ultrasound.

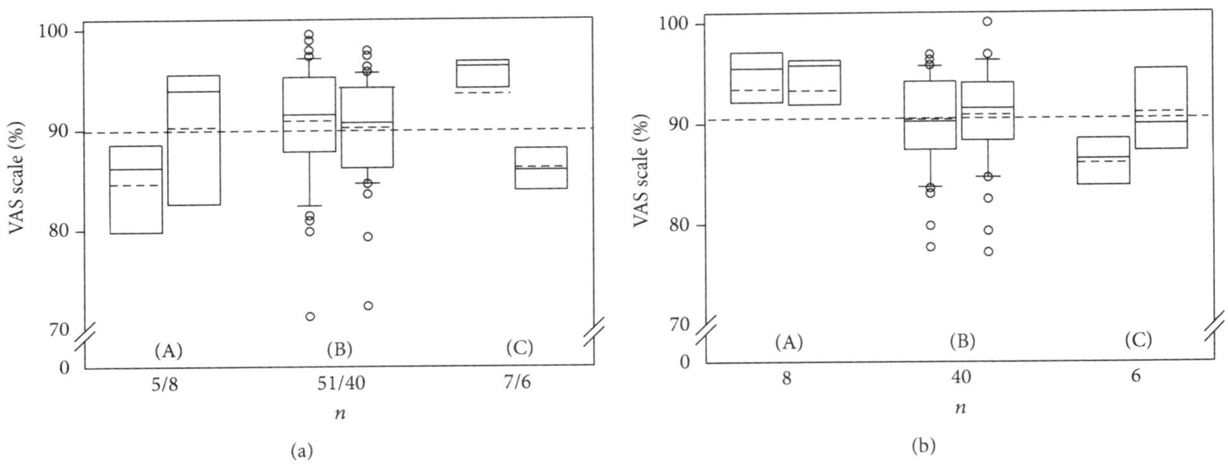


FIGURE 2: Physician assessment of diagnostic quality, ultrasound-guided interventions, and reproducibility when using a personalized ultrasound device (VAS scale; substudy 2). (A): pericardial effusion; (B): pleural effusion; (C): urinary bladder. (a) Each left boxplot shows diagnostic ultrasound, each right boxplot ultrasound-guided punctures. (b) Physician assessment of feasibility in ultrasound-guided interventions with a personalized device (VAS scale): inclination to use PersUS in future examinations (each left boxplot) and inclination to use PersUS for other anatomical regions (each right boxplot).

consumption. Although PersUS was integrated easily into this physical exam, it caused a marked prolongation of the examination time to a mean of 154 ± 6 seconds (95% CI 13.2) in Group B (Figure 3(a)). However, in Group B, a change of management in 6/22 (27%) cases as well as valuable additional information for immediate recognition of underlying disease in 19/22 (86%) patients (10 with dyspnoea/thorax pain; 9 with abdominal pain) was registered by the examiner.

*3.4. Substudy 4: Integration into Critical Care Ward Rounds.* PersUS was integrated into 53 regular ward rounds with a total of 1007 patients on two wards. Mean ward round operation time was 142 ± 33 minutes with 18 ± 3 patients per ward.

In 194 of 1007 (19%) patient visits, an ultrasound exam was requested due to one or more indications per patient (Figure 3(b), Table 2). According to the randomization, 133 questions regarding 95 patients in Group A remained unanswered as a result of a strict removal of the PersUS. In Group B, when focused PersUS was available, 134 questions regarding 99 patients could be answered while focused PersUS exams were applied at each respective patient contact. The average PersUS examination time was 3.6 ± 2 minutes per patient and was rated 2.4 ± 0.9 (good to satisfactory). Interestingly, this PersUS integration into the ward rounds management effected a significant reduction of the time needed per patient from a mean of 8.9 minutes to 7.2 minutes (Figure 3(b)). Patient referral to the echo lab for further examination was deemed necessary for 95 of 473 patients

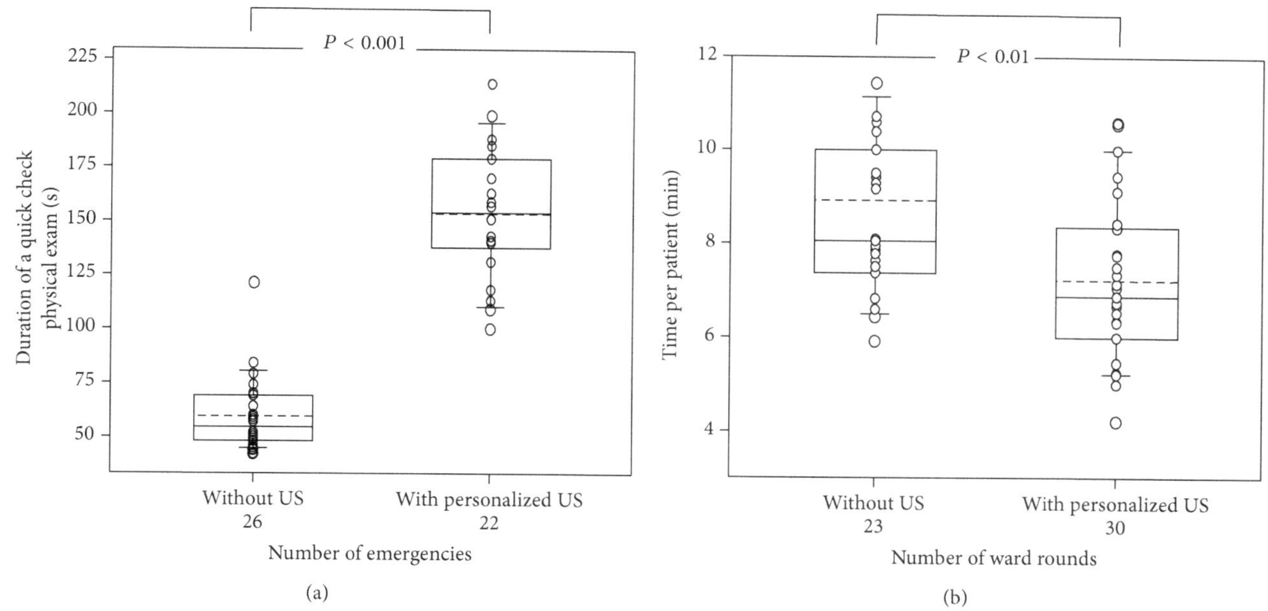


FIGURE 3: Influence of personalized ultrasound on time when integrated into the physical examination of emergency admissions or within regular ward rounds (substudies 3 and 4). Although mean examination time per emergency patient increased (a), average time consumption per patient on ward rounds markedly decreased (b).

(20.1%) in Group A; however, only 12 of 534 patients (2.2%) in Group B with 16 distinct questions were referred. This was mainly the case in request for Doppler examination of diastolic function, which is not yet available in PersUS.

Based on clinical context, ten categories of focused ultrasound examinations were established. (Table 2).

There were no adverse results or effects during any patient exams or interventions with PersUS or MobUS in all substudies.

## 4. Discussion

The main findings of our studies were that personalized ultrasound was safe, feasible, of good quality, and easily implementable into routine critical care work. The availability of personalized ultrasound increased the requests for focused ultrasound exams and offered an image quality comparable to high-quality mobile ultrasound, allowing targeted decision-making. While PersUS extended the examination time in emergency admissions it positively influenced patient management, increased information gain about the underlying disease, reduced the contact times per patient in ward rounds, and lowered the request for patient referral to an echo lab.

*4.1. Feasibility of Integration into Clinical Operating Processes.* Ultrasound and echocardiography in critical care medicine were considered for widespread use [8] and recommended in a recent guideline as a complement to a physical examination in coronary and intensive care units [3]. It has been shown that ultrasound in the ED or ICU supports the early finding of main diagnoses and has the potential to eliminate other differential diagnoses [9, 10]. However, clinical integration concepts are lacking [3, 5]. PersUS allows a more sophisticated integration into the daily workflow and clinical pathways so that ad hoc procedures can be realized.

However, PersUS offers more options: it can complement [11] or replace a complete physical exam while screening [12] or be interwoven with the physical exam or algorithm-like procedures such as the focused assessment of abdominal sonography (FAST). It can be utilised in triage [13, 14] or integrated into the advanced life support as focused echocardiography (FEEL exam) [15–17]. Furthermore, a PersUS could be incorporated into more complex operating procedures such as work shifts and ward rounds.

The ready availability of PersUS increased the number of requests for focused ultrasound examinations. These were not referred to another operator or echo lab but executed as point-of-care exams in real time or shortly thereafter by the same physician determining the indication. The types of indications were related to cardiac chamber dimensions and function as well as pericardial and pleural effusions and reflect recent recommendations for focused echocardiography in cardiology [18]. In critical care and ventilated patients, effusion diagnostic and interventions were the main reasons for the increase of requests, thus reflecting a real need for transcutaneous ultrasound exams in critical care practice.

*4.2. Is a 3.5-Inch Screen Sufficient to Make Decisions or Guide Punctures?* The PersUS screen size raises concerns about image quality [19], although similar devices have been demonstrated to provide the same accuracy in cardiac sonoanatomy (endo-/pericardial effusion) as high-end echocardiography [20, 21]. We observed a highly reliable image quality for evaluation of effusions and basic cardiac

TABLE 2: Indications for clinical context-based ultrasound requests within routine ward rounds without or with personalized ultrasound (PersUS). Randomized determination of availability of PersUS. Group A did not receive ultrasound within a ward round and indications regularly determined a systematic echocardiography in a laboratory. In contrast, Group B received personalized ultrasound during the ward round.

| Category number | Indication for request of a focused exam within ward round | Group A No US | Group B PersUS | Total | Decision for referral to echo lab Group A versus B |
|---|---|---|---|---|---|
| No. of patients in ward round | | 473 | 534 | 1007 | 95 versus 12 |
| No. of patients receiving indications for echocardiography | | 95 | 99 | 194 | 95 versus 12 |
| 1 | Focused echo (1) | 22 | 16 | 38 | 22/1 |
| 2 | EF of both ventricles | 41 | 37 | 78 | 41/6 |
| 3 | Pleural effusion (both hemithoraces) including quantification | 37 | 42 | 83 | 37/4 |
| 4 | Ascites, marking for later puncture or puncture (2) | 11 | 8 | 18 | 11/1 |
| 5 | Valve function (3) | 3 | 4 | 7 | 3/2 |
| 6 | Mitral insufficiency (focused assessment prior TOE) | 4 | 0 | 4 | 4/0 |
| 7 | Resuscitation (FEEL protocol) | 0 | 1 | 1 | — |
| 8 | Urinary bladder filling state, postrenal failure | 1 | 2 | 3 | 1/0 |
| 9 | Pericardial effusion (exclusion, or size and clinical course) | 22 | 18 | 40 | 22/0 |
| 10 | Pulmonary valve replacement, postinterventional check | 2 | 6 | 8 | 2/0 |
| Indications total | | 133 | 134 | 267 | 133/14 |

(1) Combined focused TTE including EF, oriented valve morphology and function, left and right ventricular dimensions. Clinical contexts contained focus on hypertension (LV-hypertrophy), right heart pressure overload, NSTEMI (LVEF), atrial fibrillation (valves, LVEF), postintervention (EF, pericardial effusion), pulmonary vein isolation therapy in case of atrial fibrillation (EF, pericardial effusion).
(2) Including 3 cases per group of the request soft tissue or musculoskeletal assessment for hematoma in the groin after coronary angiography or after pacemaker/defibrillator implantation in the anterior chest or shoulder area.
(3) Main issues were focused assessment of aortic valve opening in the elderly.

anatomy and function in critical care. Our data suggests that the size itself has little impairment on decision making in real time. In agreement with recent studies of the same type of device [20, 21] we found that this quality was sufficient for real-time punctures of various targets. However, for more advanced examinations, such as diastolic function, MobUS seems to be the better choice.

*4.3. Time Constraints.* One concern of PersUS integration in our study was the investment of up to 10 minutes per ultrasound exam. Time is an essential component in acute care. Early application of ultrasound has been shown to reduce the number of viable diagnoses in the emergency setting [9] and determine outcome [13, 16, 17, 22], leading to calls for documentation of focused ultrasound examination length [18]. For goal-directed echocardiography, mean acquisition time was 10.5 ± 4.2 min [23]. Duration depends on the type of focused exam [3] and the body region (cardiac, lung, abdomen, and multiple regions). Exam times can vary from seconds up to 10 min [23–30]. The screening capability of PersUS allows effusions, for example, to be examined faster in triage [12, 13, 26] or within Advanced Life Support (maximum 10 seconds for a subxiphoidal view) during pauses between chest compressions [25]. In contrast, it was estimated that the comprehensive cardiac or abdominal exams would take more than 20 min [4, 18, 29, 31]. Although we found similar results in our substudies of cardiac diagnostic ultrasound, the integration of a quick-check ultrasound exam such as the one in the acute setting was considerably faster. The PersUS exam in our study was not restricted to cardiac indications [30], contained fewer than 5 questions per patient, and required much less time than was expected [32].

*4.4. Future Remarks.* We suggest combining the physical and PersUS exams into a standard clinical exam protocol [33]. This would yield increased implementation in the clinical context of acute and critical care medicine and cost-effective analysis as calculated for other settings [34–36].

*4.5. Limitations.* Due to the prospective design and the broad number of patients examined in different substudies and hospitals, we did not have the possibility to review all examinations by blinded experts. In addition, blinding of the pictures/movies according to the US device was technically not possible. Therefore, comparison between different US devices might be subjective according to the examiners observation. Moreover, this study does not intend to suggest that focused and personal ultrasound examinations are sufficient to understand the patient's complete physiological state. Complete evaluation of dyspnoea, for example, requires comprehensive echocardiography [18]; however, this is rarely achievable in all critical care units in real time, leaving the treating physician to obtain additional information for a specific clinical problem before the more specialised practitioner is involved. Our study required neither comparison with findings using a standard ultrasound machine and a comprehensive exam nor confirmation of findings from a second expert sonographer. It is not generalisable to other hospitals. However, there is, to our knowledge, no existing gold standard for focused ultrasound combined with clinical examination.

## 5. Conclusions and Key Message

The integration of personalized ultrasound in the daily acute and critical care workflow is safe and easily applied to patient admissions, routine procedures, and ward rounds with little additional time requirement. It will accelerate and improve decision making and interventions. We propose the development of novel ultrasound-based clinical pathways, standard operation procedures, and workflow protocols by integration of PersUS.

## Abbreviations

ED: Emergency department
PersUS: Personalized ultrasound
MobUS: Mobile ultrasound.

## Conflict of Interests

The authors have no conflict of interests to declare.

## Authors' Contribution

Raoul Breitkreutz planned the study and analyzed the data. Marco Campo dell' Orto (substudies 1 and 2), Peter M. Zechner (substudy 3), and Florian H. Seeger (substudy 4) were responsible for study planning and execution, participated in the respective substudy protocols, and completed data acquisition. Tanja Stenger checked statistical accuracy. Felix Walcher provided oversight to the study. Raoul Breitkreutz drafted the paper, which was revised by Marco Campo dell'Orto, Florian H. Seeger, Felix Walcher, Peter M. Zechner, and Colleen Cuca and reviewed and approved by all the coauthors. Raoul Breitkreutz and Marco Campo dell'Orto contributed equally to the study.

## Acknowledgments

The authors thank T. O'Neill, K.-U. Lempertz, and S. Müller from GE Healthcare for their support. They are indebted to the Department of Cardiology of the Goethe University Hospital, in particular to H. Fox and S. Heyl as well as T. Schwietz, W. Weihs, G. Geyer, H. V. Groesdonk, and A. Meiser from the University of the Saarland for partial data acquisition of substudies 1 and 2 and H. Wurzer from the Department of Internal Medicine, LKH Graz West. This study was based on a clinical evaluation agreement by GE Medical Systems/Ultrasound and Primary Care Diagnostics LLC, Wauwatosa, WI, USA, and RB and supported with a fund explicitly to RB. There was a partial fund by SonoABCD.org, acute and critical care ultrasound regional network.

## References

[1] American College of Emergency Physicians, "ACEP emergency ultrasound guidelines–2001," *Annals of Emergency Medicine*, vol. 38, no. 4, pp. 470–481, 2001.

[2] Expert Round Table on Ultrasound in ICU, "International expert statement on training standards for critical care ultrasonography," *Intensive Care Medicine*, vol. 37, no. 7, pp. 1077–1083, 2011.

[3] R. Sicari, M. Galderisi, J.-U. Voigt et al., "The use of pocket-size imaging devices: a position statement of the European association of echocardiography," *The European Journal of Echocardiography*, vol. 12, no. 2, pp. 85–87, 2011.

[4] J. B. Seward, P. S. Douglas, R. Erbel et al., "Hand-carried cardiac ultrasound (HCU) device: recommendations regarding new technology. A report from the echocardiography task force on new technology of the nomenclature and standards committee of the American Society of Echocardiography," *Journal of the American Society of Echocardiography*, vol. 15, no. 4, pp. 369–373, 2002.

[5] J. Roelandt, J. W. Wladimiroff, and A. M. Baars, "Ultrasonic real time imaging with a hand-held-scanner. Part II. Initial clinical experience," *Ultrasound in Medicine and Biology*, vol. 4, no. 2, pp. 93–97, 1978.

[6] J. Kluger, "The 50 Best Inventions of 2009," *Time*, 2009.

[7] K. Skjetne, T. Graven, B. O. Haugen, Ø. Salvesen, J. O. Kleinau, and H. Dalen, "Diagnostic influence of cardiovascular screening by pocket-size ultrasound in a cardiac unit," *The European Journal of Echocardiography*, vol. 12, no. 10, pp. 737–743, 2011.

[8] B. P. Cholley, A. Vieillard-Baron, and A. Mebazaa, "Echocardiography in the ICU: time for widespread use!," *Intensive Care Medicine*, vol. 32, no. 1, pp. 9–10, 2006.

[9] A. E. Jones, V. S. Tayal, D. M. Sullivan, and J. A. Kline, "Randomized, controlled trial of immediate versus delayed goal-directed ultrasound to identify the cause of nontraumatic hypotension in emergency department patients," *Critical Care Medicine*, vol. 32, no. 8, pp. 1703–1708, 2004.

[10] M. X. Joseph, P. J. Disney, R. da Costa, and S. J. Hutchison, "Transthoracic echocardiography to identify or exclude cardiac cause of shock," *Chest*, vol. 126, no. 5, pp. 1592–1597, 2004.

[11] S. L. Kobal, S. Atar, and R. J. Siegel, "Hand-carried ultrasound improves the bedside cardiovascular examination," *Chest*, vol. 126, no. 3, pp. 693–701, 2004.

[12] A. C. Sisley, G. S. Rozycki, R. B. Ballard, N. Namias, J. P. Salomone, and D. V. Feliciano, "Rapid detection of traumatic

effusion using surgeon-performed ultrasonography," *Journal of Trauma*, vol. 44, no. 2, pp. 291–297, 1998.

[13] D. Plummer, D. Brunette, R. Asinger, and E. Ruiz, "Emergency department echocardiography improves outcome in penetrating cardiac injury," *Annals of Emergency Medicine*, vol. 21, no. 6, pp. 709–712, 1992.

[14] A. W. Kirkpatrick, M. Sirois, K. B. Laupland et al., "Hand-held thoracic sonography for detecting post-traumatic pneumothoraces: the extended focused assessment with sonography for trauma (EFAST)," *Journal of Trauma*, vol. 57, no. 2, pp. 288–295, 2004.

[15] R. Breitkreutz, F. Walcher, and F. H. Seeger, "Focused echocardiographic evaluation in resuscitation management: concept of an advanced life support-conformed algorithm," *Critical Care Medicine*, vol. 35, no. 5, pp. S150–S161, 2007.

[16] J. P. Nolan, J. Soar, D. A. Zideman et al., "European Resuscitation Council guidelines for resuscitation 2010 section 1. Executive summary," *Resuscitation*, vol. 81, no. 10, pp. 1219–1276, 2010.

[17] C. D. Deakin, J. P. Nolan, J. Soar et al., "European Resuscitation Council guidelines for resuscitation 2010 section 4. Adult advanced life support," *Resuscitation*, vol. 81, no. 10, pp. 1305–1352, 2010.

[18] A. J. Labovitz, V. E. Noble, M. Bierig et al., "Focused cardiac ultrasound in the emergent setting: a consensus statement of the American society of echocardiography and American college of emergency physicians," *Journal of the American Society of Echocardiography*, vol. 23, no. 12, pp. 1225–1230, 2010.

[19] M. Blaivas, L. Brannam, and D. Theodoro, "Ultrasound image quality comparison between an inexpensive handheld emergency department (ED) ultrasound machine and a large mobile ED ultrasound system," *Academic Emergency Medicine*, vol. 11, no. 7, pp. 778–781, 2004.

[20] C. Prinz and J. U. Voigt, "Diagnostic accuracy of a hand-held ultrasound scanner in routine patients referred for echocardiography," *Journal of the American Society of Echocardiography*, vol. 24, no. 2, pp. 111–116, 2011.

[21] M. J. Liebo, R. L. Israel, E. O. Lillie, M. R. Smith, D. S. Rubenson, and E. J. Topol, "Is pocket mobile echocardiography the next-generation stethoscope? a cross-sectional comparison of rapidly acquired images with standard transthoracic echocardiography," *Annals of Internal Medicine*, vol. 155, no. 1, pp. 33–38, 2011.

[22] N. P. Symbas, P. F. Bongiorno, and P. N. Symbas, "Blunt cardiac rupture: the utility of emergency department ultrasound," *Annals of Thoracic Surgery*, vol. 67, no. 5, pp. 1274–1276, 1999.

[23] A. R. Manasia, H. M. Nagaraj, R. B. Kodali et al., "Feasibility and potential clinical utility of goal-directed transthoracic echocardiography performed by noncardiologist intensivists using a small hand-carried device (SonoHeart) in critically ill patients," *Journal of Cardiothoracic and Vascular Anesthesia*, vol. 19, no. 2, pp. 155–159, 2005.

[24] P. Ferrada, R. J. Anand, J. Whelan et al., "Limited transthoracic echocardiogram: so easy any trauma attending can do it," *Journal of Trauma*, vol. 71, no. 5, pp. 1327–1331, 2011.

[25] R. Breitkreutz, S. Price, H. V. Steiger et al., "Focused echocardiographic evaluation in life support and peri-resuscitation of emergency patients: a prospective trial," *Resuscitation*, vol. 81, no. 11, pp. 1527–1533, 2010.

[26] F. Walcher, M. Weinlich, G. Conrad et al., "Prehospital ultrasound imaging improves management of abdominal trauma," *The British Journal of Surgery*, vol. 93, no. 2, pp. 238–242, 2006.

[27] M. Dijos, Y. Pucheux, and M. Lafitte, "Fast track echo of abdominal aortic aneurysm using a real pocket-ultrasound device at bedside," *Echocardiography*, vol. 29, no. 3, pp. 285–290, 2012.

[28] C. A. Frederiksen, P. Juhl-Olsen, U. T. Larsen, D. G. Nielsen, B. Eika, and E. Sloth, "New pocket echocardiography device is interchangeable with high-end portable system when performed by experienced examiners," *Acta Anaesthesiologica Scandinavica*, vol. 54, no. 10, pp. 1217–1223, 2010.

[29] F. Lapostolle, T. Petrovic, G. Lenoir et al., "Usefulness of hand-held ultrasound devices in out-of-hospital diagnosis performed by emergency physicians," *The American Journal of Emergency Medicine*, vol. 24, no. 2, pp. 237–242, 2006.

[30] N. Cardim, C. Fernandez Golfin, D. Ferreira et al., "Usefulness of a new miniaturized echocardiographic system in outpatient cardiology consultations as an extension of physical examination," *Journal of the American Society of Echocardiography*, vol. 24, no. 2, pp. 117–124, 2011.

[31] J. Reuss, H. Weiss, T. Wanner, and H.-G. Leser, "Time requirements of medical and non-medical personnel for ultrasound studies," *Ultraschall in der Medizin*, vol. 19, no. 3, pp. 126–129, 1998.

[32] M. Rugolotto, B. S. Hu, D. H. Liang, and I. Schnittger, "Rapid assessment of cardiac anatomy and function with a new hand-carried ultrasound device (OptiGo): a comparison with standard echocardiography," *The European Journal of Echocardiography*, vol. 2, no. 4, pp. 262–269, 2001.

[33] T. Xie, A. J. Chamoun, M. McCulloch, N. Tsiouris, Y. Birnbaum, and M. Ahmad, "Rapid screening of cardiac patients with a miniaturized hand-held ultrasound imager—comparisons with physical examination and conventional two-dimensional echocardiography," *Clinical Cardiology*, vol. 27, no. 4, pp. 241–245, 2004.

[34] K. Greaves, P. Jeetley, M. Hickman et al., "The use of hand-carried ultrasound in the hospital setting-A cost-effective analysis," *Journal of the American Society of Echocardiography*, vol. 18, no. 6, pp. 620–625, 2005.

[35] E. C. Vourvouri, L. Y. Koroleva, F. J. Ten Cate et al., "Clinical utility and cost effectiveness of a personal ultrasound imager for cardiac evaluation during consultation rounds in patients with suspected cardiac disease," *Heart*, vol. 89, no. 7, pp. 727–730, 2003.

[36] G. Giannotti, S. Mondillo, M. Galderisi et al., "Hand-held echocardiography: added value in clinical cardiological assessment," *Cardiovascular Ultrasound*, vol. 3, article 7, 2005.

# 21

# Minimizing ED Waiting Times and Improving Patient Flow and Experience of Care

**Assaad Sayah,**[1] **Loni Rogers,**[2,3] **Karthik Devarajan,**[2,3]
**Lisa Kingsley-Rocker,**[1] **and Luis F. Lobon**[1]

[1] *Department of Emergency Medicine, Cambridge Health Alliance, 1493 Cambridge Street, Cambridge, MA 02139, USA*
[2] *Tufts University School of Medicine, Boston, MA, USA*
[3] *Heller School of Social Policy and Management, Brandeis University, Waltham, MA, USA*

Correspondence should be addressed to Assaad Sayah; asayah@cha.harvard.edu

Academic Editor: Chak W. Kam

We conducted a pre- and postintervention analysis to assess the impact of a process improvement project at the Cambridge Hospital ED. Through a comprehensive and collaborative process, we reengineered the emergency patient experience from arrival to departure. The ED operational changes have had a significant positive impact on all measured metrics. Ambulance diversion decreased from a mean of 148 hours per quarter before changes in July 2006 to 0 hours since April 2007. ED total length of stay decreased from a mean of 204 minutes before the changes to 132 minutes. Press Ganey patient satisfaction scores rose from the 12th percentile to the 59th percentile. ED patient volume grew by 11%, from a mean of 7,221 patients per quarter to 8,044 patients per quarter. Compliance with ED specific quality core measures improved from a mean of 71% to 97%. The mean rate of ED patients that left without being seen (LWBS) dropped from 4.1% to 0.9%. Improving ED operational efficiency allowed us to accommodate increasing volume while improving the quality of care and satisfaction of the ED patients with minimal additional resources, space, or staffing.

## 1. Introduction

At the intersection of diagnosis, treatment, and immense patient volumes, the Emergency Department (ED) is arguably the most operationally complex clinical setting of the modern hospital. Unfortunately, it may also be the least understood. From 1995 to 2009, annual ED visits in the US increased by 41% (from 96.5 million to 136.1 million). At the same time, however, the number of hospital Emergency Departments decreased by 27% (from 2,446 to 1,779) [1–3]. Long ED waiting and turnaround times have been shown to decrease both quality outcomes and patient satisfaction [4–6]. Among US Emergency Departments in 2010, only 31% achieved the appropriate triage targets for their patients, while only 48% admitted their patients within 6 hours [7].

Like many other EDs around the country, The Cambridge Hospital (TCH) ED suffered from similar patient flow issues including long waits, inefficient processes, and poor patient satisfaction. This paper describes the changes implemented at TCH and the resulting impact on quality, patient flow, and experience of care.

## 2. Methods

We conducted a pre- and postintervention analysis to assess the impact of a patient flow improvement project at TCH, an academic public institution located in Cambridge Massachusetts with an annual ED census of approximately 30,000 patients. Every patient that entered the ED from January 2005 to December 2011 was included as a study participant. The protocol received an Exempt Status from the Cambridge Health Alliance IRB.

In mid-2006, we committed to a system-wide process improvement project aimed at optimizing the ED patient experience by expediting throughput and flow. The Patient

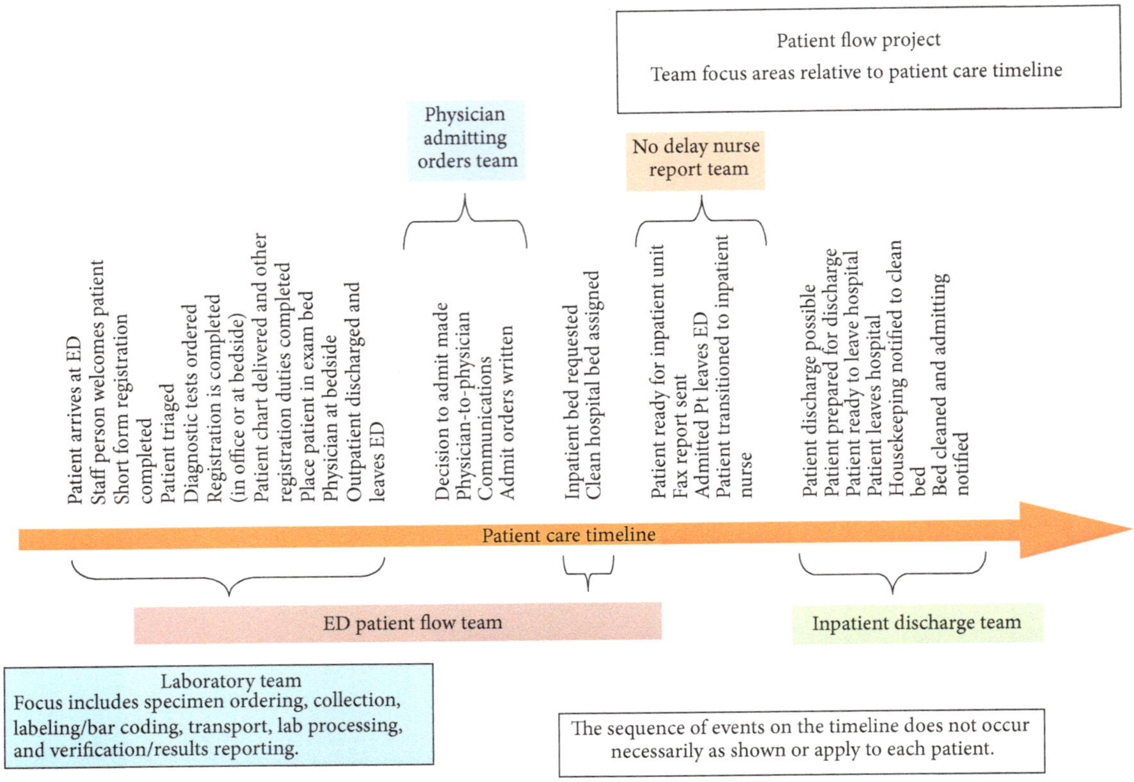


FIGURE 1: Patient flow diagram.

Flow Project used modern quality improvement operational methodologies and sought to achieve the following goals:

(i) to improve patient flow in an effective and patient centered manner;

(ii) to implement evidence-based best practices;

(iii) to utilize improvement methodologies, tools, and measures;

(iv) to utilize a multidisciplinary, multicampus single solution approach;

(v) to explore the reasons for ED leakage.

To accomplish this, we developed a patient care timeline for each ED visit (Figure 1) and created five interdisciplinary teams to focus on evaluating and improving different areas of care. The teams and their missions are outlined as follows.

(1) *ED Patient Flow.* Minimizing the time that patients spend in the ED through the application of best practices.

(2) *Laboratory Turnaround Time.* Managing the ordering, collecting, testing, and verification of lab work through improved and standardized procedures.

(3) *No Delay Nurse Report.* Transfer of admitted patients to inpatient unit within 30 minutes of ED Nurse's report.

(4) *Physician Admitting Orders.* Expediting completion of admitting orders by inpatient team for admitted patients.

(5) *Inpatient Discharges.* Decreasing inpatient length of stay through effective discharge planning activities.

Each team studied the patient's experience at different points in the care timeline, identified the bottlenecks, and developed a plan of action. Teams met weekly and reported to the project leadership biweekly. We organized quarterly daylong summits for teams to present their findings, progress, and recommendations. Every team's plan of action recommendation was vetted by all five teams and implemented immediately after majority approval. Eighteen months after the start of the project, we held a final summit which marked the end of the analysis and recommendation phase.

The overall recommendations from the teams were to implement front-end reengineering, improve throughput and expedite patient disposition. Reengineering the arrival phase of the ED patient experience included the creation of the "Patient Partner" role, establishing a rapid assessment (RA) unit, and instituting bedside registration.

Due to the diversity of our patient population, we hired nonclinical multilingual persons with customer service background to fulfill this important role. Our Patient Partners welcomed and greeted patients, performed a miniregistration, generated a patient encounter in the electronic medical record, and escorted the patient immediately to a RA bed.

We simplified our initial registration process to the bare minimum in order to identify the patient's electronic health record (EHR) or create one for a new patient in the most expeditious way. This new miniregistration consisted of three questions: name, social security number (or date of birth), and chief complaint. Eventually, during downtime between tests and procedures, full bedside registration was performed after nursing and physician assessment, patient stabilization, and initiation of patient care.

After arrival and miniregistration, patients were immediately escorted into the RA unit where they met our clinicians. The RA unit combined the space, resources, and personnel of the previous registration, triage, and express care areas. The purpose of this unit was to facilitate rapid assessment and treatment at the point of entry to the ED. We augmented space and staffing, minimized redundancies, and created parallel functions without adding any new resources. Our plan was to triage patients in accordance with the national average of 7 minutes using emergency severity index (ESI) triage protocol. In the RA unit, low acuity patients (ESI 4 and 5) would get their complete care in the RA unit, without ever entering the acute ED area. Patients triaged with the more concerning ESI levels (1, 2, and 3) would be immediately moved to the acute ED areas where they could be evaluated and treated by the clinical team.

Improving ED throughput involved keeping all beds full while allowing specialized areas to be flexible. To this end, all beds became telemetry capable and we loosened up the rigid designations of specialized areas (adult, pediatric, trauma, psychiatric, etc.) so that any patient could be evaluated in any bed during high census intervals in order to maximize bed utilization. We also empowered the Charge Nurse to be the gatekeeper for patient flow in the department by problem solving during volume surges, expediting bed access for new patients, and coordinating timely assessment, treatment, and disposition of patients with the clinical teams.

As we examined the ED work processes for inefficiencies, we found a lack of clarity in staff roles including many gaps and overlap in their responsibilities. While this was probably a consequence of the need to multitask and collaborate in the ED, we found that this led to unclear accountability, which in turn resulted in redundancies, poor communication, medical errors, and delay of care. Consequently, we defined and clarified the roles of all ED personnel. We also trained them to perform tasks that were otherwise done by visiting specialized staff like phlebotomy and respiratory therapy. The laboratory team additionally focused on improving diagnostic turnaround times.

It is common knowledge that Emergency Department crowding is directly related to the total length of stay and boarding of admitted patients. To that end, we had a high focus on expediting the disposition of admitted patients and reducing their ED total length of stay. One of the interventions that we implemented was early identification of patients with high likelihood of being admitted even before all ancillary data was available. We created a special status for these patients on our electronic ED tracking board and made it accessible to the hospital admitting service, the hospitalists, the residents, and nurses on the inpatient floors, housekeeping, and transport. This provided an early warning process to all stakeholders that could affect the flow of admitted patients and allowed the admitting service time to prepare and receive the admission.

We also developed methods to facilitate nursing and physician handoffs of admitted patients. For nursing, we implemented a faxed nursing report handoff. This report format was developed jointly by the ED and inpatient nurses and included all pertinent clinical and nonclinical information and was used on all noncritical patients. Once the patient was ready to be sent to the inpatient floor, several actions occur in order: the ED nurse would hand the completed nursing report to the ED secretary who would in turn fax it to the inpatient unit and call to verify that it had been received. The nurse on the inpatient unit receiving the patient would review the report and call the ED with any questions or concerns. The patient was then transported to the floor within 30 minutes of faxing the report unless valid concerns were communicated by the inpatient staff. The faxed report was ultimately eliminated in 2011 when the inpatient service implemented the electronic medical record (EPIC) and was able to visualize the ED record in real-time.

Physician hand-off was reduced to one call from the ED to a single lead hospitalist who was designated on a daily basis to receive all communications from the ED regarding medical admissions. At the end of the call, the ED provider and hospitalist agreed on the patient diagnosis and designated an admitting attending and resident who were responsible for patient care, the level of care necessary (e.g., ICU, telemetry, or medical), the admission status (e.g., "inpatient" or "observation"), and any other special needs for the patient (e.g., "isolation" or "watch"). The lead hospitalist would communicate the information to the chosen admission team. This team was encouraged to call the ED with any questions or concerns otherwise they would complete the admission workup once the patient was transported to the inpatient unit.

Other interventions included early recognition and discharge of patients from the inpatient units to create beds for the ED particularly during high census periods. These interventions were supported by an institution wide escalation process to notify all stakeholders and leaders of critical ED boarding situations and recruit their assistance to find solutions in real-time. Additionally, we instituted an institutional internal rapid response plan (Code Help) to provide the ED with additional resources to safely care for patients during high ED volume times and decompress the ED policy that allows inpatient units to receive ED patients. When activated, Code Help requires that all ED admitted patients would be transported to the inpatient units within 30 minutes even if they have to be temporarily treated in inpatient unit hallways.

*2.1. Data Collection and Processing.* The data was collected using the electronic medical record systems (Meditech and EPIC). Timestamps were used to compute the total length of stay time. Flags and patient records were used to determine whether a patient left without being seen (LWBS). Patient records were reviewed to access if acute myocardial infarction (AMI) and community acquired pneumonia (CAP) patients met the appropriate quality core measures. Patient Satisfaction Surveys were sent and data compiled by Press Ganey associates.

Table 1: Raw data used for statistical analysis, collected from January 2005 to December 2011.

| Time | Median patient satisfaction per quarter (Press Ganey percentile) | Median door-to-provider time per quarter (in minutes) | Median total length of stay per quarter (in minutes) | Total hours on diversion per quarter | Percentage successfully meeting core measures per quarter | Left without being seen median rate per quarter (%) | ED Volume per quarter |
|---|---|---|---|---|---|---|---|
| Before | | | | | | | |
| FY05-Q1 | 6 | 69 | 212 | 165.79 | 66 | 4.15 | 7,293 |
| FY05-Q2 | 9 | 64 | 198 | 189.78 | 68 | 4.12 | 7,008 |
| FY05-Q3 | 15 | 62 | 205 | 172.33 | 66 | 4.09 | 7,411 |
| FY05-Q4 | 9 | 58 | 208 | 185.42 | 72 | 4.1 | 7,367 |
| FY06-Q1 | 15 | 67 | 205 | 104.31 | 78 | 4.35 | 7,394 |
| FY06-Q2 | 16 | 58 | 197 | 70.21 | 76 | 3.82 | 6,852 |
| During | | | | | | | |
| FY06-Q3 | 41 | 62 | 195 | 76.53 | 80 | 4.1 | 7,051 |
| FY06-Q4 | 23 | 59 | 201 | 61.70 | 82 | 3.9 | 7,184 |
| FY07-Q1 | 22 | 53 | 191 | 40.99 | 81 | 3.37 | 7,240 |
| FY07-Q2 | 27 | 49 | 185 | 0.00 | 95 | 2.4 | 6,922 |
| FY07-Q3 | 31 | 52 | 187 | 0.00 | 94 | 2.16 | 7,274 |
| FY07-Q4 | 43 | 46 | 185 | 0.00 | 96 | 1.86 | 7,360 |
| FY08-Q1 | 43 | 37 | 172 | 0.00 | 94 | 1.05 | 7,394 |
| After | | | | | | | |
| FY08-Q2 | 46 | 29 | 162 | 0.00 | 94 | 1.14 | 7,283 |
| FY08-Q3 | 41 | 23 | 169 | 0.00 | 95 | 1.79 | 7,859 |
| FY08-Q4 | 49 | 23 | 164 | 0.00 | 99 | 1.25 | 7,805 |
| FY09-Q1 | 53 | 25 | 128 | 0.00 | 97 | 1.29 | 8,007 |
| FY09-Q2 | 57 | 27 | 122 | 0.00 | 97 | 0.77 | 7,155 |
| FY09-Q3 | 46 | 19 | 125 | 0.00 | 94 | 0.72 | 7,761 |
| FY09-Q4 | 49 | 18 | 128 | 0.00 | 97 | 1.13 | 8,942 |
| FY10-Q1 | 72 | 18 | 126 | 0.00 | 94 | 1.04 | 8,500 |
| FY10-Q2 | 71 | 19 | 122 | 0.00 | 99 | 0.87 | 8,386 |
| FY10-Q3 | 58 | 13 | 130 | 0.00 | 98 | 0.67 | 8,025 |
| FY10-Q4 | 71 | 14 | 126 | 0.00 | 96 | 0.89 | 8,492 |
| FY11-Q1 | 43 | 13 | 128 | 0.00 | 98 | 0.8 | 8,116 |
| FY11-Q2 | 63 | 14 | 126 | 0.00 | 96 | 0.52 | 7,797 |
| FY11-Q3 | 80 | 14 | 128 | 0.00 | 99 | 0.69 | 7,859 |
| FY11-Q4 | 78 | 14 | 130 | 0.00 | 98 | 0.49 | 7,913 |

FY: Fiscal year; Q: quarter.

*2.2. Primary Data Analysis.* For our data analysis, we used a two-sample independent $t$-test to compare the mean of the "before" data, from January 2005 (FY05-Q1) to June 2006 (FY06-Q2) to the mean of the "after" data, from April 2008 (FY08-Q2) to December 2011 (FY11-Q4), of the following parameters: (1) median ambulance hours on diversion per fiscal quarter, (2) Press Ganey Patient Satisfaction Percentile scores, (3) median ED total length of stay time, (4) median door-to-provider time (or "ED wait time"), (5) quality core measurements (such as AMI and CAP), and (6) percent of volume that left without being seen (LWBS). The data generated between May 2006 (FY06-Q3) and March 2008 (FY08-Q1) (i.e., the "during data") was not included in the analysis to decrease confounding; as during this time, the patient flow project was being implemented, and there were many changes occurring simultaneously. The "after" data collection began once all changes had been completely implemented. Equal variances were not assumed. We used the SPSS program for this analysis.

## 3. Results

Table 1 summarizes the quarterly data for the study duration. The ED operational changes have had a significant positive impact on all measured metrics (Table 2). Ambulance diversion decreased from a record high

Table 2: Summary of results and statistical analysis.

| Metric | Mean | | $P$ value | Mean difference | 95% Confidence interval of the mean difference |
|---|---|---|---|---|---|
| | Before* ($N = 6$) | After** ($N = 14$) | | | |
| Door-to-provider time | 63 | 18.14 | <0.001 | 44.86 | (39.83, 49.89) |
| Total length of stay | 204.17 | 132.29 | <0.001 | 71.88 | (62.24, 81.52) |
| ED hours on diversion | 147.97 | 0 | <0.001 | 147.97 | (96.53, 199.41) |
| Core measures (%) | 71 | 96.93 | <0.001 | 25.93 | (20.15, 31.35) |
| Left without being seen (%) | 4.11 | 0.92 | <0.001 | 3.18 | (2.94, 3.43) |
| Quarterly volume | 7220.83 | 8044.07 | <0.001 | 823.24 | (506.93, 1139.55) |
| Patient satisfaction Press Ganey (%ile) | 11.67 | 59.36 | <0.001 | 47.69 | (38.44, 55.95) |

*Before: FY05-Q1 to FY06-Q2.
**After: FY08-Q3 to FY11-Q4.

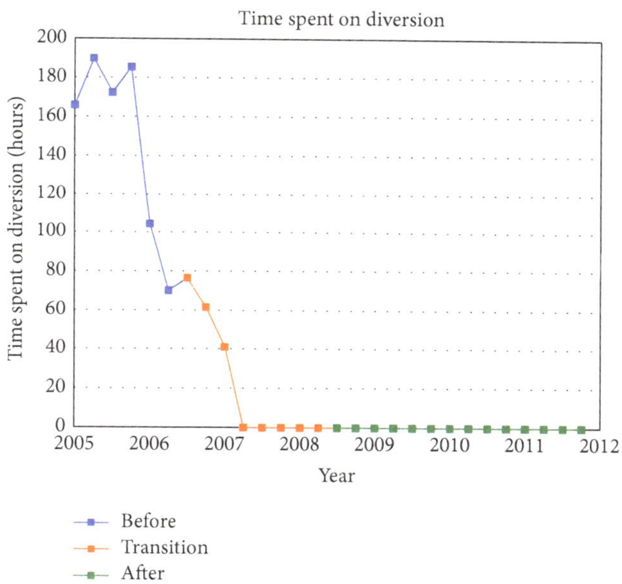


Figure 2: Hours of ambulance diversion. The quarterly number of hours the ED spent on diversion (refusing to receive ambulances).

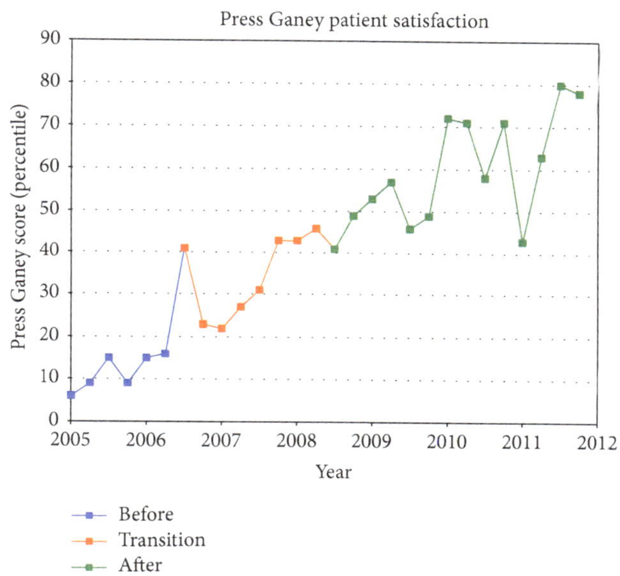


Figure 3: Quarterly patient satisfaction percentile scores based on Press Ganey report.

mean of 148 hours per fiscal quarter before changes to 0 hours since April 2007 (Figure 2). Press Ganey Patient satisfaction scores rose from 12th percentile in 2005 to 59th percentile after implementation (Figure 3). ED total length of stay decreased from a mean of 204 minutes to mean of 132 minutes (Figure 4). Door-to-provider time decreased from a mean of 63 minutes to mean of 18 minutes (Figure 5). Compliance with ED specific quality core measures improved from a mean of 71% to 97% (Figure 6). The mean rate of ED patients that left without being seen (before treatment) treatment was completely dropped from 4.1% to 0.9% (Figure 7). All improvements were statistically significant with a $P \leq 0.001$ (Table 2). More importantly these improvements occurred and were sustained amidst an 11% increase (from a mean of 7221 to 8044) in quarterly patient volume between 2005 and 2011 (Figure 8).

## 4. Discussion

TCH struggled with ED operations for many years and continued to fall short on many performance metrics. Prior to this initiative, diversions were routine, patient satisfaction scores were among the worst in the state, and there was a culture of inefficiency. In 2005, TCH spent more than 700 hours on diversion, scored in the 6th percentile in Patient Satisfaction, and had more than 4% of patients leave prior to receiving care (LWBS). Meanwhile, the ED was meeting quality core indicator rates for acute myocardial

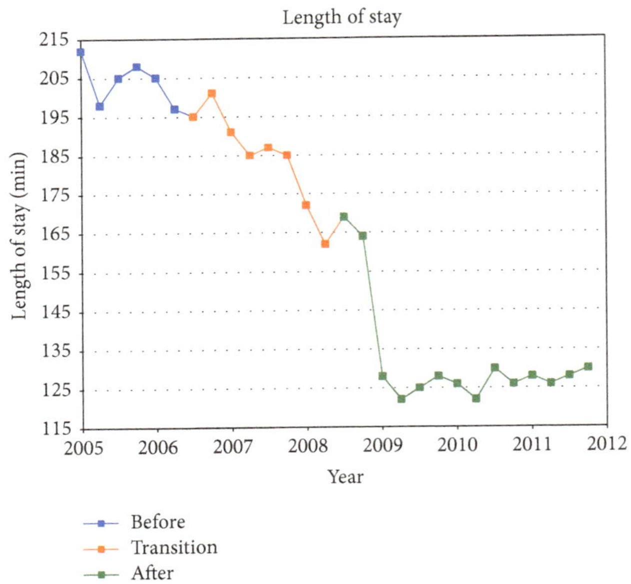


FIGURE 4: CHA ED total length of stay: the median time a patient spent from arrival to discharge.

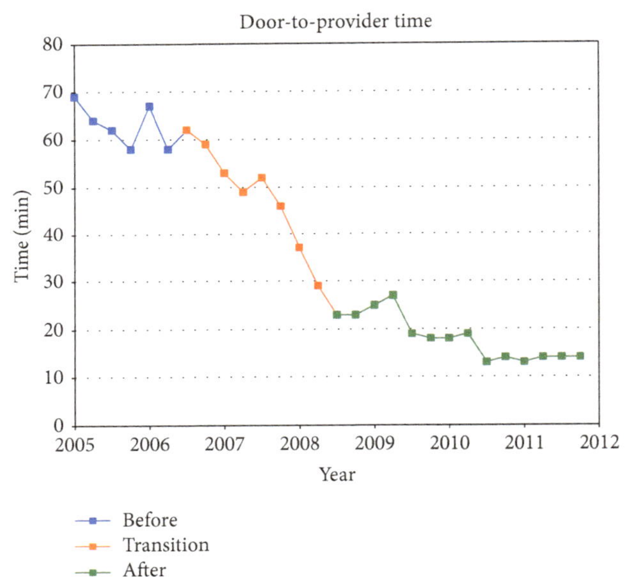


FIGURE 5: Median quarterly door-to-provider time: the median time patients spent waiting before being seen by a provider.

infarction (aspirin and a beta-blocker on arrival) and community acquired pneumonia (blood culture and appropriate antibiotics within 4 hours) less than 70% of the time.

Since the ED often served as first interaction between the hospital and its patients, poor ED performance affected institutional reputation and contributed to the stagnant ED volume levels. Since the ED accounts for more than 60% of all inpatient admissions, operational struggles were impacting the total patient experience for admitted patients. Improving the patient experience and quality of care in the ED was essential.

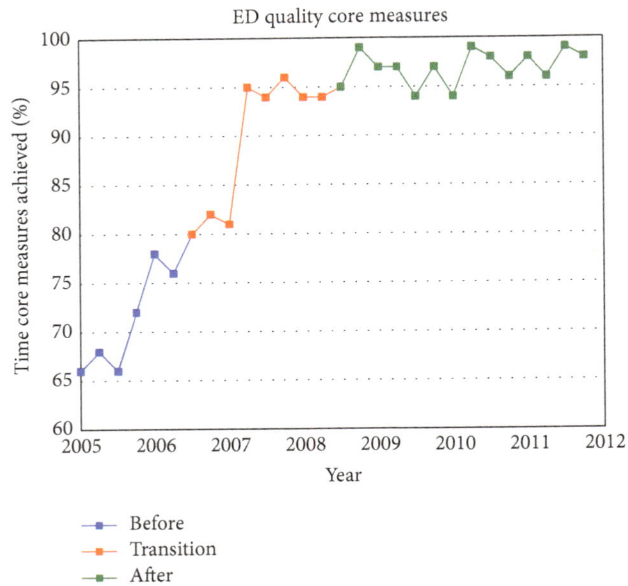


FIGURE 6: Core Measures: average ED sensitivity quality core measures indicator rates for two conditions. (1) Acute myocardial infarction (AMI): percent of time in which the patient received aspirin and beta-blocker on arrival. (2) Community acquired pneumonia (CAP): percent of time in which the patient received antibiotics within 4 hours and a blood culture prior to administration of antibiotics.

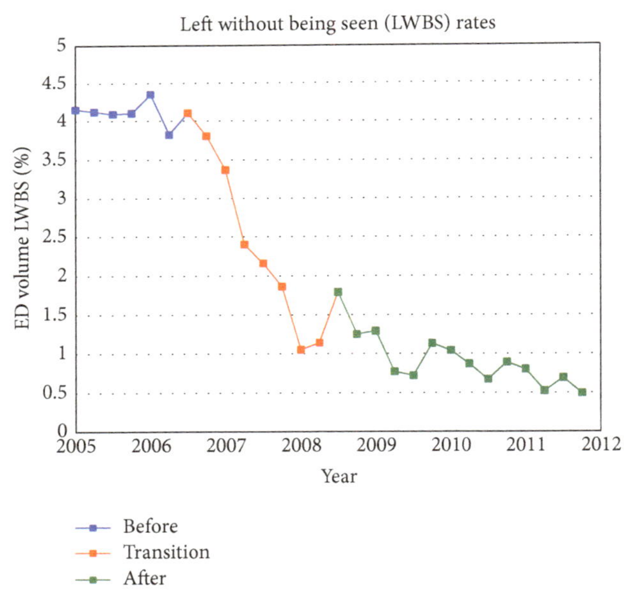


FIGURE 7: Left without being seen (LWBS) rate: percentage of patients who arrived at the ED but then left without receiving medical care.

Recent publications regarding improving ED flow have shown that rapid assessment zone (RAZ), advanced triage protocols, and tracking systems/whiteboards resulted in a significant reduction in both total length of stay and left without being seen rates [8–14]. Furthermore, the utilization of the "Lean" principles of the Toyota Production system greatly enhanced efforts to improve throughput time and quality assurance [9–11]. A cohesive staffing strategy and concrete flow targets were also crucial components of the ED redesign [15–20].

Through a comprehensive assessment process, the ED management team decided to address these issues by optimizing front-end operations and utilizing a team-wide approach to improve patient throughput and disposition. In our front end reengineering, we effectively eliminated our sequential intake process where patients went through extended triage and a comprehensive registration before entering the ED and receiving care. Instead, we created a process where the patient was greeted by a customer service expert and placed in an ED bed immediately after a three-question miniregistration to identify the patient's electronic health record (EHR) or create one for a new patient in the most expeditious way. Once inside, patients were evaluated by any member of the care team that was available and their care was initiated. Full registration took place after nursing and physician assessment, stabilization, and initiation of care. Currently over 70% of ED patients in both RA and main ED stay in the same room and are cared for by the same physician/nursing team throughout their ED stay. We found that this approach served to limit the number of times a patient was moved, the number of times they had to present their story, the number of nursing and physician handoffs, the likelihood of miscommunication and errors, and the total length of stay. After implementation of these initiatives, we saw statistically significant improvement in all metrics including zero diversion since April 2007, two years before diversion was banned in Massachusetts. With collaboration and inclusion, we were able to make strides in staff alignment and performance achievements in a system that included 14 distinct unions representing various disciplines.

Emergency Department patient flow is difficult to transform for many reasons including culture and history. Traditionally, patient flow is based on inefficient processes leading staff to become myopic on single tasks, causing patients to repeat information to multiple clinicians, and producing undesirable outcomes like boarding, diversion, and long waits which all work to increase the number of patients leaving without being seen. Part of the reason why so many hospital EDs follow such hopelessly inefficient patient flow standards has been the ambivalence thinking that ED patterns are intractable and cannot be solved without substantial capital infusion to expand facilities and the addition of staff. We have discovered that ED transformation is manageable, strategic, and inexpensive. Along with the new operational changes came new structures for accountability and communication that allowed our team to manage in fundamentally different ways. We followed a plan that allowed for quick victories while continuing a gradual trend of overall change to improve our operations.

We believe the three main factors that led to our success were gaining administrative support, aligning a leadership team, and stakeholder inclusion. The Emergency Department is unique in that it interfaces with all other departments within the institution and even some services offered outside of the institution. Before we began to tackle the Emergency

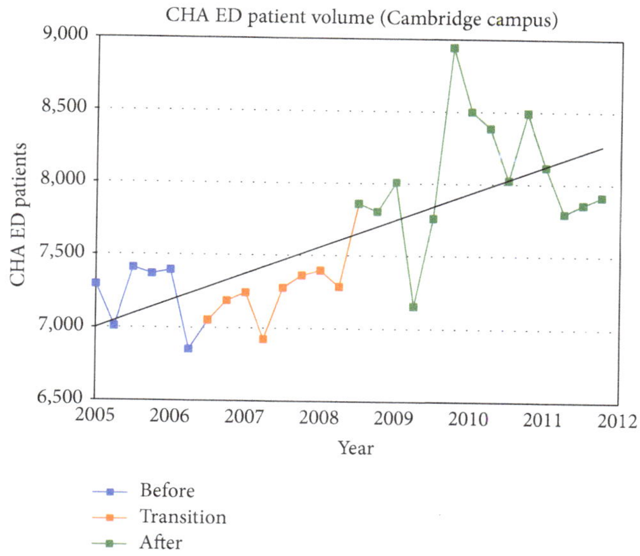


FIGURE 8: ED volume.

Department pitfalls, it was necessary to gain administrative support for such a project. This support was crucial to resolve ED throughput obstacles surrounding physician and nursing handoff of admitted patients and the ability to institute our Code Help policy to decompress the ED at times of high volume. The creation of Code Help and the knowledge that a full inpatient unit will be receiving admitted patients to its hallways motivated the staff in receiving units to work harder on their discharges.

During times of change, confusion among staff and unclear leadership is a recipe for failure. The key to any success is to have a well-developed mission that has the total support of the physician, nursing, and administrative ED leadership. We created a concrete mission statement and made certain that every person in the department, administrators, nurses, and physicians alike, across all three locations, knew what we wanted to accomplish and why changes were necessary. We also realized that a frontline staff participation and inclusion of all stakeholders was critical to the adoption and acceptance of any new initiative.

In summary, inefficiencies in the ED throughput process and delays of care may negatively impact patient satisfaction and patient outcomes [20–24]. During our operations overhaul we tackled this problem by improving the ED flow process, changing the staff culture, and placing the patient first. Ultimately, the Cambridge ED was able to meet and sustain our target outcomes and goals. We became a best practice institution based on patient satisfaction, reduced the door-to-provider time, and increased total ED volume and capacity. Improving ED operational efficiency allowed us to accommodate increasing volume while at the same time improving the quality of care and satisfaction of ED patients. This implementation serves to demonstrate that outcomes and cultural traditions can be improved through strategy rather than heavy capital investment.

## Abbreviations and Acronyms

AMI: Acute myocardial infarction
TCH: The Cambridge Hospital
CAP: Community acquired pneumonia
ED: Emergency Department
FY: Fiscal year
LWBS: Left without being seen
RA: Rapid assessment
TLOS: Total length of stay.

## Limitations

These changes were implemented in a medium-sized, urban ED and some of the initiatives described and results derived may not be applicable to EDs operating under different constraints and with different patient populations. The institution of the electronic health record in the ED was another confounding factor. However, we feel that the changes implemented in the TCH ED would be beneficial to many EDs facing the challenges of crowding in times of limited resources.

## Conflict of Interests

The authors declare that there is no conflict of interests regarding the publication of this paper.

## References

[1] K. D. Johnson and C. Winkelman, "The effect of emergency department crowding on patient outcomes: a literature review," *Advanced Emergency Nursing Journal*, vol. 33, no. 1, pp. 39–54, 2011.

[2] M. Bullard, C. Villa-Roel, X. Guo et al., "The role of a rapid assessment zone/pod on reducing overcrowding in emergency departments: a systematic review," *Emergency Medicine Journal*, vol. 29, no. 5, pp. 372–378, 2012.

[3] M. Bell and J. Parisi, "ED slashes average wait time by more than an hour," *ED Management*, vol. 21, no. 3, pp. 30–31, 2009.

[4] "D-to-D slashed 85% in seven weeks," *ED Management*, vol. 21, no. 8, pp. 90–91, 2009.

[5] J. C. Moskop, D. P. Sklar, J. M. Geiderman, R. M. Schears, and K. J. Bookman, "Emergency department crowding. Part 1. Concept, causes, and moral consequences," *Annals of Emergency Medicine*, vol. 53, no. 5, pp. 605–611, 2009.

[6] "Comprehensive emergency department and inpatient changes improve emergency department patient satisfaction, reduce bottlenecks that delay admissions," 2011, http://www.innovations.ahrq.gov/content.aspx?id=1757.

[7] J. L. Wiler, C. Gentle, J. M. Halfpenny et al., "Optimizing emergency department front-end operations," *Annals of Emergency Medicine*, vol. 55, no. 2, pp. 142–160, 2010.

[8] L. I. Horwitz, J. Green, and E. H. Bradley, "US emergency department performance on wait time and length of visit," *Annals of Emergency Medicine*, vol. 55, no. 2, pp. 133–141, 2010.

[9] R. J. Holden, "Lean thinking in emergency departments: a critical review," *Annals of Emergency Medicine*, vol. 57, no. 3, pp. 265–278, 2011.

[10] R. C. Dart, "Can lean thinking transform American health care?" *Annals of Emergency Medicine*, vol. 57, no. 3, pp. 279–281, 2011.

[11] D. Ng, G. Vail, S. Thomas, and N. Schmidt, "Applying the Lean principles of the Toyota Production System to reduce wait times in the emergency department," *Canadian Journal of Emergency Medicine*, vol. 12, no. 1, pp. 50–57, 2010.

[12] P. Jones and K. Schimanski, "The four hour target to reduce emergency department waiting time": a systematic review of clinical outcomes," *Emergency Medicine Australasia*, vol. 22, no. 5, pp. 391–398, 2010.

[13] E. Weber, S. Mason, A. Carter, and R. L. Hew, "Emptying the corridors of shame: organizational lessons from England's 4-hour emergency throughput target," *Annals of Emergency Medicine*, vol. 57, no. 2, pp. 79–88, 2011.

[14] J. C. Moskop, D. P. Sklar, J. M. Geiderman, R. M. Schears, and K. J. Bookman, "Emergency department crowding. Part 2- barriers to reform and strategies to overcome them," *Annals of Emergency Medicine*, vol. 53, no. 5, pp. 612–617, 2009.

[15] T. Chan, J. Killeen, D. Kelly, and D. A. Guss, "Impact of rapid entry and accelerated care at triage on reducing emergency department patient wait times, lengths of stay, and rate of left without being seen," *Annals of Emergency Medicine*, vol. 46, no. 6, pp. 491–497, 2005.

[16] "Doctor in triage slices door-to-discharge times," *ED Management*, vol. 18, no. 5, pp. 54–55, 2006.

[17] J. Travers and F. Lee, "Avoiding prolonged waiting time during busy periods in the emergency department: is there a role for the senior emergency physician in triage?" *European Journal of Emergency Medicine*, vol. 13, no. 6, pp. 342–348, 2006.

[18] P. Patel and D. Vinson, "Team assignment system: expediting emergency department care," *Annals of Emergency Medicine*, vol. 46, no. 6, pp. 499–506, 2005.

[19] R. W. Derlet and J. R. Richards, "Overcrowding in the nation's emergency departments: complex causes and disturbing effects," *Annals of Emergency Medicine*, vol. 35, no. 1, pp. 63–68, 2000.

[20] S. Bernstein, D. Aronsky, and B. Asplin, "The effect of emergency department crowding on clinically oriented outcomes," *Academic Emergency Medicine*, vol. 16, no. 1, pp. 1–10, 2009.

[21] J. M. Pines, C. V. Pollack Jr., D. B. Diercks, A. M. Chang, F. S. Shofer, and J. E. Hollander, "The association between emergency department crowding and adverse cardiovascular outcomes in patients with chest pain," *Academic Emergency Medicine*, vol. 16, no. 7, pp. 617–625, 2009.

[22] R. Cowan and S. Trzeciak, "Clinical review: emergency department overcrowding and the potential impact on the critically ill," *Critical Care*, vol. 9, no. 3, pp. 291–295, 2005.

[23] M. R. Sills, D. Fairclough, D. Ranade, and M. G. Kahn, "Emergency department crowding is associated with decreased quality of care for children with acute asthma," *Annals of Emergency Medicine*, vol. 57, no. 3, pp. 191–198, 2011.

[24] "Improved flow aids patient safety," *ED Management*, vol. 23, no. 1, pp. 10–11, 2011.

# 22

# Recent Advances of Hemorrhage Management in Severe Trauma

**Mohamed El Sayad[1] and Hussein Noureddine[2]**

[1] *Trauma and Orthopaedics, Wishaw General Hospital, Wishaw, UK*
[2] *Trauma and Orthopaedics, Ninewells Hospital, Dundee, UK*

Correspondence should be addressed to Mohamed El Sayad; msayad1@hotmail.com

Academic Editor: Chak W. Kam

Trauma is one of the most common causes of mortality worldwide with a substantial percentage of deaths resulting secondary to haemorrhages, which are preventable and treatable when adequately managed. This paper offers a review of the current literature on how to successfully resuscitate patients with major haemorrhage.

## 1. Introduction

Trauma is the third most common cause of mortality worldwide and is the leading cause of death in the age group ranging between 1 and 44 years [1]. Among those trauma patients, major haemorrhage is responsible for 30 to 40% of mortality, with up to half of them dying prior to their arrival to hospital [1]. Whilst injuries to the central nervous system are the leading cause of mortality, haemorrhagic shock ranks second despite the fact that it could be preventable and reversible. Within hospital settings, it accounts for more than 80% of the mortality in operating theatres and 50% of the overall mortality in the first 24 hours of admission [1]. Major haemorrhage is defined as the loss of 100% of total blood volume within 24 hours, loss of 50% within four hours, or the loss of 150 mL per minute. Given the above, the importance of successful resuscitation of major haemorrhage becomes paramount [2].

## 2. Early Identification

Early identification of patients with major haemorrhage is a necessity and the diagnosis should be established promptly. Suffering from hypovolemia due to haemorrhage presents with a variety of clinical features. The American College of Surgeons through their ATLS protocols have traditionally provided a classification for haemorrhagic shock that is divided according to the amount of blood loss; see Table 1 [3]. However, there are limitations to this classification. For example, the clinical signs might be masked in young fit individuals with larger physiological reserves, as well as elderly patients on medications such as beta-blockers that manipulate normal physiological responses.

Introduction of new methods of shock assessment has shown to be more sensitive compared to conventional monitoring of vital signs. The shock index is the ratio of heart rate to systolic blood pressure. Birkhahn et al. proved that the shock index was a more useful tool in diagnosing early haemorrhage. They performed an observational study that included 46 healthy blood-donating individuals; each patient had 450 mLs of blood taken over 20 minutes. Their vital signs were measured before donation, immediately after donation while lying down, and after one and five minutes of standing. The results showed a significant increase in the mean shock index, whilst the vital signs remained within the normal limits despite revealing some extent of variation from predonation readings [4].

Cannon et al. performed a retrospective review of 2445 trauma patients to examine the correlation between shock index and mortality rates. Results showed that patients with a shock index ratio of more than 0.9 had a higher mortality rate of 15.9% compared to a rate of 6.9% in those with a normal shock index. Furthermore, patients whose shock indices measured in the emergency department were higher than those measured in the field had a mortality rate of 9.3% compared to only 5.7% in those who had unchanged shock indices [5].

Table 1: Classification of haemorrhagic shock (ATLS manual American College of Surgeons).

| | Class of haemorrhagic shock | | | |
|---|---|---|---|---|
| | I | II | III | IV |
| Blood loss (mL) | Up to 750 | 750–1500 | 1500–2000 | >2000 |
| Blood loss (% blood volume) | Up to 15 | 15–30 | 30–40 | >40 |
| Pulse rate (per minute) | <100 | 100–120 | 120–140 | >140 |
| Blood pressure | Normal | Normal | Decreased | Decreased |
| Pulse pressure (mm Hg) | Normal or increased | Decreased | Decreased | Decreased |
| Respiratory rate (per minute) | 14–20 | 20–30 | 30–40 | >35 |
| Urine output (mL/hour) | >30 | 20–30 | 5–15 | Negligible |
| Central nervous system/mental status | Slightly anxious | Mildly anxious | Anxious/confused | Confused/lethargic |

ROPE is another method of assessment that has also been described; it involves the division of pulse rate by pulse pressure (pulse rate/systolic blood pressure-diastolic blood pressure). Ardagh et al. assessed ROPE as a mean to predict the risk of decompensation in patients with compensated haemorrhagic shock, by undergoing a retrospective study on a cohort of 184 trauma victims. Their results showed that a ROPE value of less than 3.0 was predictive of patients remaining stable while a ROPE value of more than 3.0 was predictive of patients that may develop decompensated haemorrhagic shock [6].

Both methods were assessed by Campbell et al. [7] who carried out a prospective observational study of one hundred and sixteen healthy individuals that donated one unit of blood (420 mLs); both their heart rate and blood pressure were measured immediately before and after donating the blood. Their shock index and ROPE measurements were calculated and the mean of both measurements increased significantly by 12.2%. This study showed that the rope and shock indices correlated with blood loss better than conventional observation monitoring and that they are suitable methods to detect early blood loss.

Subsequent to diagnosing hypovolemia due to haemorrhage, it becomes imperative to identify the source of bleeding. This can be achieved by clinical examination (reduced breath sounds, abdominal or pelvic tenderness, deformed limbs, etc.), bedside investigations in the emergency department (trauma series X-rays, fast scan), or radiological investigation most notably whole body CT scan which is very helpful in rapid diagnosis after patient stabilization [8].

## 3. Damage Control Resuscitation (Prevention and Treatment of the Lethal Triad)

Our approach to major haemorrhage mainly stems from experiences accumulated during periods of war. The conflicts in both Afghanistan and Iraq have inspired us to implement changes to current practice. The military has developed a trauma resuscitation protocol of their own similar to the ATLS called Battlefield Advanced Trauma Life Support (BATLS). This is applied to the management of military trauma victims where the starting point is stopping catastrophic haemorrhage, ensued by the conventional ABCDE ATLS algorithm [9].

For appropriate resuscitation to be established, it is important to understand the severe pathophysiological derangements of the exsanguinating patients, in terms of hypothermia, coagulopathy, and acidosis also known as the lethal triad. Bleeding patients with these findings have up to 90% mortality rate requiring massive transfusion [10]. We will discuss each of the elements of the lethal triad in turn.

*3.1. Hypothermia.* Hypothermia secondary to trauma is a common occurrence; it is due to the inability of the body to generate heat, because of altered central thermoregulation, blocked shivering response, and reduction of metabolic activity at the cellular level. Resuscitation is also a common reason for hypothermia. Cold intravenous fluid administration and patient exposure during initial evaluation as well as peritoneal exposure during laparotomies in the operating theatres are all major contributors. Hypothermia is clinically significant when the core temperature is less than 36 degrees for more than 4 hours.

Hypothermia exacerbates coagulopathy by affecting platelet function; the imbalance of thromboxane and prostacyclin reduces the response of platelet activation. Hypothermia also reduces the enzyme activation pathway of the coagulation cascade. At 35°C, factors eleven and twelve would only function at 65% of normal [11]. Trauma victims with a core temperature below 35°C have a poor prognosis, and those with a core temperature of 32°C have a 100% mortality rate [11]. Recent data from the 31st Combat Support Hospital in Iraq showed that 18% of 2848 trauma patients were hypothermic and that hypothermia is significantly correlated with admission GCS, tachycardia, hypotension, low hematocrit, and acidosis thus making it an independent contributor to overall mortality [12].

Treatment of the hypothermic patient could be carried out passively or actively. Passive warming entails preventing further heat loss, by means such as covering the patients and warming the operating or resuscitation room. Active warming involves covering the trauma victims with warming blankets and administering warmed intravenous fluid or blood and warm body cavity lavage, aiming to keep core temperature at 36 degrees.

*3.2. Acidosis.* Metabolic acidosis is due to the prolonged inadequate tissue perfusion. This leads to cellular metabolism converting from aerobic to anaerobic and the increased production of lactate causing a reduction in pH. This reduction in pH has a negative effect on cardiac contractility.

The effect of the acidosis on the coagulation cascade was shown by Meng et al. They measured the activity of recombinant factor VIIa on phospholipids and platelets, and the results showed that it was reduced by 90% when the pH was reduced from 7.4 to 7 [13]. Martini et al. showed the effect of acidosis on coagulation by infusing 12 pigs with 0.2 mol/L of hydrochloric acid until their pH was 7.1. Ringer lactate was continually transfused to maintain that pH. Blood samples were taken at baseline and at 15 minutes after acidosis induction. Coagulation function was assessed by measuring the prothrombin time (PT), partial thromboplastin time (PTT), and thrombin generation. They concluded that acidosis reduced fibrinogen concentration to 66% ± 2%, decreased platelet counts to 49% ± 4%, and decreased thrombin generation to 60% ± 4%. Acidosis also prolonged PT and PTT by about 20% [14].

A sensitive means of assessing tissue oxygenation is by measuring the base deficit, which is a measure of the number of millimoles of base required to correct the pH of one liter of whole blood to 7.4 and its normal value is −3 to +3. Davis et al. demonstrated that measurement of the base deficit was more accurate in deciding the clearance of the acidosis after trauma shock than PH measurement. They performed a retrospective analysis of 674 trauma victims that had both their pH and base deficits measured during their admission to hospital. The base deficit was significantly different between the survivors and the nonsurvivors at all of the time intervals at which it was measured. However, the same differences were not noted when the pH was assessed making it a less reliable predictor of outcome [15].

Treatment of acidosis mainly constitutes restoration of the circulation to maintain tissue perfusion. Lier et al. provided a comprehensive review of the effect of acidosis on coagulation and recommended neutralization of the acidosis to improve the coagulopathy especially when the trauma victim is receiving a massive transfusion. The recommendation was that buffering could be established by using either sodium bicarbonate or trishydroxymethylaminomethane (THAM), with the latter recording superior results. This is due to its effect on coagulation, as it did not inhibit thrombin formation when compared to sodium bicarbonate, but they both had a negative effect on the conversion of fibrinogen to fibrin [16].

*3.3. Coagulopathy.* Hess et al. reviewed the reasons for the development of acute coagulopathy following trauma. They identified 6 initiators: (1) tissue damage which leads to the exposure of endothelium and initiates the coagulation cascade and fibrinolysis; (2) shock, which is dose dependent to the degree of coagulopathy; this mechanism is not clearly understood; (3) haemodilution from the shift of cellular and interstitial fluid that is deficient in clotting factors into the plasma, and the administration of intravenous fluid, which also interrupts clot formation and the transfusion of red blood cells, (4) inflammation which interferes in coagulation as it causes monocytes to adhere to platelets, activation of the thrombomodulin-protein C pathway, and the binding of C4b to protein S [17], finally the last 2 initiators which are (5) hypothermia and (6) acidosis as discussed previously.

Acute coagulopathies are found in one in four trauma patients as shown by Brohi et al. They underwent a retrospective review of 1088 patients that were admitted to their trauma centre between the years of 1993 and 1998. These patients had their coagulation profile measured on admission, including PT, APTT, and thrombin time. The results showed that 24.4% of patients had a coagulopathy and that these patients had a mortality of 46%. This was significantly different to the mortality of 10.9% for those with normal clotting [18].

Currently, there are no accurate methods to assess acute trauma coagulopathy. The traditional investigations of PT, PTT, fibrinogen, and platelet count are of limited value during massive hemorrhage as they do not provide enough information about clot formation. Additionally, the platelet count is usually normal during the initial stage of haemorrhage. The current treatment of coagulopathy is by the early empirical transfusion of blood and clotting factors [19].

*3.4. Massive Transfusion and Fluid Resuscitation.* Massive transfusion is defined as transfusion of more than ten units of packed red cells over 24 hours or four units within one hour. Administering blood should be initiated at the scene of the accident, thus avoiding the rapid administration of iv fluids (filler fluid) that has been traditionally promoted by the ATLS guidelines. This involves giving two liters of crystalloids and continuing with packed red blood cells (PRBCs) and fresh-frozen plasma (FFP) if there was transient or no response, with the aim of achieving normotension.

Duke et al. provided data from a retrospective analysis of 307 patients that were admitted to a level one-trauma centre between January 2007 and May 2011. The inclusion criteria were patients with penetrating torso injuries and a systolic blood pressure less than 90 mmHg who were managed by damage control resuscitation and surgery. 175 patients received standard fluid resuscitation (SFR) which was 150 mLs of crystalloid or more; 132 patients received restricted fluid resuscitation (RFR) which was less than 150 mLs of crystalloid before damage control surgery. The results showed that the first group (SFR) received more preoperative fluid then the (RFR) group (2,275 mLs versus 129 mLs) and that they had a higher intraoperative mortality rate (32% versus 9%) and overall mortality rate (37% versus 21%). The higher mortality rate was attributed to the effect of large volume of fluids in diluting clotting factors and reducing blood viscosity and the increase of blood pressure. RFR was beneficial to these patients as it provided them with permissive hypotension (systolic blood pressure of 90) until damage control surgery was achieved [20].

Serious attempts at challenging the clinical validity of the widely accepted concept of conventional fluid resuscitation first surfaced in the mid-1990s. In 1996, Dries published a mini review of summaries in his paper “hypotensive resuscitation” suggesting that “Limited attempts to restore blood pressure improve cardiac output, tissue perfusion, and survival while attempts to restore normal tension with crystalloid result in increased hemorrhage volume and higher mortality”

[21]. However, some of the earlier randomized controlled trials did not concur with those findings. For instance, Dutton et al. [22] underwent a study where a cohort of 110 patients presenting in hemorrhagic shock, more than half of which were victims of penetrating trauma, was randomized to one of two fluid resuscitation protocols: target SBP > 100 mm Hg or target SBP of 70 mm Hg. And fluid therapy was titrated to this endpoint until definitive hemostasis was achieved. His results showed similar survival rates in both groups suggesting that resorting to hypotensive resuscitation did not affect mortality [22]. Nevertheless, since then, more evidence has emerged favoring the concept of hypotensive resuscitation. Morrison et al. performed a randomized controlled study on 90 patients that required a laparotomy or thoracotomy following trauma; they were divided into 2 groups; the first group was resuscitated aiming for a mean arterial blood pressure of 65 mm Hg with standard fluid protocol, while the second group was managed by hypotensive resuscitation to a mean blood pressure of 50 mm Hg. The results showed that the second group had a lower requirement of fluid and blood product transfusion, lower postoperative mortality, and reduced postoperative bleeding. And in those of them who did develop a coagulopathy, it was less severe compared to coagulopathic patients of the first group as evidenced by INR measurements [23].

The ratio of packed RBC (PRBC) : fresh frozen plasma (FFP) : platelets (plt) should be 1 : 1 : 1. Two studies showed that there was an increase in survival rate by increasing the ratio of FFP to RBC [24] and platelets to RBC [25]. This is the current military guidelines in massive transfusion [9].

*3.5. Antifibrinolytics.* Crash 2 was a randomized controlled trial, that was performed in 274 hospitals in 40 different countries and involved 20,211 patients to assess the effect of tranexamic acid on death, vasoocclusive events, and blood transfusion in trauma patients. The patients had to be above the age of 16 years, exposed to trauma, and had to have evidence of bleeding in the form of systolic blood pressure of less than 90 mm Hg or a pulse rate of 110 beats per minute. 10,060 patients received tranexamic acid and 10,067 were randomized to the placebo group. The results yielded that tranexamic acid reduced the mortality rate to 14.5% compared to 16% in the placebo group. The conclusion of this trial was that tranexamic acid reduced the risk of death in trauma patients that were at risk of hemorrhage [26].

This conclusion was also echoed by Morrison et al. in the Military Application of Tranexamic Acid in Trauma Emergency Resuscitation study (MATTER) in 2012. The study was designed as a retrospective observational study that looked at a cohort of 896 patients admitted with combat injuries; the cohort was primarily divided into two groups the first included 293 patients who received TXA, and the second included the rest of the cohort who did not receive TXA. Both groups were further subdivided based on whether patients received massive transfusion (identified as 10 or more units of PRBCs within 24 hours). The outcomes that were measured were mortality at 24 hours, 48 hours, and 30 days, as well as the influence of TXA administration on postoperative coagulopathy and the rate of thromboembolic complications. The results showed an absolute reduction of in-hospital mortality by 6.5% in the TXA group compared to the non-TXA group and an absolute reduction of 49% in the TXA massive transfusion group compared to the massive transfusion non-TXA group. This was not completely cost-free though, as the study established that there was a higher rate of thromboembolic events in the TXA and TXA massive transfusion groups compared to their non-TXA counterparts, but it was noteworthy that there were no increased fatalities due to those events.

## 4. Hemorrhage Control and Damage Control Surgery

Despite taking all the above measures, if hemorrhage control is not achieved these resuscitation efforts would be futile. Hemorrhage control should be achieved in a timely fashion, initially by temporary measures such as direct compression, hemostatic dressings, tourniquets or the application of pelvic binders, and finally by definitive surgical control of the source of bleeding.

Temporary measures like the tourniquet, is well recognized and was first documented in 1674. Bellamy believed that 38% of the patients in the Vietnam War that died from extremity hemorrhage could have been salvaged by appropriate application of a tourniquet [27]. Pelvic binders help stabilize exsanguinating patient with open pelvic fractures by reducing their pelvic volume thus increasing intrapelvic pressure providing a tamponade effect to the catastrophic bleeding that is associated with these injuries. Extreme caution needs to be taken with both of these methods as they are both associated with grave complications due to prolonged application; tourniquets can cause neuropraxia, limb ischemia muscle injury, and compartment syndrome. On the other hand, pelvic binders can lead to skin necrosis.

Damage control surgery is a concept that emerged because the physiological derangements of hemorrhagic shock are more important than definitive surgery. It was described by Feliciano et al. as a 3-stage procedure in which the first is to control the bleeding, the second stage is where the patient is transferred to ITU for correction of the lethal triad and stabilization, and the 3rd stage is for definitive surgical repair [28].

## 5. Conclusion

Whilst massive hemorrhage continues to be a major cause of mortality, it is often reversible, and it can be adequately managed by early identification of these patients and the source of their bleeding, approaching them with (CABC) protocol and prevention and treatment of the lethal triad and damage control surgery to stop the bleeding.

## Conflict of Interests

The authors declare that there is no conflict of interests regarding the publication of this paper.

## References

[1] D. S. Kauvar, R. Lefering, and C. E. Wade, "Impact of hemorrhage on trauma outcome: an overview of epidemiology, clinical presentations, and therapeutic considerations," *Journal of Trauma*, vol. 60, no. 6, pp. S3–S11, 2006.

[2] R. L. Gruen, G. J. Jurkovich, L. K. McIntyre, H. M. Foy, and R. V. Maier, "Patterns of errors contributing to trauma mortality: lessons learned from 2594 deaths," *Annals of Surgery*, vol. 244, no. 3, pp. 371–378, 2006.

[3] The American College of Surgeons, "Shock," in *Advanced Trauma Life Support*, The American College of Surgeons, Ed., pp. 59–73, 1990.

[4] R. H. Birkhahn, T. J. Gaeta, D. Terry, J. J. Bove, and J. Tloczkowski, "Shock index in diagnosing early acute hypovolemia," *American Journal of Emergency Medicine*, vol. 23, no. 3, pp. 323–326, 2005.

[5] C. M. Cannon, C. C. Braxton, M. Kling-Smith, J. D. Mahnken, E. Carlton, and M. Moncure, "Utility of the shock index in predicting mortality in traumatically injured patients," *Journal of Trauma*, vol. 67, no. 6, pp. 1426–1430, 2009.

[6] M. W. Ardagh, T. Hodgson, L. Shaw, and D. Turner, "Pulse rate over pressure evaluation (ROPE) is useful in the assessment of compensated haemorrhagic shock," *Emergency Medicine*, vol. 13, no. 1, pp. 43–46, 2001.

[7] R. Campbell, M. W. Ardagh, and M. Than, "validation of pulse rate over pressure evaluation index as a detector of early occult hemorrhage," *Journal of Trauma and Acute Care Surgery*, vol. 73, no. 1, pp. 286–288, 2012.

[8] C. W. Kam, C. H. Lai, S. K. Lam, F. L. So, C. L. Lau, and K. H. Cheung, "What are the ten new commandments in severe polytrauma management?" *World Journal of Emergency Medicine*, vol. 1, no. 2, 2010.

[9] R. Dawes and G. R. Thomas, "Battlefield resuscitation," *Current Opinion in Critical Care*, vol. 15, no. 6, pp. 527–535, 2009.

[10] A. Ferrara, J. D. MacArthur, H. K. Wright, I. M. Modlin, and M. A. McMillen, "Hypothermia and acidosis worsen coagulopathy in the patient requiring massive transfusion," *American Journal of Surgery*, vol. 160, no. 5, pp. 515–518, 1990.

[11] L. M. Gentilello and D. J. Pierson, "Trauma critical care," *American Journal of Respiratory and Critical Care Medicine*, vol. 163, no. 3, pp. 604–607, 2001.

[12] Z. Arthurs, D. Cuadrado, A. Beekley et al., "The impact of hypothermia on trauma care at the 31st combat support hospital," *American Journal of Surgery*, vol. 191, no. 5, pp. 610–614, 2006.

[13] Z. H. Meng, A. S. Wolberg, D. M. Monroe III, and M. Hoffman, "The effect of temperature and pH on the activity of factor VIIa: implications for the efficacy of high-dose factor VIIa in hypothermic and acidotic patients," *Journal of Trauma*, vol. 55, no. 5, pp. 886–891, 2003.

[14] W. Z. Martini, M. A. Dubick, A. E. Pusateri, M. S. Park, K. L. Ryan, and J. B. Holcomb, "Does bicarbonate correct coagulation function impaired by acidosis in swine?" *Journal of Trauma*, vol. 61, no. 1, pp. 99–106, 2006.

[15] J. W. Davis, K. L. Kaups, and S. N. Parks, "Base deficit is superior to pH in evaluating clearance of acidosis after traumatic shock," *Journal of Trauma*, vol. 44, no. 1, pp. 114–118, 1998.

[16] H. Lier, H. Krep, S. Schroeder, and F. Stuber, "Preconditions of hemostasis in trauma: a review. The influence of acidosis, hypocalcemia, anemia, and hypothermia on functional hemostasis in trauma," *Journal of Trauma*, vol. 65, no. 4, pp. 951–960, 2008.

[17] J. R. Hess, K. Brohi, R. P. Dutton et al., "The coagulopathy of trauma: a review of mechanisms," *Journal of Trauma*, vol. 65, no. 4, pp. 748–754, 2008.

[18] K. Brohi, J. Singh, M. Heron, and T. Coats, "Acute traumatic coagulopathy," *Journal of Trauma*, vol. 54, no. 6, pp. 1127–1130, 2003.

[19] R. Davenport and S. Khan, "Management of major trauma haemorrhage: treatment priorities and controversies," *British Journal of Haematology*, vol. 155, no. 5, pp. 537–548, 2011.

[20] M. D. Duke, C. Guidry, J. Guice et al., "Restrictive fluid resuscitation in combination with damage control resuscitation: time for adaptation," *Journal of Trauma and Acute Care Surgery*, vol. 73, no. 3, pp. 674–678, 2012.

[21] D. J. Dries, "Hypotensive resuscitation," *Shock*, vol. 6, no. 5, pp. 311–316, 1996.

[22] R. P. Dutton, C. F. Mackenzie, and T. M. Scalea, "Hypotensive resuscitation during active hemorrhage: impact on in-hospital mortality," *Journal of Trauma*, vol. 52, no. 6, pp. 1141–1146, 2002.

[23] C. A. Morrison, M. M. Carrick, M. A. Norman et al., "Hypotensive resuscitation strategy reduces transfusion requirements and severe postoperative coagulopathy in trauma patients with hemorrhagic shock: preliminary results of a randomized controlled trial," *Journal of Trauma*, vol. 70, no. 3, pp. 652–663, 2011.

[24] M. A. Borgman, P. C. Spinella, J. G. Perkins et al., "The ratio of blood products transfused affects mortality in patients receiving massive transfusions at a combat support hospital," *Journal of Trauma*, vol. 63, no. 4, pp. 805–813, 2007.

[25] J. G. Perkins, A. P. Cap, and P. C. Spinella, "An evaluation of the impact of apheresis platelets used in the setting of massively transfused trauma patients," *Journal of Trauma*, vol. 66, no. 4, pp. S77–S85, 2009.

[26] CRASH II, "Clinical randomisation of an antifibrinolytic in significant haemor- rhage," http://www.crash2.lshtm.ac.uk.

[27] R. F. Bellamy, "The causes of death in conventional land warfare: implications for combat casualty care research," *Military Medicine*, vol. 149, no. 2, pp. 55–62, 1984.

[28] D. V. Feliciano, J. M. Burch, V. Spjut-Patrinely, K. L. Mattox, and G. L. Jordan Jr., "Abdominal gunshot wounds. An urban trauma center's experience with 300 consecutive patients," *Annals of Surgery*, vol. 208, no. 3, pp. 362–370, 1988.

# Coca: The History and Medical Significance of an Ancient Andean Tradition

**Amy Sue Biondich and Jeremy David Joslin**

*Department of Emergency Medicine, SUNY Upstate Medical University, 550 E. Genesee Street, Suite 103, Syracuse, NY 13202, USA*

Correspondence should be addressed to Amy Sue Biondich; amybee@mac.com

Academic Editor: Jeffrey R. Avner

Coca leaf products are an integral part of the lives of the Andean peoples from both a cultural and traditional medicine perspective. Coca is also the whole plant from which cocaine is derived. Coca products are thought to be a panacea for health troubles in regions of South America. This review will examine the toxicology of whole coca and will also look at medicinal applications of this plant, past, present, and future.

## 1. Introduction

Coca is an indigenous plant of South America with numerous alkaloid components, the most well-known one of which is the psychoactive component, cocaine. Its leaves have been a staple in the Andean lifestyle for thousands of years. Strong interest in coca use has existed in the anthropological world for decades. Areas of study have not only attempted to understand traditional use during the Incan empire and coca's role in folk medicine, but also focused on factors that influence the ability of this native tradition to continue in the face of increasingly strict regulations of coca production. Efforts have been made to understand the long-term Andean use of coca, with subsequent research examining the scientific basis behind local beliefs. This review will examine the history of coca production, its toxicity profile, and its varied uses throughout the centuries. It is important to note that although coca continues to be valuable to native Andean people for religious and cultural reasons, travelers to these regions need to be aware that there is a paucity of medical data supporting the safe use of coca. The astute toxicologist should maintain an understanding of the cultural pressures experienced by contemporary travelers.

## 2. Coca Species

The Aymara people are an indigenous population of the Andes and Altiplano regions of South America. "Khoka" is an Aymara word that means "the tree." This is the origin for our modern usage of "coca" [1]. The coca shrub is indigenous to South America, Mexico, Indonesia, and the West Indies. It is one of the oldest cultivated plants of South America [2]. Cultivated coca plants belong to two distinct species of the genus *Erythroxylum* (family Erythroxylaceae): *Erythroxylum coca* Lam. and *Erythroxylum novogranatense* (Morris) Hieron [3]. There are two varieties to be found within each of the cultivated species of coca. *E. coca* Lam. var. *coca* is also known as "Bolivian" or "Huanuco" coca. This is the best-known variety and continues to be widely cultivated throughout the Andean region for both legal uses and the illegal production of cocaine [2]. Other varieties are found in smaller areas and are mainly cultivated for coca chewing or other traditional uses by local peoples [4].

Cocaine is the principal alkaloid found in the cultivated varieties of coca. Cocaine was first isolated in 1860 by Dr. Albert Nieman from leaves of cultivated cocaine [5]. It is also the most studied and discussed alkaloid in the scientific literature. *E. coca* var. *coca*, the most widely cultivated variety, has been found to contain approximately 0.6% cocaine in its dried leaves [6]. However, there are a number of other biologically active alkaloids that have been studied. The four cultivated *Erythroxylum* varieties contain eighteen alkaloids, belonging to the tropanes, pyrrolidines, and pyridines [2].

An extensive review by Novák et al. details the previously studied biological activity of several of the alkaloids found in coca. Compounds reviewed include cinnamoylcocaine, benzoylecgonine, methylecgonine, pseudotropine, benzoyltropine, tropacocaine, $\alpha$- and $\beta$-truxilline, hygrine, and cuscohygrine. All compounds were found to be considerably less toxic than cocaine with a lack of the euphoric effects that cocaine is known to have. The reader is referred to the articles by Jenkins et al. and Rivier for identification and quantitation of the alkaloids found in whole coca [7, 8]. However, in agreement with Novák et al. conclusion, the overall effect gained from using whole coca products may be in fact from the sum total of all plant constituents, rather than just cocaine alone. In addition, coca leaves include calories, carbohydrates, minerals, and vitamins which could also lend a source of energy and nutrients to its user.

## 3. Toxicity and Other Medical Concerns

The bulk of toxicology research is based on the pure isolate, cocaine, from coca leaves; therefore the extrapolation to the toxicity of whole coca is somewhat limited. However, of the studied biologically active alkaloids in coca, cocaine is the limiting factor in reaching a toxic dose. The physiologic effects of other alkaloids are considerably less than that of cocaine [2]. A toxicity study performed on rats found that the alkaloids benzoylecgonine and ecgonine methyl ester did not produce toxic manifestations when infused at rates that were found to be toxic for cocaine [9]. In fact, 30- and 60-fold higher doses of these alkaloids were necessary to produce any neurobehavioral changes, which ultimately proved to be mild. Benzoylecgonine did not prove to be lethal even when given in doses greater than 100 times that of cocaine [9].

In comparison to modern usage of cocaine isolates, the amount of the drug used by native peoples was and remains quite low with an estimated 60 grams of coca leaf chewed per day [1]. A coca leaf typically contains between 0.1 and 0.9% cocaine [10]. Another study that examined over 3,000 coca users found that mine workers, typically the largest consumers of coca products, chew roughly 13 ounces (368.5 grams) per week which is a similar consumption rate to previously referenced studies [11]. This would mean that an average user would extract approximately 3.9 net grams of the alkaloids contained in coca per week. This would give a maximal total dosage of roughly 200–300 mg per a 24-hour period. The actual dosage is likely much less as the user will not absorb 100% of the alkaloid. The amount of cocaine to be found in coca tea products has also been assessed. Depending on the origin of the tea bags (Bolivia versus Peru), after exhaustive extraction, an average of 4.86–5.11 mg of cocaine was found per tea bag [8]. An investigation conducted in Bolivia found that after chewing 30 g of coca leaves, whole blood cocaine levels reach around 98 ng [12].

In contrast, there is a large difference in what an average cocaine user is exposed to in modern times. A "line" of cocaine bought on the street contains an estimated 20–50 mg of cocaine hydrochloride [13]. Modern users may administer cocaine through several routes: insufflation, intravenous injection, smoking, ingestion, or mucosal application. The half-life of cocaine is 0.7–1.5 hours [14, 15]. Cocaine is rapidly cleared from the plasma but can be detected in the brain, ocular fluid, and liver for 8 hours after initial usage [16]. Following single doses of cocaine, plasma concentrations typically average 200,000–400,000 ng or 4890 ng in whole blood [17, 18]. The whole blood concentration of cocaine is almost 50 times greater after using the pure isolate in comparison to chewing whole coca. Plasma half-life and blood concentrations are both known to be dose dependent.

The estimated minimum lethal dose of cocaine is 1.2 g [19]. However, there have been case studies where individuals have died from as little as 30 mg applied to mucous membranes, and there are also addicts who may tolerate up to 5 g daily [20, 21]. The LD50 of cocaine or the dose determined to be lethal in 50% of the test population has been found to be 95.1 mg/kg in mice. For whole coca, the LD50 is considered to be 3450 mg/kg [22]. In rats, the accepted LD100 is 100 mg/kg [22]. Extrapolating these numbers to humans is not entirely generalizable; however if this data is applied to the standard 70 kg human, it can be seen that these would be very large amounts of coca.

The pharmacology of cocaine is complex with several organ systems affected simultaneously by the drug. Systems affected by acute and chronic use of cocaine include psychological, neurological, renal, cardiac, pulmonary, gastrointestinal, obstetrical, and otolaryngological ones. As mentioned in the toxicology data, medical and physiologic effects in the literature concentrate on the pure isolate cocaine. As outlined above, coca is quite different from cocaine, including common dosages and safety profiles. Local use patterns of coca are also quite different from that of individuals using the purer isolate, cocaine. Because of this, it is thought that cocaine studies have limited generalizability to coca. It is interesting to note that coca tea ingestion has resulted in a positive urine assay for cocaine metabolite [23]. It is worth noting that there is no evidence in the literature to support habitual whole coca use causing addiction or withdrawal physiology in contrast to that of cocaine users.

Cocaine serum concentrations are determined by the following: (1) dose; (2) route of administration; (3) binding to plasma proteins; and (4) rate of metabolism [13]. Most pharmacologic effects of cocaine are neuroexcitatory in nature, with resultant agitation, combativeness, hyperactivity, and seizures [24]. Cocaine is sought out for its euphoric effects, but it can also cause agitation, anxiety, panic, and psychosis [25]. Both hemorrhagic and ischemic stroke are known consequences of cocaine use [16]. Because of the potent vasoconstrictive effects on vascular smooth muscle, cocaine leads to widespread vascular dysfunction. This vasoconstriction and its anesthetic properties are the mechanisms behind the widespread effects of cocaine on multiorgan systems. In addition to vasoconstrictive effects, cocaine is also an inhibitor of tPA. This is the mechanism for accelerated atherosclerosis in users [16]. Cocaine also acts as a sodium channel blocker which can result in dysrhythmias [16]. Physiologic consequences of cocaine in a medical context are well described in the literature.

## 4. Historical Background

The antiquity of coca use is well established through archaeological studies in South and Central America. Analysis of mummified human remains from Northern Chile indicates the use of coca as early as 1000 BC [26]. These records establish that the use of coca has been ongoing for over 3,000 years in the native peoples of the Andes.

Under Incan rule, coca was used for numerous purposes, including ritual, social, and physiological uses [27]. In 1532, a Spanish expedition conquered the Inca. The Spanish conquerors then attempt to eradicate the use of coca in the native cultures [28]. However, after the elimination of coca proved unsuccessful, the Spanish then decided to exploit coca growth. Subsequently, coca use became more widespread throughout the former Incan empire, and the custom of giving agricultural workers a ration of coca leaves along with their daily wage began [28, 29]. Coca use continues to be a daily staple in the life of many Andean workers.

Interest in coca was prompted in the nineteenth century in Europe and the United States as discussed in an article by Dr. Weil [30]. Mantegazza spent years practicing medicine in Peru. Based on his experience with the local peoples, he became convinced of the widespread benefits of coca including reduction of fatigue, improvements to one's mood, and even the increase of sexual vigor [31]. Editorials on coca made their way into the British Medical Journal [32], and even writings of Sigmund Freud reflected the belief that whole coca could be a psychological cure-all [33]. The interest in whole coca quickly diminished after the isolation of cocaine. The bulk of research has been conducted on the cocaine isolate rather than the fourteen other alkaloids known to be contained in the coca plant [34]. This has led to a paucity of scientific knowledge of whole coca along with any potential medicinal effects that it may have.

## 5. Use in Contemporary Medicine

The Euro-American enthusiasm for coca quickly cooled in the early twentieth century with the increasing concerns of the addictive properties and poor side effect profiles witnessed with the use of cocaine [29]. Coca importation has since been banned in the United States.

*5.1. Gastrointestinal Symptom Treatment.* The South American Indians continue to rely on coca as a medicinal remedy in addition to its general usages for stimulant and social purposes [35]. One of the more traditional roles that coca plays in Andean life is for the relief of gastrointestinal upset. Coca leaf tea is taken to combat stomach pain, intestinal spasm, nausea, indigestion, and even constipation and diarrhea [30]. It is essentially viewed as a comprehensive remedy that restores balance to the digestive system. Coca is masticated or held in the mouth for relief of painful oral sores and also to aid in the healing of oral lesions [30]. Similarly, this plant is used for toothaches as well.

*5.2. Environmental Stress Treatment.* One of the usages of coca that continues to intrigue the medical community is as a remedy for dealing with the stresses of life at high altitude [36]. Given the strong belief in the inherent energizing effects of coca, this could explain the benefit of using this leaf in the high stress environment of high altitude. Coca is also believed to possess properties that help the user withstand hypoxia, cold, and hunger. A series of experiments in the 1970s aimed to test the hypothesis of whether coca chewing was associated with the feeling of warmth. Hanna and Little found that hand and foot temperatures were lowered in Andean people who used coca [37, 38]. Although the thermal difference between control and experimental subjects was not great, this small difference could be advantageous in decreasing the amount of heat loss in extreme environments.

*5.3. Hunger Treatment.* Coca chewing is thought to decrease the feeling of hunger in Andean peoples. Further investigation of this phenomenon has discovered that coca has effects on glucose homeostasis. Chewing coca leaves has been found to elevate blood glucose above the fasting level [39]. This finding led Bolton to believe that coca has a fundamental metabolic function for those Indians with difficulties in glucose homeostasis. This finding of elevated glucose after coca chewing also lends scientific credibility to the native belief that coca staves off hunger pains [40].

*5.4. Altitude Illness Treatment.* As the drive to understand coca's place in Andean culture increased, there was a flurry of work to pin down the mechanism in which the benefits of taking coca existed. Specific to the realm of high altitude medicine, coca chewers report less head pain and dizziness associated with working at high altitudes [41, 42]. Fuchs et al. used available ethnographic and physiologic data to propose a working hypothesis of how coca chewing was aiding individuals who lived and worked in high altitude settings [43]. Through collation of data, it was shown that the percentage of native peoples using coca increases with altitude. This generalization extends to other cultural groups and the female gender, which typically do not exhibit the high acceptance and use of coca as Quechua or other high altitude cultural groups.

Although previous work had shown that physiological adaptations to cold may be enhanced by coca use [37, 38], Fuchs et al. noted that the frequency of coca use does not necessarily correlate with climate. Mineworkers use coca extensively, and yet this is an environment not solely defined by frigid temperatures or high altitude [44]. An interesting new hypothesis was that coca's beneficial properties may lie in the mitigation of effects of hypoxia. Polycythemia is a standard response to the sustained hypoxia of high altitude environments [45]. However, controversy now exists as to whether this beneficial physiologic change can become a maladaptation when taken to the extreme. A detrimental effect of polycythemia is increased blood viscosity, thought to be the mechanism in chronic mountain sickness. Ultimately, Fuchs et al. proposed that the alkaloids present in whole leaf coca pharmacologically inhibit the stimulation of excessive red blood cell production caused by hypoxia. The decreased polycythemic stress decreases the symptoms of mountain sickness and alters the mechanisms by which the body adjusts to the high altitude environment [43].

The belief in coca as an uplifting agent for those individuals working in a high altitude environment is not without its naysayers. Many have argued that it is merely a "spurious correlation" between coca chewing and high altitude [46]. Other theories propose that coca use is thought to be a function of how "Indian" a given society is or that it is used for its general stimulant properties rather than as a specific treatment for symptoms related to high altitude [46]. It remains to be seen if any consensus will be arrived at in the anthropological quest to integrate traditional patterns of coca consumption within a biological or physiological framework.

## 6. Conclusions

Anthropologists continue to examine patterns of coca use among natives to the Andean regions of South America in order to assist in the preservation of this ancient practice. Possession of coca is illegal in many countries due to one of its products, cocaine. International treatises have called for the destruction of all coca farming. Barring Bolivia and Peru, coca is now banned, even for indigenous use. Despite this ongoing controversy, some practitioners who span the cultural and medical divide have proposed the use of coca for contemporary ailments. Due to consumer demand for more natural forms of treatment, folk medicine may be considered in modern pharmacologic contexts. Possible uses could include gastrointestinal conditions, fast-acting antidepressant, treatment for acute mountain sickness, as an energizer for persons involved in physical labor, and symptomatic treatment of toothache and oral lesions [30]. Because the known toxicity and pharmacologic profiles almost exclusively pertain to the pure isolate of cocaine, and not whole coca, controlled trials would need to be undertaken prior to any recommendation for coca in a medical context.

Although most of the theories produced by these scientists are based on observational and not experimental data, merit is to be given for attempting to understand a custom that has been ongoing for thousands of years. The pursuit of continued research from a physiologic or medical perspective will add to the respect of cultural traditions by trying them to give them a venue in which to thrive in our modern world.

## Competing Interests

The authors declare that they have no competing interests.

## References

[1] S. B. Karch, "The history of cocaine toxicity," *Human Pathology*, vol. 20, no. 11, pp. 1037–1039, 1989.

[2] M. Novák, C. A. Salemink, and I. Khan, "Biological activity of the alkaloids of *Erythroxylum coca* and *Erythroxylum novogranatense*," *Journal of Ethnopharmacology*, vol. 10, no. 3, pp. 261–274, 1984.

[3] T. Plowman, "The identification of coca (Erythroxylum species): 1860–1910," *Botanical Journal of the Linnean Society*, vol. 84, no. 4, pp. 329–353, 1982.

[4] T. Plowman, "The identity of amazonian and trujillo Coca," *Botanical Museum Leaflets, Harvard University*, vol. 27, no. 1-2, pp. 45–68, 1979.

[5] F. Wöhler, "Ueber eine organische Base in der Coca," *Archiv der Pharmazie*, vol. 152, no. 1, pp. 29–32, 1860.

[6] T. Plowman, "Botanical perspectives on coca," *Journal of Psychedelic Drugs*, vol. 11, no. 1-2, pp. 103–117, 1979.

[7] L. Rivier, "Analysis of alkaloids in leaves of cultivated *Erythroxylum* and characterization of alkaline substances used during coca chewing," *Journal of Ethnopharmacology*, vol. 3, no. 2-3, pp. 313–335, 1981.

[8] A. J. Jenkins, T. Llosa, I. Montoya, and E. J. Cone, "Identification and quantitation of alkaloids in coca tea," *Forensic Science International*, vol. 77, no. 3, pp. 179–189, 1996.

[9] H. O. Morishima, R. A. Whittington, A. Iso, and T. B. Cooper, "The comparative toxicity of cocaine and its metabolites in conscious rats," *Anesthesiology*, vol. 90, no. 6, pp. 1684–1690, 1999.

[10] R. A. Goldstein, C. DesLauriers, and A. M. Burda, "Cocaine: history, social implications, and toxicity—a review," *Disease-a-Month*, vol. 55, no. 1, pp. 6–38, 2009.

[11] M. Carter, "Chapter II, coca leaves: scientific aspects," in *Cocaine the Legend*, J. H. Gumuciol, Ed., Hisbol, La Paz, Bolivia, 1995.

[12] G. Lanza, *Coca Prohibited*, HISBOL, La Paz, Bolivia, 1995.

[13] K. Heard, R. Palmer, and N. R. Zahniser, "Mechanisms of acute cocaine toxicity," *The Open Pharmacology Journal*, vol. 2, no. 1, pp. 70–78, 2008.

[14] E. A. Warner, "Cocaine abuse," *Annals of Internal Medicine*, vol. 119, no. 3, pp. 226–235, 1993.

[15] R. Baselt, *Disposition of Toxic Drugs and Chemicals in Man*, Biomedical, Foster City, Calif, USA, 6th edition, 2002.

[16] M. S. Boghdadi and R. J. Henning, "Cocaine: pathophysiology and clinical toxicology," *Heart & Lung*, vol. 26, no. 6, pp. 466–483, 1997.

[17] C. van Dyke, P. Jatlow, J. Ungerer, P. G. Barash, and R. Byck, "Oral cocaine: plasma concentrations and central effects," *Science*, vol. 200, no. 4338, pp. 211–213, 1978.

[18] J. I. Javaid, M. W. Fischman, C. R. Schuster, H. Dekirmenjian, and J. M. Davis, "Cocaine plasma concentration: relation to physiological and subjective effects in humans," *Science*, vol. 202, no. 4364, pp. 227–228, 1978.

[19] R. E. Mittleman and C. V. Wetli, "Death caused by recreational cocaine use. An update," *Journal of the American Medical Association*, vol. 252, no. 14, pp. 1889–1893, 1984.

[20] K. Blaho, B. Logan, S. Winbery, L. Park, and E. Schwilke, "Blood cocaine and metabolite concentrations, clinical findings, and outcome of patients presenting to an ED," *The American Journal of Emergency Medicine*, vol. 18, no. 5, pp. 593–598, 2000.

[21] F. J. Peretti, D. S. Isenschmid, B. Levine, Y. H. Caplan, and J. E. Smialek, "Cocaine fatality: an unexplained blood concentration in a fatal overdose," *Forensic Science International*, vol. 48, no. 2, pp. 135–138, 1990.

[22] P. E. Heckelman, M. J. O'Neil, and C. B. Kock, *The Merck Index: An Encyclopedia of Chemicals, Drugs, and Biologicals*, Merck, Kenilworth, NJ, USA, 2006.

[23] S. S. Mazor, M. B. Mycyk, B. K. Wills, L. D. Brace, L. Gussow, and T. Erickson, "Coca tea consumption causes positive urine

cocaine assay," *European Journal of Emergency Medicine*, vol. 13, no. 6, pp. 340–341, 2006.

[24] J. Glauser and J. R. Queen, "An overview of non-cardiac cocaine toxicity," *The Journal of Emergency Medicine*, vol. 32, no. 2, pp. 181–186, 2007.

[25] U. D. McCann and G. A. Ricaurte, "Neuropathology of cocaine abuse," *Current Opinion in Psychiatry*, vol. 12, no. 3, pp. 277–280, 1999.

[26] M. A. Rivera, A. C. Aufderheide, L. W. Cartmell, C. M. Torres, and O. Langsjoen, "Antiquity of coca-leaf chewing in the south centralandes: a 3,000 year archaeological record of coca-leaf chewing from Northern Chile," *Journal of Psychoactive Drugs*, vol. 37, no. 4, pp. 455–458, 2005.

[27] B. Cobo, *History of the Inca Empire: An Account of the Indian's Customs and their Origin, Together with a Treatise on Inca Legend*, University of Texas Press, Austin, Tex, USA, 1979.

[28] E. Carroll, "Coca: the plant and its use," in *Cocaine*, NIDA Research Monograph #13, pp. 35–46, National Institute on Drug Abuse, 1977.

[29] V. B. Stolberg, "The use of coca: prehistory, history, and ethnography," *Journal of Ethnicity in Substance Abuse*, vol. 10, no. 2, pp. 126–146, 2011.

[30] A. T. Weil, "The therapeutic value of coca in contemporary medicine," *Journal of Ethnopharmacology*, vol. 3, no. 2-3, pp. 367–376, 1981.

[31] P. Mantegazza, *Sulle Virtio Igieniche e Medicinale della Coca*, Annali Universali di Medicina, Milan, Italy, 1859.

[32] A. Bennett, "The physiological action of coca," *BMJ*, vol. 1, no. 694, p. 510, 1874.

[33] B. Robert, S. Freud, and A. Freud, *Cocaine Papers*, Stone Hill, 1974.

[34] D. Streatfeild, *Cocaine: An Unauthorized Biography*, Picador/St. Marten's Press, New York, NY, USA, 2001.

[35] R. T. Martin, "The role of coca in the history, religion, and medicine of South American Indians," *Economic Botany*, vol. 24, no. 4, pp. 422–438, 1970.

[36] T. Torchetti, "Coca chewing and high altitude adaptation," *Totem*, vol. 1, no. 1, article 16, 2011.

[37] J. M. Hanna, "Responses of Quechua Indians to coca ingestion during cold exposure," *American Journal of Physical Anthropology*, vol. 34, no. 2, pp. 273–277, 1971.

[38] M. A. Little, "Effects of alcohol and coca on foot temperature responses of highland Peruvians during $\alpha$ localized cold exposure," *American Journal of Physical Anthropology*, vol. 32, no. 2, pp. 233–242, 1970.

[39] R. Bolton, "Andean coca chewing: a metabolic perspective," *American Anthropologist*, vol. 78, no. 3, pp. 630–634, 1976.

[40] R. Bolton, "On coca chewing and high-altitude stress," *Current Anthropology*, vol. 20, no. 2, pp. 418–420, 1979.

[41] C. Monge, "Chronic mountain sickness," *Physiological Reviews*, vol. 23, no. 2, pp. 166–184, 1943.

[42] W. G. Mortimer, *Peru: History of Coca, "the Divine Plant" of the Incas*, J. H. Vail, New York, NY, USA, 1901.

[43] A. Fuchs, R. E. Burchard, C. C. Curtain et al., "Coca chewing and high-altitude stress: possible effects of coca alkaloids on erythropoiesis [and comments and reply]," *Current Anthropology*, vol. 19, no. 2, pp. 277–291, 1978.

[44] E. Galeano, *Open Veins of Latin America: Five Centuries of the Pillage of a Continent*, Monthly Review Press, New York, NY, USA, 1973.

[45] A. Hurtado, "Influence of anoxemia on the hemopoietic activity," *Archives of Internal Medicine*, vol. 75, no. 5, pp. 284–323, 1945.

[46] W. Bray, C. Dollery, G. Barnett et al., "Coca chewing and high-altitude stress: a spurious correlation [and comments and reply]," *Current Anthropology*, vol. 24, no. 3, pp. 269–282, 1983.

# 24

# Drug Utilization Study in Medical Emergency Unit of a Tertiary Care Hospital in North India

**Sharonjeet Kaur,[1] Sujit Rajagopalan,[1] Navjot Kaur,[1] Nusrat Shafiq,[1] Ashish Bhalla,[2] Promila Pandhi,[1] and Samir Malhotra[1]**

[1] *Department of Pharmacology, PGIMER, Chandigarh 160012, India*
[2] *Department of Internal Medicine, PGIMER, Chandigarh 160012, India*

Correspondence should be addressed to Nusrat Shafiq; nusha.pgi2302@yahoo.com

Academic Editor: Òscar Miró

*Objective.* To generate data on the drug utilization pattern and cost of drug treatment and to determine the rationality of prescriptions. *Methods.* A retrospective cross-sectional drug utilization study was conducted in the medical emergency unit of our hospital. Patient case records were reviewed to extract data on the pattern of drug use. Cost of drug treatment for the emergency visit was calculated by referring to the cost mentioned in Monthly Index of Medical Specialties and the rationality of prescriptions was evaluated using WHO core indicators of drug utilization. *Results.* 1100 case records were reviewed. Majority of patients received proton pump inhibitors followed by multivitamins. The median cost per prescription was 119.23$ (7.32$–7663.46$). Majority (49.9%) of drug cost was driven by antibiotics alone. An average of 4.9 drugs was prescribed per prescription. There were 14.89% encounters with antibiotics. 75.17% of the drugs were given as injectables and only 29.27% of the drugs were prescribed as generics. *Conclusion.* There is need to rationalize the drug therapy in terms of increasing prescribing of drugs by generic name and to avoid overuse of PPIs and multivitamins in emergency unit. Also the hospital pharmacy should be encouraged to procure more cost effective alternative antibiotics in future.

## 1. Introduction

The World Health Organization (WHO) defines drug utilization research as "*the marketing, distribution, prescription and use of drugs in a society, with special emphasis on the resulting medical, social, and economic consequences*" [1]. Thus, inherent in the definition, such studies provide logical background for determining the rationality of drug use as well as providing evidence based guidance for making policy decisions at various levels of healthcare. Drug utilization research studies conducted in the inpatient settings are effective tools that help in evaluating the drug prescribing trends, efficiency, and cost-effectiveness of hospital formularies. There is always a variation in drug utilization among different countries and even among health institutions within a country and sometimes within the same institute at different point of time probably because of changing disease trends over a period of time [2]. Conducting periodic studies of pattern of drug use in various hospital settings or patient populations is therefore essential to critically analyse the current hospital drug policies and to make recommendations based on various guidelines to improve upon the current drug usage pattern in the future, if needed. This is more importantly required in resource poor countries like ours so as to ensure that the scarce resources are utilized in the best possible manner. Though there have been various drug utilization studies conducted on specific populations and in varied settings in India [3, 4], only a few have been conducted in emergency settings [5–7]. Previous studies conducted by the authors in our hospital emergency department were primarily safety utilization studies [8, 9].

The emergency department represents an important platform for conducting drug utilization studies as patients present with a wide range of diseases in acute form and the drug use is quite extensive. Therefore, evaluating the drug prescribing behaviour and usage patterns in the emergency settings has the potential of determining the rationality of drug therapy being given in the particular region to a broader extent. Keeping this in view, we conducted a drug utilization study in our tertiary care hospital with the objective of studying pattern of drug use and cost of drug treatment and determining the rationality of prescriptions so as to identify priority areas that need to be targeted for further improvement in patient care.

## 2. Methods

We conducted a retrospective cross-sectional drug utilization study at the Medical Emergency Department of Postgraduate Institute of Medical Education and Research, Chandigarh, India, over a period of six months. Our institute is a premier tertiary care hospital which caters to needs of a large patient pool from both urban and rural areas of North India. Medical emergency unit has 44 beds and has a turnover of about 3000 patients per month. All adult patients presenting with any emergency medical need are attended by internal medicine specialists in the emergency department for initial management.

For studying the drug utilization pattern, following data were collected-(i) age, (ii) gender, (iii) average stay in the emergency department, (iv) diagnosis of the patient, (v) comorbid conditions. Detailed information on drugs used including name of the drug, dosage schedule (form, route, and frequency), and duration of treatment was recorded from the patient medical records.

For cost assessment, we considered only those drugs which were prescribed in the emergency department for the presenting acute condition. Cost of individual drugs was calculated according to the pricing of drugs given in Monthly Index of Medical Specialists (MIMS). We summed up the costs for each group of drugs. Cost of individual prescriptions was also calculated. The currency we used for cost calculations was INR, which was later converted to US dollars (2011).

Rationality of prescriptions was evaluated by using the WHO core drug prescribing indicators, that is, (a) average number of drugs per encounter, (b) percentage of encounters with an antibiotic, (c) percentage of encounters with an injection, (d) percentage of drugs prescribed from the essential drugs list or formulary, and (e) percentage of drugs prescribed by generic names. Indian National List of Essential Medicines, 2003, was used for assessing the number of drugs prescribed from the essential list. The term antibiotic was inclusive of antitubercular, antiprotozoal, and antihelminthic agents in addition to antibacterial, antiviral, and antifungal agents.

Statistical analysis—continuous data are expressed as mean ± S.D. Nominal data were expressed as percentages. No formal statistical hypothesis was tested.

## 3. Results

*3.1. Analysis of Drug Utilization Pattern.* A total of 1100 case records were reviewed. Among the cases, 736 were males and 364 were females. The mean age group of patients admitted was 46 ± 17.4 years. Among the different age groups of the patients admitted, maximum patients ($n$ = 452) were in the age group of 40 to 59 yrs. The average stay of patients in the emergency department was 2.23 ± 1.3 days.

Majority of the patients presented with diseases of cardiovascular system (26.5%), followed by central nervous system (23.5%), gastrointestinal system (20%), and respiratory system (10.7%). The rest of the cases were related to other organ systems as given in Figure 1. Acute coronary syndrome (13.67%), seizures (7.14%), acute cerebrovascular accidents (5.45), acute gastroenteritis (5.09), and epigastric pain presenting as acid peptic disease (5%) followed by hypertensive disease and respiratory disorders like acute exacerbation of chronic obstructive pulmonary disease and asthma constituted the majority of the total cases. Hypertension and diabetes mellitus (49.69%) accounted for the majority of the underlying comorbid conditions, followed by chronic kidney disease, coronary artery disease, tuberculosis, COPD, liver disease, dilated cardiomyopathy, cancer, and arrhythmias (Table 1).

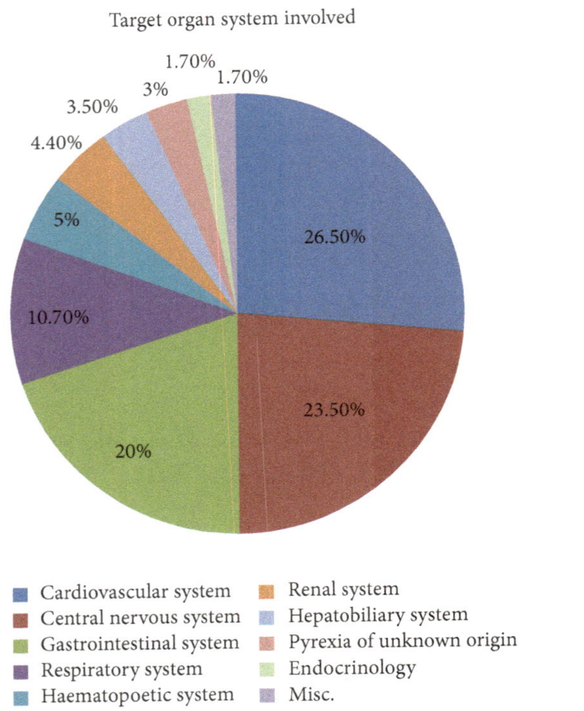


FIGURE 1: Pie chart showing the distribution of various target organ systems involved.

Most of the drugs prescribed were for cardiovascular system (36%) followed by gastrointestinal system (20.8%) and other systems (Figure 2). Among the drugs prescribed, majority of the patients ($N$ = 646) received proton pump inhibitors, followed by multivitamins ($N$ = 567), antibiotics ($N$ = 462), diuretics ($N$ = 265), and antiplatelet drugs ($N$ = 224) (Table 2). 1.44% of the total prescribed drugs were given as fixed dose combinations (FDCs). The commonly prescribed FDCs were amoxicillin-clavulanic acid (0.83%), antitubercular therapy (0.20%), piperacillin-tazobactam (0.16%), and trimethoprim-sulphamethoxazole (0.08%). Among the injectable preparations proton pump inhibitors (41.8%) were the most commonly prescribed agents followed by other agents as shown in Figure 3.

TABLE 1: Various comorbid conditions in the cases studied.

| S. number | Underlying disease | Number of cases (%) |
|---|---|---|
| 1 | Hypertension | 86 (26.06) |
| 2 | Diabetes mellitus | 78 (23.63) |
| 3 | Chronic kidney disease | 29 (8.78) |
| 4 | Coronary artery disease | 19 (5.75) |
| 5 | Tuberculosis | 16 (4.84) |
| 6 | Chronic obstructive pulmonary disease | 15 (4.54) |
| 7 | Chronic liver disease | 13 (3.93) |
| 8 | Dilated cardiomyopathy | 12 (3.63) |
| 9 | Cerebrovascular accidents | 10 (3.03) |
| 10 | Cancer | 6 (1.81) |
| 11 | Arrhythmias | 1 (0.30) |

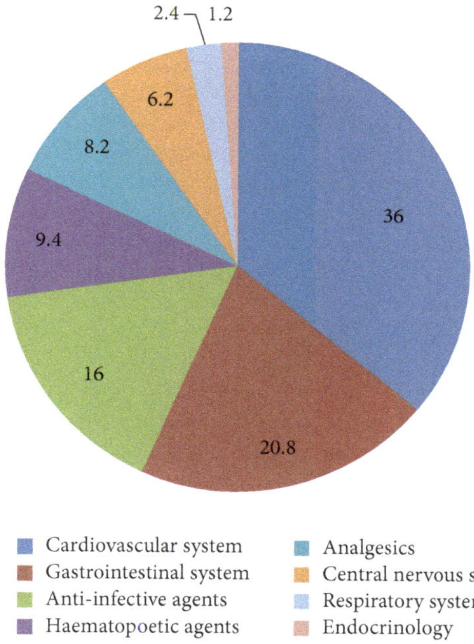


FIGURE 2: Pie chart showing various classes of drugs prescribed.

TABLE 2: Most commonly prescribed drugs.

| Drug class | Number of patients | ATC |
|---|---|---|
| Proton pump inhibitors | 646 | A02BC |
| Multivitamins | 567 | A11 |
| Antibiotic | 462 | J01 |
| Diuretics | 265 | C03 |
| Antiplatelet drug | 224 | B01AC |

ATC: Anatomical Therapeutic and Chemical Classification drug class coding (as per WHO).

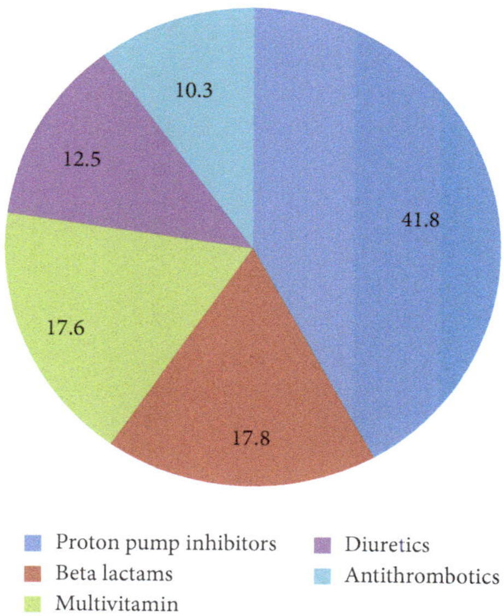


FIGURE 3: Percentage of the drugs used as injectables.

*3.2. Cost of Drug Treatment.* Cost of individual drug classes varied widely. The summed-up costs for each group of drugs towards out-of-pocket expenses are presented in Table 3. Among the different drugs prescribed, anti-infectives (49.9%) accounted for the maximum cost followed by the drugs acting on the cardiovascular system (25.8%), drugs acting on the gastrointestinal system (11%), nutritional supplements (4.7%), analgesic/anti-inflammatory drugs (4.3%), and hormones (2.8%).

*3.3. Analysis of Prescription Indicators.* Analysis of prescriptions using WHO core indicators revealed that the average number of drugs prescribed per prescription was 4.9. There were 610 (14.89%) encounters with antibiotics. 75.17% of the drugs were prescribed as injectables. 64.94% of the total drugs were prescribed from the national essential medicine list, 2003. Branded drugs constituted 70.73% and generic drugs constituted 29.27% of the total drugs prescribed (Table 4).

## 4. Discussion

The emergency department of a tertiary care unit of a developing country is faced with the problem of heavy patient load and relative paucity of human and economic resources. Specifically, our hospital is a premier tertiary care hospital which caters to a large population pool of the North Indian region. The drugs are prescribed by the attending internal medicine physician. The emergency drugs are provided within the hospital but the majority of the drug expenses have to be borne by the patients themselves.

The average stay of the patients in the emergency was $2.23 \pm 1.3$ days. This indicates a rapid and efficient management of patients after which they were discharged or they were transferred to a medical ward. The most commonly involved organ systems were cardiovascular system and CNS and the top five diseases were acute coronary syndrome, seizures, acute cerebrovascular accidents, acute gastroenteritis, and acute epigastric pain. This picture is representative of our medical emergency set-up which caters to wide range of diseases presenting in acute forms. The most common

Table 3: Cost of various drug classes.

| Drug class | Cost of drugs (USD) |
|---|---|
| Sulphonamide | 0.261 |
| Cholinergic | 0.53 |
| ARBs | 1.59 |
| Anticholinergic | 7.32 |
| H2 blockers | 7.33 |
| Tetracyclines | 9.49 |
| Antifungal | 12.5 |
| Beta blockers | 14.56 |
| Bronchodilators | 15.12 |
| NSAIDS | 16.14 |
| Aminoglycosides | 21.42 |
| Opioids | 52.93 |
| ACE inhibitors | 55.49 |
| Sedative hypnotics | 69.78 |
| Antitubercular drugs | 85.22 |
| CCBs | 85.42 |
| Statins | 92.33 |
| Antiplatelet | 95.55 |
| Inotropic agents | 97.84 |
| Misc. GIT drugs | 119.23 |
| Antiemetics | 167.82 |
| Antiviral | 180.48 |
| Misc. CVS drugs | 196.86 |
| Nitrates | 199.54 |
| Antifibrinolytic | 220.28 |
| Antiepileptic | 236.81 |
| Antiarrhythmics | 298.44 |
| Antidiabetic | 316.57 |
| Antiprotozoal | 375.99 |
| Fluoroquinolones | 382.14 |
| Fibrinolytic drugs | 492.91 |
| Hormones | 575.51 |
| Corticosteroids | 792.1 |
| Multivitamins | 956.68 |
| Diuretics | 1032.46 |
| PPIs | 1913.61 |
| Antithrombotic | 2312.24 |
| Macrolides | 3605.81 |
| Beta lactams | 7663.46 |

Table 4: Analysis of prescriptions using WHO core prescribing indicators.

| WHO core indicators | *N* (%) |
|---|---|
| Average number of drugs per prescription | 4.9 |
| Encounter with antibiotics | 610 (14.89) |
| Encounter with injectables | 3079 (75.17) |
| Drug prescribed from essential medicine list | 2660 (64.94) |
| Drug prescribed as generic | 1199 (29.27) |

underlying comorbid conditions were hypertension and diabetes mellitus which adds to the existing body of evidence that these diseases are assuming epidemic proportions in developing countries as well.

Analysis of case records for drug utilization pattern revealed that most of the drug classes were prescribed for appropriate indication. However, prescription of multivitamins appears largely irrational as they are not indicated for the management of emergency conditions. Moreover, a large number of these agents were prescribed as injectables and since these are expensive, they would have definitely increased costs associated with the emergency visit. Similarly, proton pump inhibitors were also found to be used for some patients where there was no appropriate indication, for example, in a patient of fever under evaluation, in a patient of right thigh cellulitis, and in a patient of bronchiectasis. The rationality of use of proton pump inhibitors and multivitamins is thus questionable.

We considered only the direct drug costs for those agents that were prescribed for the presenting emergency condition. Cost of chronic medications was not considered in the analysis nor was that of the other hospital charges. The median cost per prescription was 119.23$ (7.32$–7663.46$). This is very high, especially in our setting where most of the patients are from the lower socioeconomic strata and cannot afford such expensive therapy. Analysis of the data revealed that majority of the cost was driven by antimicrobials. This is probably because, in an emergency setting, there is a dire need to give broad spectrum antibiotics as empirical therapy, which is usually very expensive. But what is essential is to narrow down the therapy as soon as we have a sensitivity report for the infecting organism. Apart from the benefit of reduced cost, this will also help combat drug resistance due to inadvertent use of antibiotics. In our hospital set-up, the culture sensitivity report usually becomes available within 48–72 hrs. So, for most of the patients de-escalation did not happen in the emergency visit but was advised at the time of discharge from emergency unit where it was required.

Average number of drugs per prescription was 4.9 which is more than double the average number (i.e., 2) recommended by WHO [10]. However, this cannot be considered irrational polypharmacy practice as there is need of empirical therapy till definitive diagnosis becomes clear and secondly for management of acute life threatening conditions most of the patients would usually require more than two drugs. Different studies conducted in India have given varied results, but all of them point to higher incidence of multiple drug usage in emergency set-ups. For example, one reports this incidence to be 3.3, whereas another study has reported the use of drugs to be as high as $9.9 \pm 2.5$ drugs per prescription [6, 11]. Similarly number of encounters with injectables was on the higher end (75.17%), which again seems justifiable on account of need of immediate drug action. Drugs prescribed from the WHO essential medicine list comprised only 64.94% of drugs. This proportion should have been higher since this list of drugs is prepared with regard to public health relevance, evidence on efficacy and safety of the drugs, and comparative cost effectiveness. Also, another area of concern was the lower proportion of drugs prescribed as generics (only 29.27%). There are several benefits of prescribing drugs as generics such as increased patient compliance and lower cost of drug therapy [12, 13]. American Academy of Family Physicians recommends prescribing drugs in generic forms as a strategy to avoid high cost of drug therapy [14].

Our study has some limitations. We are not certain if our sample size of 1100 patients was truly representative of total population visiting emergency, but nevertheless our sample size is much larger as compared to previous studies conducted in India [7, 11]. Another limitation was that we have not analysed the data for the disorders managed differently (e.g., acute coronary syndrome with or without ST segment elevation). This would have given a clearer picture on the cost of drug treatment.

## 5. Conclusion

This study highlights the need for rationalising drug therapy in the emergency settings with regard to increasing adherence to national essential medicine list and increasing prescription of drugs by generic name. Also there is need to prevent inappropriate overuse of PPI and multivitamins where it is not indicated. Since the drug cost is mostly driven by prescription of broad spectrum antibiotics, therefore hospital pharmacy should be encouraged to procure more cost effective alternative antibiotics in future.

## Conflict of Interests

The authors declare no conflict of interests and no relationships with the industry.

## References

[1] 2014, http://apps.who.int/medicinedocs/en/d/Js4876e.

[2] U. Bergman, I. Christenson, B. Jansson, and B. E. Wiholm, "Auditing hospital drug utilisation by means of defined daily doses per bed-day. A methodological study," *European Journal of Clinical Pharmacology*, vol. 17, no. 3, pp. 183–187, 1980.

[3] R. Sharma, B. Kapoor, and U. Verma, "Drug utilization pattern during pregnancy in North India," *Indian Journal of Medical Sciences*, vol. 60, no. 7, pp. 277–287, 2006.

[4] P. R. Jadhav, V. V. Moghe, and Y. A. Deshmukh, "Drug utilization study in ophthalmology outpatients at a tertiary care teaching hospital," *ISRN Pharmacology*, vol. 2013, Article ID 768792, 22 pages, 2013.

[5] S. R. Pendhari, D. R. Chaudhari, S. R. Burute, and B. M. Bite, "A study on the drug utilization trends in the cardiovascular emergencies in a tertiary care hospital," *Journal of Clinical and Diagnostic Research*, vol. 7, no. 4, pp. 666–670, 2013.

[6] P. A. Barot, S. D. Malhotra, D. A. Rana, V. J. Patel, and K. P. Patel, "Drug utilization in emergency medicine department at a tertiary care teaching hospital: a prospective study," *Journal of Basic and Clinical Pharmacy*, vol. 4, pp. 78–81, 2013.

[7] K. A. Al Balushi, S. Al-Shibli, and I. Al-Zakwani, "Drug utilization patterns in the emergency department: a retrospective study," *Journal of Basic and Clinical Pharmacy*, vol. 5, pp. 1–6, 2014.

[8] S. Malhotra, S. Jain, and P. Pandhi, "Drug-related visits to the medical emergency department: a prospective study from India," *International Journal of Clinical Pharmacology and Therapeutics*, vol. 39, no. 1, pp. 12–18, 2001.

[9] S. Malhotra, R. S. Karan, P. Pandhi, and S. Jain, "Drug related medical emergencies in the elderly: role of adverse drug reactions and non-compliance," *Postgraduate Medical Journal*, vol. 77, no. 913, pp. 703–707, 2001.

[10] J. D. Quick, H. V. Hogerzeil, G. Velásquez, and L. Rägo, "Twenty-five years of essential medicines," *Bulletin of the World Health Organization*, vol. 80, no. 11, pp. 913–914, 2002.

[11] C. Cheekavolu, R. M. Pathapati, K. Babasaheb Laxmansingh et al., "Evaluation of drug utilization patterns during initial treatment in the emergency room: a retroprospective pharmacoepidemiological study," *ISRN Pharmacology*, vol. 2011, Article ID 261585, 3 pages, 2011.

[12] J. S. Haas, K. A. Phillips, E. P. Gerstenberger, and A. C. Seger, "Potential savings from substituting generic drugs for brand-name drugs: medical expenditure panel survey, 1997–2000," *Annals of internal medicine*, vol. 142, no. 11, pp. 891–897, 2005.

[13] W. H. Shrank, T. Hoang, S. L. Ettner et al., "The implications of choice: Prescribing generic or preferred pharmaceuticals improves medication adherence for chronic conditions," *Archives of Internal Medicine*, vol. 166, no. 3, pp. 332–337, 2006.

[14] P. Gardiner and L. Dvorkin, "Promoting medication adherence in children," *The American Family Physician*, vol. 74, no. 5, pp. 793–798, 2006.

# 25

# Tranexamic Acid (TXA) in Trauma Patients: Barriers to Use among Trauma Surgeons and Emergency Physicians

**Abdulaziz Alburaih**

*Department of Emergency Medicine, University of Maryland Shore Regional Health, Easton, MD, USA*

Correspondence should be addressed to Abdulaziz Alburaih; azizalburaih@gmail.com

Academic Editor: Joe Nemeth

*Objective.* Tranexamic Acid (TXA) is currently the only drug with prospective clinical evidence supporting its use in bleeding trauma patients. We sought to better understand the barriers preventing its use and elicit suggestions to further its use in trauma patients in the state of Maryland. *Methods.* This is a cross-sectional study. *Results.* The overall response rate was 38%. Half of all participants reported being familiar with the CRASH-2 trial and MATTERs study. Half reported being aware of TXA as part of their institution's massive transfusion protocol. The majority of participants felt that TXA would have a significant positive impact on the survival of trauma patients. A majority also felt that the use of TXA would increase if its administration was the responsibility of both trauma surgeons and emergency physicians. *Conclusion.* Only half of responders reported being aware of TXA as being part of their institution's massive transfusion protocol. Lack of awareness of the clinical data supporting its use is a major barrier. However, most trauma providers and emergency physicians do have a favorable view of TXA and support its incorporation into massive transfusion protocols. We believe that more studies of this kind on both state and national level are needed.

## 1. Introduction

Bleeding contributes to about one-third of trauma-related deaths [1]. It is a major contributing factor to other causes of death such as head injury and multiorgan failure in trauma patients [2]. In a retrospective cohort study conducted at level I trauma center in Toronto, massive bleeding resulting from blunt pelvic injury was the leading cause of preventable death among trauma patients [3]. Coagulopathy is one component of the lethal triad of trauma, in addition to hypothermia and acidosis. In the setting of massive bleeding, trauma-related coagulopathy occurs through a myriad of mechanisms, including consumption and subsequent acute deficiency of clotting factors and platelets, concomitant acidosis, hypothermia and dysregulation of mediatory pathways leading to fibrinolysis, and systemic activation of thrombin [4]. The activation of fibrinolysis accompanying the massive generation of thrombin in the period immediately following trauma has been well described and is indicated by the elevated levels of D-dimers, fibrin split products, and plasmin-antiplasmin complexes found in the blood samples drawn from trauma patients on presentation [5]. Tranexamic Acid (TXA) is a synthetic lysine derivative that acts as a competitive inhibitor of plasminogen activation, whereas at higher concentration it acts as a noncompetitive inhibitor of plasmin. It is believed that its main action is to improve coagulation through stabilization of clot [6]. The CRASH-2 trial was an international randomized, placebo controlled trial of the early administration of TXA to bleeding trauma patients. CRASH-2 enrolled 20,211 patients from 274 hospitals in 40 countries. The investigators reported that all-cause mortality was significantly lower among patients who received TXA than in a placebo group (4.5% versus 16.0%; relative risk 0.91, 95% CI, 0.85–0.97; $P = 0.0035$), with number needed to treat (NNT) of 67, importantly, with no apparent increase in side effects [7]. Early treatment with TXA (within 1 hour of injury) significantly reduced the risk of death due to bleeding (5.3% in TXA group versus 7.7% in placebo group; RR 0.68; $P < 0.0001$). TXA given between 1 and 3 hours also reduced the risk of death due to bleeding (4.8% versus 6.1%; RR 0.79, $P = 0.03$). TXA given after 3 hours seemed to increase the risk of death due to bleeding (4.4% versus 3.1%; RR 1.44, 0.004) [8]. Early administration of TXA may decrease mortality due to bleeding in trauma patients but late administration of TXA is less effective and could be harmful. The Military Application of Tranexamic Acid for Trauma Emergency Resuscitation (MATTERs) trial results showed an absolute reduction in mortality of 6.7% (14.4% in TXA group versus 28.1% in no TXA group; $P = 0.004$), and number needed to treat (NNT) was 1:7. All patients in the MATTERs trial received blood transfusion: those who received TXA required less blood products [9]. MATTERs trial addressed some of the critiques of CRASH-2 trail including its use of civilian hospitals that lacked modern trauma systems, its lack of laboratory testing to determine coagulopathy, its inclusion of a small number of penetrating traumas, and, most importantly, its uncertainty concerning the need for an antifibrinolytic in a group in which only half required blood transfusion and an equally small amount required surgery [10]. In 2011, the US Army reviewed the evidence from the CRASH-2 trial and included TXA into its trauma treatment protocols [11]. A recent prospective cohort study of severely injured adult patients (injury severity score > 15) admitted to a civilian trauma system showed that TXA was independently associated with a reduction in multiorgan failure (odds ratio [OR] = 0.27, $P = 0.01$) and was protective for adjusted all-cause mortality (OR = 0.16 CI: 0.03–0.86, $P = 0.03$) among patients in shock. The authors concluded that TXA as part of a major hemorrhage protocol within a mature civilian trauma system provides outcome benefits specifically for severely injured shocked patients [12]. Tranexamic Acid (TXA) has been shown to reduce bleeding in many surgical and medical settings. Since the 1970s, its applications were expanded to dysfunctional uterine bleeding, refractory thrombocytopenia, hemophilia, and von Willebrand's disease [13]. Tranexamic Acid (TXA) has been used effectively to reduce bleeding and the concomitant need for blood transfusions in nontrauma patients; for example, a systematic review of randomized trial showed that TXA reduced the number of patients receiving blood transfusion by third [13]. A meta-analysis of randomized controlled trials suggested that TXA might reduce the amount of blood transfusions in patients undergoing total knee replacement [14]. Two other randomized controlled trials suggested a benefit of TXA in patients undergoing liver transplantation and cesarean sections [15, 16]. Despite all the current evidence supporting its use in these settings, TXA is underutilized. We aimed to better understand why this is so by surveying the opinions of providers who deal directly with trauma patients, trauma surgeons and emergency physicians in the states of Maryland.

## 2. Material and Methods

*2.1. Study Design.* This is a cross-sectional study using an online and paper based survey. A representative sample of trauma providers and emergency physicians in the state of Maryland were asked to complete the survey. No identifying information, including IP addresses, was collected from participants. Trauma providers at trauma centers in the state of Maryland were identified through records maintained by Committee of Trauma of the American College of Surgeon (ACS) Maryland Chapter. Members received an e-mail (from

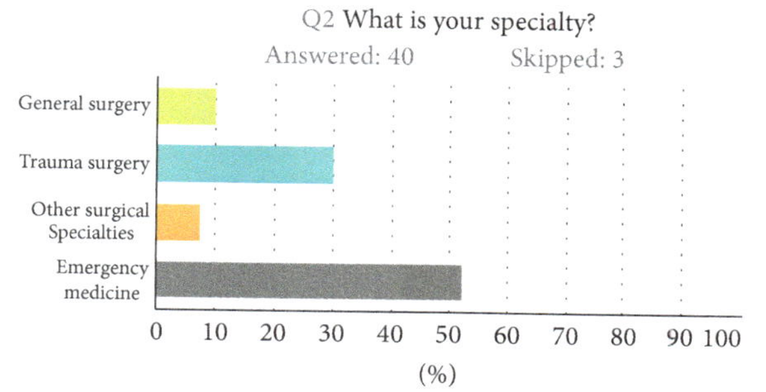


FIGURE 1: Participants by specialty.

May to July 2015) with an invitation to participate in the study and a unique link to the online version of the survey. A similar paper version of the survey was distributed to emergency physicians during Maryland American College of Emergency Physician (ACEP) 2015 Annual Educational Conference. Participation was voluntary and all responses were collected anonymously. Electronic safeguards were implemented to prevent multiple replies from respondents. Results from the questionnaire were compiled using a password-protected database.

*2.2. Methods.* This anonymous survey was designed to (1) assess baseline knowledge and awareness of the evidence for the use of TXA in bleeding trauma patients, (2) identify the perceived barriers to use of TXA among trauma surgeons and ER physicians, and (3) elicit suggestions on ways to incorporate TXA into trauma protocols and increase its use in bleeding trauma patients. Demographic data were collected regarding trauma designation and specialty of participants. University of Maryland Shore Health Institutional Review Board (IRB) exempted the study from review and waived informed consent requirement for this study.

## 3. Results

An online and printed survey version were distributed to 60 trauma surgeons and 54 emergency physicians at the Maryland ACEP 2015 Annual Educational Conference. The overall response rate was 38% (49% trauma surgeons, 51% emergency physicians). The survey was divided into four main sections: demographics, knowledge of the literature, barriers to TXA use, and suggestions on ways to implement TXA in trauma protocols.

*3.1. Demographics.* Half of respondents (51%) worked at one of the two level I trauma centers in Maryland; 20% and 15% of respondents worked at level II and III centers, respectively. Among survey respondents, 30% were trauma surgeons; 10% were general surgeons; 7.5 were from other surgical specialties; and 52.5% were emergency physicians (Figure 1).

*3.2. Knowledge of the Literature.* Half of the participants (50%) reported being familiar with the results of the CRASH-2 trial and the MATTERs study. Among those who were not

Table 1

| Question | Strongly agree | Somewhat agree | Unsure | Strongly disagree | Somewhat disagree |
|---|---|---|---|---|---|
| What position do you hold to implementing Tranexamic Acid in trauma or massive transfusion protocol for exsanguinating trauma patients? | 20% | 53.33% | 23.33% | 0% | 3.33% |
| What is your opinion regarding the following statement? The use of Tranexamic Acid (TXA) as part of a massive transfusion protocol will have a significant positive impact on the survival of those trauma patients upon whom it is used. | 10% | 53.33% | 30% | 0% | 6.67% |

familiar with those studies, 33% were trauma care providers working in designated trauma centers. Almost two-thirds of respondents (62.5%) thought that CRASH-2 trial conclusions applied to US trauma patients. In contrast 37.5% thought the conclusions of CRASH-2 did not apply to US trauma patients because the study was conducted in the developing world. Half of the participants agreed that the MATTERs study supported the use of TXA in American trauma patients, and the other half were unsure. Sixty-two percent of participants thought that both the CRASH-2 trial and MATTERs study presented strong evidence supporting the use of TXA in trauma patients. Only 19% thought that both studies provided weak evidence regarding that use in trauma patients.

*3.2.1. Barriers to TXA Use in Trauma Patients.* Half of all participants reported being aware of TXA being part of their institutions' massive transfusion protocol for exsanguinating trauma patients. Twenty-nine percent of participants were not aware of TXA being part of a massive transfusion protocol at their institution, whereas 20.8% where unsure (28.5% of trauma surgeons reported either "no" or "unsure" if TXA is part of their massive transfusion protocols). Three-fourths (75%) of participants state that they would feel comfortable giving TXA to exsanguinating patients if TXA were to be incorporated in their institution's massive transfusion protocols (35% of them are trauma surgeons) (Figure 2). In terms of barriers to adopting a protocol-based approach to giving TXA to trauma patients, 44% of participants pointed to a lack of unawareness of the evidence as the greatest barrier, 19% to a lack of knowledge regarding the time sensitivity of TXA administration, 15% to its absence in massive transfusion protocols, and 11% to doubts about CRASH-2 trail findings (Figure 3).

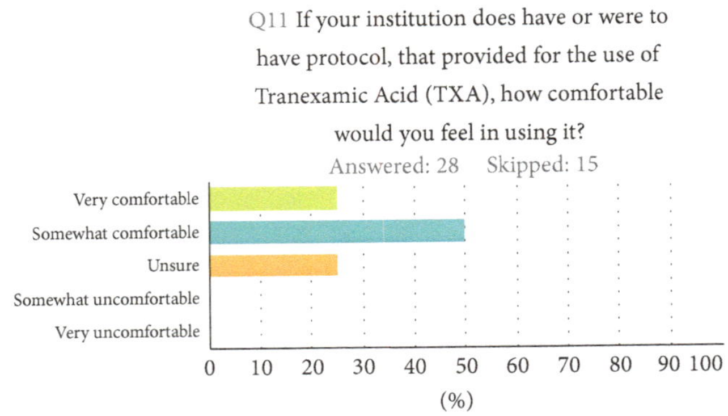


Figure 2: How comfortable would you feel to use TXA in exsanguinating trauma patients if TXA were incorporated in your institution massive transfusion protocols.

*3.2.2. Suggestions on Ways to Implement TXA in Trauma Protocols.* Almost three-quarters (73%) of the participants agreed that TXA should be included in massive transfusion protocols for exsanguinating trauma patients. Sixty-three percent felt that use of TXA as part of a massive transfusion protocol would have a significant impact on the survival of trauma patients who received it (Table 1).

About half of the respondents (53%) thought that making TXA administration the responsibility of both trauma surgeons and emergency physicians would most likely lead to a protocol-based approach for administering TXA to patients with acute coagulopathy of trauma. About a quarter (26%) thought a recommendation from ACS Committee on Trauma would likely lead to a protocol-based approach for administering TXA to trauma patient (Figure 4).

## 4. Discussion

About half of the participants (51%) worked at one of the two level I trauma centers in Maryland. Participants were balanced by specialty (52% were emergency physicians and 48% were trauma care providers). Data from this cross-sectional survey reveal that only half of the respondents were familiar with either the CRASH-2 trial or the MATTERs study. A third of those who reported being unfamiliar with these studies were trauma care providers (72% from surgical subspecialties and 28% trauma surgeons, all working in level II and III trauma centers). This high degree of a lack of awareness is alarming. At the same time 44.4% of respondents felt that unawareness of the evidence supporting the use of TXA is the greatest barrier to implementing a protocol-based approach to TXA administration in trauma patients.

Only 50% of study participants reported being aware of TXA as part of their institution's massive transfusion protocol in exsanguinating trauma patients. Nearly 30% of participants in this survey reported not being aware of TXA being part of massive transfusion protocol at their institution.

The results of this survey suggest that most of trauma providers and emergency physicians in this study have a favorable view of TXA for exsanguinating trauma patients.

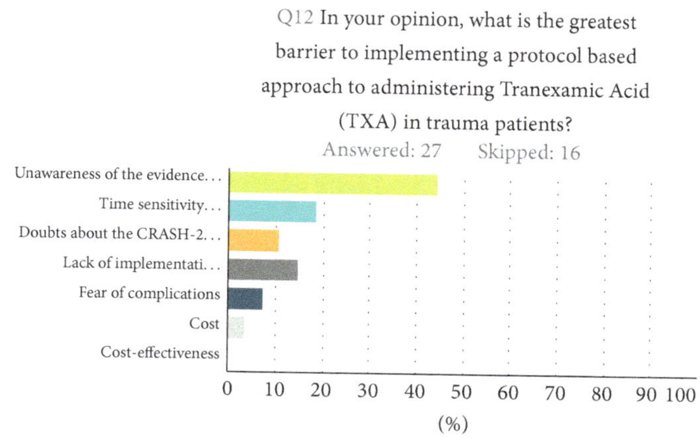


FIGURE 3: Greatest barrier to implementing TXA in trauma patients.

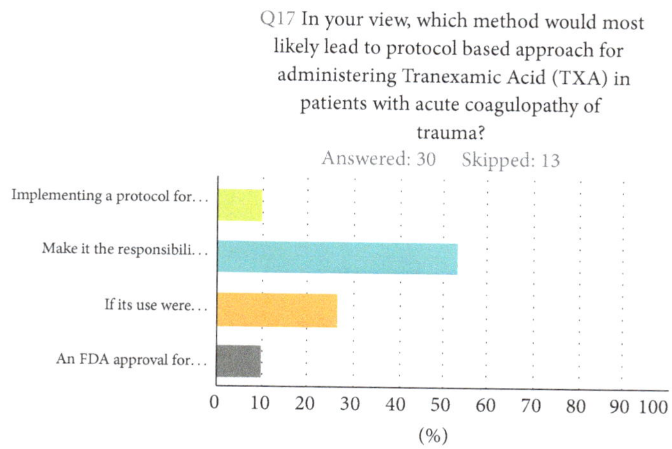


FIGURE 4: Suggestions of implementing TXA in massive transfusion protocols.

The majority of participants (63.3%) felt that use of TXA as part of a massive transfusion protocol would have a significant impact on the survival of those trauma patients who receive it. Three of every four participants were in favor of adapting TXA into trauma or massive transfusion protocols for exsanguinating trauma patients, and the same percentage reported that they would feel comfortable giving TXA to their exsanguinating patients if TXA were to be incorporated in their institution's massive transfusion protocol.

The majority of respondents (53%) thought that making TXA administration the responsibility of trauma surgeons and emergency physicians would increase its use. About one-fourth of the participants thought its use would increase if TXA were incorporated into massive transfusion protocols, especially if that inclusion would be recommended by the American College of Surgeon Committee on Trauma.

As with all survey based studies the response rate remains an important limitation of the study. However, to our knowledge, this is the first study that sought to elucidate physicians' opinions regarding barriers to the appropriate use of TXA in trauma care and also to elicit suggestions as to how its use could be increased.

## 5. Conclusion

Tranexamic Acid (TXA) has shown to be a cost effective and life-saving treatment for trauma patients. A recent economic analysis shows that it is among the most effective ways to save a life, more cost effective than antiretroviral treatment for HIV, and nearly as cost effective as bed nets for malaria prevention [12]. TXA is currently the only drug with prospective clinical evidence to support its use in bleeding trauma patients [17]. Despite the evidence, Tranexamic Acid is underutilized in trauma centers across the United States [18]. Only half of responders reported being aware of TXA as being part of their institution's massive transfusion protocol for trauma patient. Lack of awareness regarding the evidence supporting its use in patients with coagulopathy associated with trauma is a major barrier to its proper administration. Most trauma surgeons and emergency physicians who participated in this study have a favorable view regarding TXA and favor its incorporation into massive transfusion protocols. The results also suggest that making TXA administration the responsibility of trauma surgeons and emergency physicians would likely increase its use. In addition, TXA use would likely be increased if American College of Surgeon Committee on Trauma would support its inclusion in massive transfusion protocols. We believe that more studies of this kind to more fully ascertain practices and opinion on the state and national level are needed.

## Additional Points

*Hypothesis*. Tranexamic Acid (TXA) is currently the only drug with prospective clinical evidence supporting its use in bleeding trauma patients [17]. Despite the evidence, Tranexamic Acid is underutilized in trauma centers across the United States [18]. We sought to better understand barriers to the use of TXA in trauma patients by surveying the perspectives of trauma surgeons and emergency medicine physicians in the state of Maryland and elicit their suggestions as to how its appropriate use could be expanded.

## Competing Interests

The author declares that they have no competing interests.

## Acknowledgments

The author wishes to acknowledge Dr. Jeffrey Cooper and Dr. Michael Witting for their guidance and support. The manuscript was copyedited by Linda J. Kesselring, MS, ELS, the technical editor/writer in the Department of Emergency Medicine at the University of Maryland School of Medicine.

## References

[1] P. M. Mannucci and M. Levi, "Lethal injuries and time to death and time to death in a level I trauma center," *Journal of the American College of Surgeons*, vol. 186, pp. 528–533, 1998.

[2] D. S. Kauvar, R. Lefering, and C. E. Wade, "Impact of hemorrhage on trauma outcome: an overview of epidemiology, clinical presentations, and therapeutic considerations," *Journal of Trauma—Injury, Infection and Critical Care*, vol. 60, no. 6, pp. S3–S11, 2006.

[3] H. C. Tien, F. Spencer, L. N. Tremblay, S. B. Rizoli, and F. D. Brenneman, "Preventable deaths from hemorrhage at a level I Canadian trauma center," *The Journal of Trauma*, vol. 62, article 142, 2007.

[4] K. Brohi, M. J. Cohen, M. T. Ganter et al., "Acute coagulopathy of trauma: hypoperfusion induces systemic anticoagulation and hyperfibrinolysis," *Journal of Trauma - Injury, Infection and Critical Care*, vol. 64, no. 5, pp. 1211–1217, 2008.

[5] D. Frith, J. C. Goslings, C. Gaarder et al., "Definition and drivers of acute traumatic coagulopathy: clinical and experimental investigations," *Journal of Thrombosis and Haemostasis*, vol. 8, no. 9, pp. 1919–1925, 2010.

[6] M. Panteli, I. Pountos, and P. V. Giannoudis, "Pharmacological adjuncts to stop bleeding: options and effectiveness," *European Journal of Trauma and Emergency Surgery*, vol. 42, no. 3, pp. 303–310, 2016.

[7] H. Shakur, I. Roberts, R. Bautista et al., "The CRASH-2 Collaborators. Effects of tranexamic acid on death, vascular occlusive events, and blood transfusion in trauma patients with significant haemorrhage (CRASH-2): a randomised, placebo-controlled trial," *The Lancet*, vol. 376, no. 9734, pp. 23–32, 2010.

[8] I. Roberts and H. Shakur, "The importance of early treatment with tranexamic acid in bleeding trauma patients: an exploratory analysis of the CRASH-2 randomised controlled trial," *The Lancet*, vol. 377, no. 9771, p. 1096, 2011.

[9] J. J. Morrison, J. J. Dubose, T. E. Rasmussen, and M. J. Midwinter, "Military application of tranexamic acid in trauma emergency resuscitation (MATTERs) study," *Archives of Surgery*, vol. 147, no. 2, pp. 113–119, 2012.

[10] S. Binz, J. McCollester, S. Thomas et al., "CRASH-2 study of tranexamic acid to treat bleeding in trauma patients: a controversy fueled by science and social media," *Journal of Blood Transfusion*, vol. 2015, Article ID 874920, 12 pages, 2015.

[11] K. Ker, J. Kiriya, P. Perel, P. Edwards, H. Shakur, and I. Roberts, "Avoidable mortality from giving tranexamic acid to bleeding trauma patients: an estimation based on WHO mortality data, a systematic literature review and data from the CRASH-2 trial," *BMC Emergency Medicine*, vol. 12, article 3, 2012.

[12] R. Cole, K. Davenport, K. Willett, and K. Brohi, "Tranexamic Acid use in severely injured civilian patients and the effects in outcomes," *Annals of Surgery*, vol. 26, no. 2, pp. 390–394, 2015.

[13] K. Ker, P. Edward, P. Patel, H. Shakur, and I. Roberts, "Effect of tranexamic acid on surgical bleeding: systematic review and cumulative meta-analysis," *British Medical Journal*, vol. 344, Article ID e3054, 2012.

[14] J. Cid and M. Lozano, "Tranexamic acid reduces allogeneic red cell transfusions in patients undergoing total knee arthroplasty: results of a meta-analysis of randomized controlled trials," *Transfusion*, vol. 45, no. 8, pp. 1302–1307, 2005.

[15] A. Dalmau, A. Sabaté, F. Acosta et al., "Tranexamic acid reduces red cell transfusion better than ε-aminocaproic acid or placebo in liver transplantation," *Anesthesia and Analgesia*, vol. 91, no. 1, pp. 29–34, 2000.

[16] A. Movafegh, L. Eslamian, and A. Dorabadi, "Effect of intravenous tranexamic acid administration on blood loss during and after cesarean delivery," *International Journal of Gynecology and Obstetrics*, vol. 115, no. 3, pp. 224–226, 2011.

[17] A. P. Cap, D. G. Baer, J. A. Orman, J. Aden, K. Ryan, and L. H. Blackbourne, "Tranexamic acid for trauma patients: a critical review of the literature," *The Journal of Trauma: Injury, Infection, and Critical Care*, vol. 71, no. 1, pp. S9–S14, 2011.

[18] R. S. Jawa, A. Singer, J. E. Mccormack, E. C. Huang, D. N. Rutigliano, and J. A. Vosswinkel, "Tranexamic acid use in united states trauma centers: a national survey," *The American Journal of Surgery*, vol. 82, no. 5, pp. 439–447, 2016.

# 26

# Outcome of Concurrent Occult Hemothorax and Pneumothorax in Trauma Patients Who Required Assisted Ventilation

**Ismail Mahmood,[1] Zainab Tawfeek,[2] Ayman El-Menyar,[3,4,5] Ahmad Zarour,[1] Ibrahim Afifi,[1] Suresh Kumar,[1] Ruben Peralta,[1] Rifat Latifi,[1] and Hassan Al-Thani[1]**

[1] *Department of Surgery, Section of Trauma Surgery, Hamad General Hospital, P.O. Box 3050, Doha, Qatar*
[2] *Department of Emergency, Hamad Medical Corporation, P.O. Box 3050, Doha, Qatar*
[3] *Clinical Research, Section of Trauma Surgery, Hamad General Hospital, Doha, Qatar*
[4] *Clinical Medicine, Weill Cornell Medical School, P.O. Box 24144, Doha, Qatar*
[5] *Internal Medicine, Ahmed Maher Teaching Hospital, Cairo, Egypt*

Correspondence should be addressed to Ismail Mahmood; ismailyousifmah@yahoo.com

Academic Editor: Seiji Morita

*Background.* The management and outcomes of occult hemopneumothorax in blunt trauma patients who required mechanical ventilation are not well studied. We aimed to study patients with occult hemopneumothorax on mechanical ventilation who could be carefully managed without tube thoracostomy. *Methods.* Chest trauma patients with occult hemopneumothorax who were on mechanical ventilation were prospectively evaluated. The presence of hemopneumothorax was confirmed by CT scanning. Hospital length of stay, complications, and outcome were recorded. *Results.* A total of 56 chest trauma patients with occult hemopneumothorax who were on ventilatory support were included with a mean age of $36 \pm 13$ years. Hemopneumothorax was managed conservatively in 72% cases and 28% underwent tube thoracostomy as indicated. 29% of patients developed pneumonia, 16% had Acute Respiratory Distress Syndrome (ARDS), and 7% died. Thickness of hemothorax, duration of mechanical ventilation, and development of ARDS were significantly associated with tube thoracostomy in comparison to no-chest tube group. *Conclusions.* The majority of occult hemopneumothorax can be carefully managed without tube thoracostomy in patients who required positive pressure ventilation. Tube thoracotomy could be restricted to those who had evidence of increase in the size of the hemothorax or pneumothorax on follow-up chest radiographs or developed respiratory compromise.

## 1. Introduction

Patients with multiple injuries have a higher incidence of morbidity and mortality if trauma also involves the thorax. Particularly, chest injury is the cause of 10–20% of all trauma related deaths [1–3]. Computed tomography (CT) has high sensitivity for the diagnosis of clinically significant or non-significant injuries which provides accurate diagnosis of pleural blood or air in chest trauma patients. Hemopneumothorax (HPTX) is a complex problem following chest injury. The delay in diagnosis and treatment of HPTX is often associated with various complications [4]. Specifically, CT scan can efficiently diagnose HPTX in patients with normal supine chest radiographs which is defined as occult HPTX. Though HPTX is a clinical significant problem, its management is not clearly defined yet [5–7]. Rhea et al. reported 109 chest injuries to be detected by abdominal CT examination, of which 27 had pneumothorax (PTX) and 21 were defined as occult HPTX [6]. Unfortunately, the dimension of occult hemothorax (HTX) or PTX that warrants early drainage (using tube thoracostomy) on initial presentation has not been well established. de Moya et al. [8] proposed an objective scoring system for quantification of occult PTX which could potentially minimize the unnecessary tube thoracostomy for small occult PTX and supported better management decisions. Other investigators have described both qualitative and quantitative evaluation of pleural fluid with upright chest radiographs and pleural sonogram [9, 10].

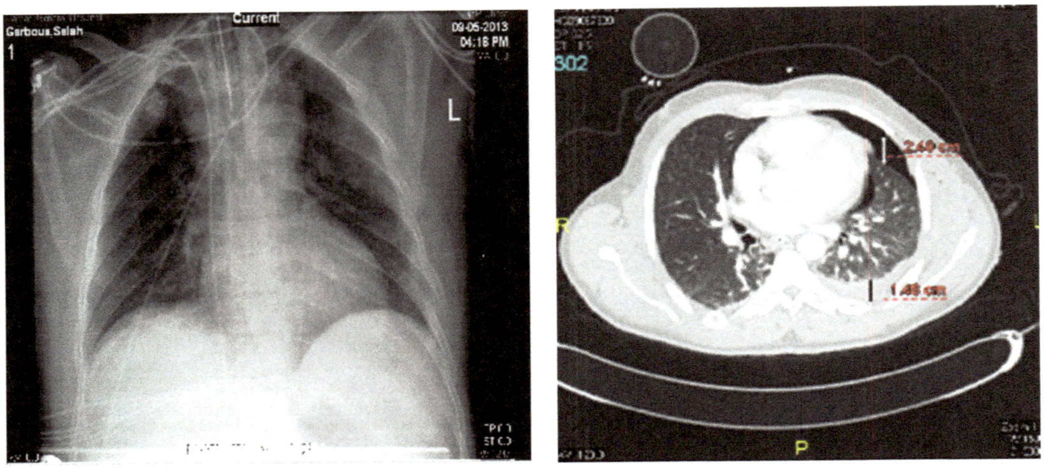


(a) (b)

FIGURE 1: : (a) Chest radiograph and (b) corresponding CT scan of patient with 24 mm pneumothorax and 14 mm hemothorax on left side not identified on chest X-ray.

In the supine position, free pleural fluid collects predominantly in the dependent posterior pleural space and appears as a sickle-shaped lamella on transverse view [9]. This lamella is also visible on chest CT scan and the greatest measured thickness of the lamella could be considered as the reflection of total effusion volume [9, 11].

In earlier practice, patients with PTX who required positive pressure ventilation (PPV) underwent tube thoracostomy to avert progression of tension PTX which might lead to serious life-threatening condition [12]. However, current literature did not clarify the management options for occult PTX particularly in patients who underwent PPV [8]. Therefore, the management of occult PTX is not well defined [12, 13]. Moreover, little is known about the treatment of concurrent occult HPTX in chest trauma patients who are subjected to PPV. Therefore, the present study aims to evaluate the management and outcomes of blunt trauma patients with occult HPTX who need PPV and to determine the role of tube thoracostomy in their management. We hypothesized that occult HPTX in patients with blunt trauma who need PPV or ventilatory support for surgical procedure can be managed conservatively.

## 2. Methods

It is a prospective observational study which included all blunt chest trauma patients who required PPV or ventilatory support for surgical procedure and presented with concurrent HPTX by chest CT (not evident on initial supine chest radiograph) from 2011 through 2013. The presence of HPTX was confirmed by CT evaluation and follow-up chest radiographs were obtained to monitor the progression of HPTX during hospital stay.

Indications for chest tube placement are respiratory compromise with oxygen desaturation and X-ray evidence of pneumothorax or hemothorax progression (increased haziness with obliteration of both costophrenic and cardiophrenic angles).

CT scan was used to quantify PTX by measuring the largest perpendicular distance in millimeters from the chest wall of the largest air pocket. Hemothorax was evaluated by measuring the deepest lamellar fluid stripe at the most dependent portion of the fluid collection (Figure 1). The ventilatory strategy used during the study was synchronized intermittent mandatory ventilation (SIMV) with pressure support mode, tidal volumes of 5 to 7 mL/kg, and controlled mechanical ventilation (CMV) for patient required surgery under general anesthesia. It is noteworthy that ventilator management during the study was not altered by the presence of an occult HPTX.

Data included demographics, mechanism of injury, injury severity score (ISS), chest abbreviated injury scale (AIS), duration of mechanical ventilation, hospital length of stay, and presence of lung contusion. Particular information regarding ventilatory mechanics (such as mode, peak inspiratory pressure, and average tidal volume), indications for tube thoracostomy, complications (pneumonia, empyema, and chest tube complications), and mortality were also recorded. The diagnosis of pneumonia was made on the basis of fever, purulent sputum, infiltrate on chest radiograph, positive culture of endotracheal secretion, and leukocytosis. In addition, all patients with occult HPTX were followed up to determine whether or not a chest tube was placed as part of management and for what indication. CT scans were performed on Siemens Medical Systems, 64-slice scanners scans with the administration of 120 mL of Omnipaque injected at 3 mL/s. Images through the chest were reconstructed at 1.2, 2.5, or 5 mm slice thickness and were analyzed by a consultant trauma radiologist. The Medical Research Center (IRB# 11112/11) at Hamad Medical Corporation, Doha, Qatar, has approved the study.

*2.1. Statistical Analysis.* The data were presented as proportions, medians, or mean ± standard deviation (SD), as appropriate. Patients were divided into two groups according to the need of chest tube insertion or no-chest tube. Differences in

Table 1: Comparison of patients with chest tube versus no-chest tube.

| | Overall ($n = 56$) | No-chest tube $n = 41$ (%) | Chest tube $n = 15$ (%) | $P$ value |
|---|---|---|---|---|
| Age (mean ± SD) | 35.8 ± 12.9 | 36 ± 12.7 | 35.3 ± 14.1 | 0.85 |
| Males $n$. (%) | 55 (98.2) | 41 (100%) | 14 (93.3) | 0.09 |
| Mechanism of injury $n$. (%) | | | | 0.13 |
| Motor vehicle crash | 25 (44.6) | 20 (48.8) | 5 (33.3) | |
| Fall from height | 16 (26.8) | 13 (31.7) | 3 (20) | |
| Pedestrian | 10 (17.9) | 6 (14.6) | 4 (26.7) | |
| Stab | 1 (1.8) | 1 (2.4) | 0 (0) | |
| Other | 4 (7.1) | 1 (2.4) | 3 (20) | |
| Lung contusion $n$. (%) | 47 (83.9) | 33 (80.5) | 14 (93.3) | 0.25 |
| Number of fractured ribs (median; range) | 4 (1–7) | 4 (1–6) | 4 (1–7) | 0.59 |
| Hemothorax thickness (median; range) | 10 (1–40) | 9 (1–21) | 13 (1–40) | 0.04 |
| Pneumothorax thickness (median; range) | 10.5 (2–80) | 10 (2–70) | 12 (2–80) | 0.12 |
| Injury severity score (mean ± SD) | 24.4 ± 8.7 | 24.3 ± 9.5 | 24.9 ± 6.5 | 0.79 |
| Chest AIS (mean ± SD) | 3 ± 2.7 | 2.98 ± 0.27 | 2.93 ± 0.25 | 0.60 |
| Surgical procedures* $n$. (%) | 19 (33.9) | 17 (41.5) | 2 (13.3) | 0.04 |
| Ventilatory days (median; range) | 3 (1–21) | 2 (1–21) | 6 (1–20) | 0.02 |
| Hospital length of stay (median; range) | 18 (3–90) | 17 (3–90) | 18 (5–90) | 0.42 |
| Ventilator-associated pneumonia $n$. (%) | 16 (28.6) | 12 (29.3) | 4 (26.7) | 0.84 |
| Acute Respiratory Distress Syndrome $n$. (%) | 9 (16.1) | 3 (7.3) | 6 (40) | 0.003 |
| Mortality $n$. (%) | 4 (7.1) | 2 (4.9) | 2 (13.3) | 0.28 |

*Orthopedic, maxillofacial, or neurosurgery.

categorical variables were analyzed using the chi-square test and the continuous variables were analyzed using Student's $t$-test. For skewed continuous data, nonparametric Mann-Whiteny $U$ test was performed. Two tailed $P$ values $< 0.05$ were considered to be significant. Data analysis was carried out using the Statistical Package for the Social Sciences version 18 (SPSS, Inc., Chicago, IL USA).

## 3. Result

A total of 56 chest trauma patients who had occult HPTX and required PPV were prospectively included in the study. The mean age of the patients was 35.8 ± 12.9 years and the majority of cases were males (98.2%). Motor vehicle crash (44.6%) and fall from height (26.8%) were the frequent mechanisms of injury (Table 1). Occult HPTX was successfully managed conservatively in 72% cases and the remaining 28% cases underwent tube thoracostomy as indicated (11 patients had progression of the HTX on follow-up chest radiographs; 2 showed PTX progression, and 2 had increased respiratory distress with oxygen desaturation). Chest tube was placed in 15 patients (13 at ICU and 2 patients needed PPV for surgical intervention within 1–6 days of admission). Lung contusion (84%) represents the most frequent chest injury and 40 (71.4%) patients had multiple rib fracture with a median of 4 (1–7) (Figure 2). On CT evaluation, 46% cases had HTX thickness of ≤9 mm, and 35% had thickness between 10 and 15 mm (Figure 3). The median HTX thickness was 10 mm (range: 1–40). Similarly, larger number of patients (42%) had PTX thickness of ≤9 mm, followed by 10 to 14 mm (32%) and the median PTX thickness was 10.5 mm (range: 2–80) (Figure 4). Seven out of 56 patients had obliteration of costophrenic angle on follow-up chest radiograph but were treated successfully expectantly.

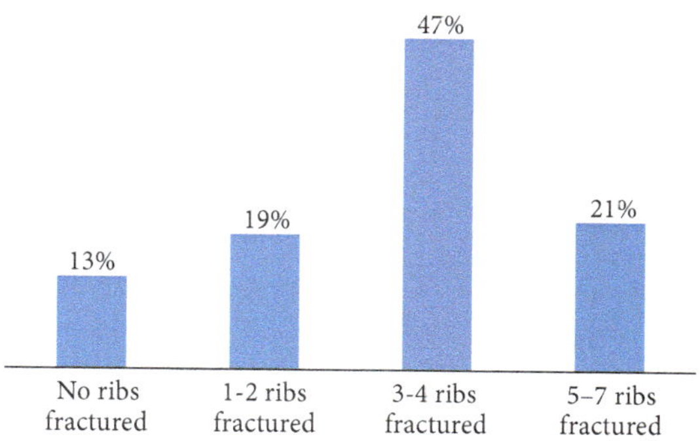


Figure 2: Number of ribs fractured.

Thirty-seven (66%) patients required intubation and mechanical ventilation due to head injury (GCS below 8) and the remaining 19 (34%) patients required general anesthesia for orthopedic, maxillofacial, or neurosurgical procedures. The ventilator strategy used for these patients was synchronized intermittent mandatory ventilation (SIMV) with pressure support mode, average peak inspiratory pressure of 18.7, and average tidal volumes (505.2 mL) together with controlled mechanical ventilation (CMV). The mean ISS was 24.4 ± 8.7 and chest AIS was 3 ± 2.7. The median mechanical ventilation was 3 (range: 1–21) days and the

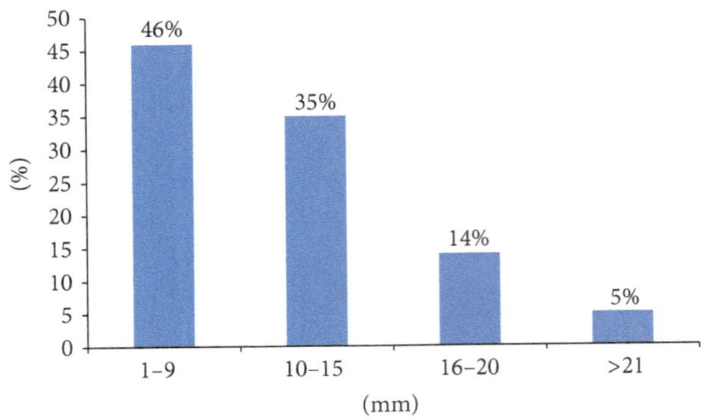


FIGURE 3: CT scan hemothorax thickness in millimeters.

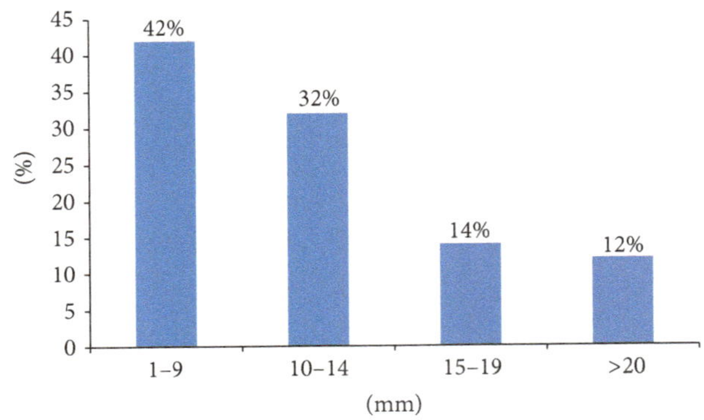


FIGURE 4: CT scan pneumothorax thickness in millimeters.

hospital length of stay was 18 (range: 3–90) days. Ventilator associated pneumonia was observed in 29% cases; 16% had developed ARDS and none of these cases were reported to have empyema. ARDS was reported to occur before tube insertion in the majority.

Table 1 showed a comparison between tube thoracostomy and conservatively treated patients. The two groups were comparable for age, number of fractured ribs, injury severity, presence of pulmonary contusions, and size of PTX. However, duration of mechanical ventilation (6 (1–20) versus 2 (1–21); $P = 0.02$), thickness of HTX (13 (1–40) versus 9 (1–21); $P = 0.04$), and rate of ARDS development (40% versus 7.3%; $P = 0.003$) were significantly higher in patients who underwent tube thoracostomy compared to no-chest tube group. In contrast, patients managed conservatively (no-chest tube) underwent significantly larger number of orthopedic, maxillofacial, or neurosurgical procedures (41.5% versus 13.3%; $P = 0.04$) than tube thoracostomy group. The overall mortality rate was 7% and the two groups were comparable with respect to mortality rate.

## 4. Discussion

To the best of our knowledge this is a unique study that focuses on the management and outcome of occult HPTX in chest trauma patients who need PPV. One of the important findings of our study is that a higher proportion (73%) of chest trauma patients with occult HPTX could be carefully managed conservatively. Our findings are consistent with an earlier prospective multicenter study that demonstrated conservative management in 94% cases of occult PTX [14]. The higher rate of successful observation in that study is due to the fact that they did not consider concurrent HTX and PTX as reported in our series.

Detection of PTX is particularly important for trauma patients who require PPV, as it is associated with the risk of progression to tension PTX and delayed life-threatening manifestations [15–17]. But, in our study, the size of PTX did not correlate with the progression or need for chest tube insertion. However, the size of HTX indicates progression on follow-up and is associated with the need of tube thoracostomy in our patients. Placement of a thoracostomy tube is not without risk and might be involved in incomplete drainage. Moreover, HTX might lead to respiratory distress/failure, retained clot, fibrothorax, empyema, and extended hospitalization [18, 19]. Ball et al. [13] reported major complications in 22% cases that had tube thoracostomy. Similarly, Bailey [20] observed an overall complication rate of 30% related to the procedure but none had insertional complication and only 2% developed major complications (e.g., empyema). Etoch et al. [21] demonstrated that the higher rate of chest tube complications is independently associated with ICU stay and need for mechanical ventilation. So it has been speculated that the selective placement of thoracostomy tubes for such patients might be useful for minimizing the risk of procedural complications.

Interestingly, the CT scan finding for the management of occult PTX remains controversial.

In 1993, Enderson et al. [12] reported the first randomized prospective study on trauma patients with occult PTX to evaluate efficacy of tube thoracostomy. The authors advocated the use of tube thoracostomy in patients with occult PTX who need PPV and also suggested that the size of the initial occult PTX could not predict the progression or formation of a tension PTX. Similarly, other investigators have recommended chest tube insertion in occult PTX patients that required PPV as these patients are at increased risk of developing tension PTX [12, 16, 17].

Over the past decade, using evidence-based practice, the strategies for mechanical ventilation have been significantly improved. An earlier study reported high tidal volumes of 8 to 10 mL/kg, limited positive end-expiratory pressure, and peak inspiratory pressure limits of 40 to 50 cm $H_2O$ [22]. However, in current practice, decreased airway pressures and tidal volumes are used in the management of critically ill patients. The management guidelines for mechanical ventilation focused on controlling peak and mean airway pressures and recommended relatively much lower pressures than used by earlier investigators [23, 24]. Consistently, lower average peak inspiratory pressure (18.7) and tidal volumes (5 to 7 mL/kg) have been used in our study. Moore et al. [14] suggested that occult PTX is not associated with the progression of respiratory distress and these patients could be safely managed conservatively regardless of the need for PPV.

Traditionally, all posttraumatic HTX cases diagnosed by chest radiograph underwent tube thoracostomy. However, the clinical significance and management of occult HTX has been investigated by several studies and the traditional practice has been changed over time [25–27]. It has been reported that small occult HTX could be managed conservatively in stable patient and the patients with HTX greater than 15 mm on CT are more likely to require drainage. However, limited information is available in the literature to address the management of concurrent occult HTX and PTX. In our series, occult HPTX patients were mainly treated conservatively and only one-third of the cases required tube thoracostomy. We also demonstrated that the size of PTX is not associated with the need of chest tube insertion in patients with PPV. Consistently, an earlier study from our institution reported no correlation between the sizes of PTX and the need for tube thoracostomy in occult HPTX patients [28]. In our series, patients with increased thickness of HTX and those who had ARDS are more likely to have chest tube insertion. Our findings are concordant with earlier studies that identified greater thickness of HTX to be an independent predictor of tube thoracotomy [25–29].

One of the limitations of our study is the small sample size that may affect the power of the study and its findings. However, we attempted to outweigh that by the prospective design. We are, to some extent, confident that our findings are important for the management of occult HPTX patients as other investigators also suggested conservative management of isolated occult PTX [14, 22] and occult HTX [25–27] patients.

In conclusion, occult HPTX can be carefully observed in patients with chest trauma who required positive pressure ventilation. Moreover, delayed tube thoracostomy is not associated with an adverse event. Though occult HPTX is infrequent, awareness of its presence is essential for the emergency physicians and care providers. Close communication with the anesthesiologist is mandatory in patients who require operative intervention. With close observation, the use of tube thoracotomy could be minimized and only restricted to those patients who had evidence of progression of hemo- or pneumothorax (increase in size) on follow-up chest radiographs or developed respiratory compromise. Therefore, the majority of HPTX patients could be spared the potential complications of tube thoracostomy and mechanical ventilation. Further prospective randomized controlled studies are needed to assess larger occult hemothorax thickness in patients who need PPV and to establish clinical guideline based on CT scan volumetric quantification.

## Disclosure

All the authors read the paper and approved it and had no financial issues to disclose. Medical Research Center (IRB# 11112/11) at Hamad Medical Corporation, Qatar, has approved the study.

## Conflict of Interests

The authors declare that there is no conflict of interests regarding the publication of this paper.

## Acknowledgments

The authors would like to thank the entire registry database team in the section of trauma surgery.

## References

[1] R. M. Shorr, M. Crittenden, M. Indeck, S. L. Hartunian, and A. Rodriguez, "Blunt thoracic trauma: analysis of 515 patients," *Annals of Surgery*, vol. 206, no. 2, pp. 200–205, 1987.

[2] D. H. Livingston and C. J. Hauser, "Trauma to the chest wall and lung," in *Trauma*, E. E. Moore, D. V. Feliciano, and K. L. Mattox, Eds., pp. 507–537, McGraw-Hill, New York, NY, USA, 5th edition, 1995.

[3] G. C. Clark, W. P. Schecter, and D. D. Trunkey, "Variables affecting outcome in blunt chest trauma: flail chest vs. pulmonary contusion," *The Journal of Trauma*, vol. 28, no. 3, pp. 298–304, 1988.

[4] N. T. Mowery, O. L. Gunter, B. R. Collier et al., "Practice management guidelines for management of hemothorax and occult pneumothorax," *Journal of Trauma-Injury, Infection and Critical Care*, vol. 70, no. 2, pp. 510–518, 2011.

[5] I. M. Tocino, M. H. Miller, P. R. Frederick, A. L. Bahr, and F. Thomas, "CT detection of occult pneumothorax in head trauma," *American Journal of Roentgenology*, vol. 143, no. 5, pp. 987–990, 1984.

[6] J. T. Rhea, R. A. Novelline, J. Lawrason, R. Sacknoff, and A. Oser, "The frequency and significance of thoracic injuries detected on abdominal CT scans of multiple trauma patients," *Journal of Trauma*, vol. 29, no. 4, pp. 502–505, 1989.

[7] S. D. Wall, M. P. Federle, R. B. Jeffrey, and C. M. Brett, "CT diagnosis of unsuspected pneumothorax after blunt abdominal trauma," *The American Journal of Roentgenology*, vol. 141, no. 5, pp. 919–921, 1983.

[8] M. A. de Moya, C. Seaver, K. Spaniolas et al., "Occult pneumothorax in trauma patients: development of an objective scoring system," *Journal of Trauma—Injury, Infection and Critical Care*, vol. 63, no. 1, pp. 13–17, 2007.

[9] K. L. Eibenberger, W. I. Dock, M. E. Ammann, R. Dorffner, M. F. Hörmann, and F. Grabenwöger, "Quantification of pleural effusions: sonography versus radiography," *Radiology*, vol. 191, no. 3, pp. 681–684, 1994.

[10] J. A. Ruskin, J. W. Gurney, M. K. Thorsen, and L. R. Goodman, "Detection of pleural effusions on supine chest radiographs," *American Journal of Roentgenology*, vol. 148, no. 4, pp. 681–684, 1987.

[11] N. L. Muller, "Imaging of the pleura," *Radiology*, vol. 186, no. 2, pp. 297–309, 1993.

[12] B. L. Enderson, R. Abdalla, S. B. Frame et al., "Tube thoracostomy for occult pneumothorax: a prospective randomized study of its use," *Journal of Trauma*, vol. 35, no. 5, pp. 726–730, 1993.

[13] C. G. Ball, J. Lord, K. B. Laupland et al., "Chest tube complications: how well are we training our residents?" *Canadian Journal of Surgery*, vol. 50, no. 6, pp. 450–458, 2007.

[14] F. O. Moore, P. W. Goslar, R. Coimbra et al., "Blunt traumatic occult pneumothorax: is observation safe?—results of a prospective, AAST multicenter study," *Journal of Trauma-Injury, Infection and Critical Care*, vol. 70, no. 5, pp. 1019–1025, 2011.

[15] N. T. Wolfman, W. S. Myers, S. J. Glauser, J. W. Meredith, and M. Y. M. Chen, "Validity of CT classification on management of

occult pneumothorax: a prospective study," *American Journal of Roentgenology*, vol. 171, no. 5, pp. 1317–1320, 1998.

[16] K. G. Bridges, G. Welch, M. Silver, M. A. Schinco, and B. Esposito, "CT detection of occult pneumothorax in multiple trauma patients," *The Journal of Emergency Medicine*, vol. 11, no. 2, pp. 179–186, 1993.

[17] A. M. Karnik and F. A. Khan, "Pneumothorax and barotrauma," in *Critical Care Medicine: Principles of Diagnosis and Management in the Adult*, J. E. Parillo and R. P. Dellinger, Eds., pp. 930–948, Mosby, St. Louis, Mo, USA, 2nd edition, 2001.

[18] J. M. Wilson, C. H. Boren Jr., S. R. Peterson, and A. N. Thomas, "Traumatic hemothorax: is decortication necessary?" *Journal of Thoracic and Cardiovascular Surgery*, vol. 77, no. 4, pp. 489–495, 1979.

[19] J. A. Watkins, D. A. Spain, J. D. Richardson, and H. C. Polk Jr., "Empyema and restrictive pleural processes after blunt trauma: an under-recognized cause of respiratory failure," *The American Surgeon*, vol. 66, no. 2, pp. 210–214, 2000.

[20] R. C. Bailey, "Complications of tube thoracostomy in trauma," *Journal of Accident and Emergency Medicine*, vol. 17, no. 2, pp. 111–114, 2000.

[21] S. W. Etoch, M. F. Bar-Natan, F. B. Miller et al., "Tube thoracostomy: factors related to complications," *Archives of Surgery*, vol. 130, no. 5, pp. 521–526, 1995.

[22] K. J. Brasel, R. E. Stafford, J. A. Weigelt, J. E. Tenquist, and D. C. Borgstrom, "Treatment of occult pneumothoraces from blunt trauma," *Journal of Trauma—Injury, Infection and Critical Care*, vol. 46, no. 6, pp. 987–991, 1999.

[23] L. Pinhu, T. Whitehead, T. Evans, and M. Griffiths, "Ventilator-associated lung injury," *The Lancet*, vol. 361, no. 9354, pp. 332–340, 2003.

[24] A. W. Kirkpatrick, M. O. Meade, and T. E. Stewart, "Lung protective ventilatory strategies in ARDS," in *Yearbook of Intensive Care and Emergency Medicine*, J. L. Vincent, Ed., pp. 398–410, Springer, Berlin, Germany, 1996.

[25] R. E. Stafford, J. Linn, and L. Washington, "Incidence and management of occult hemothoraces," *American Journal of Surgery*, vol. 192, no. 6, pp. 722–726, 2006.

[26] I. Mahmood, H. Abdelrahman, A. Al-Hassani, S. Nabir, M. Sebastian, and K. Maull, "Clinical management of occult hemothorax: a prospective study of 81 patients," *American Journal of Surgery*, vol. 201, no. 6, pp. 766–769, 2011.

[27] J. F. Bilello, J. W. Davis, and D. M. Lemaster, "Occult traumatic hemothorax: when can sleeping dogs lie?" *American Journal of Surgery*, vol. 190, no. 6, pp. 841–844, 2005.

[28] I. Mahmood, Z. Tawfeek, S. Khoschnau et al., "Occult hemopneumothorax following chest trauma does not need a chest tube," *European Journal of Trauma and Emergency Surgery*, vol. 39, no. 1, pp. 43–46, 2013.

[29] J. DuBose, K. Inaba, D. Demetriades et al., "Management of post-traumatic retained hemothorax: a prospective, observational, multicenter AAST study," *Journal of Trauma and Acute Care Surgery*, vol. 72, no. 1, pp. 11–24, 2012.

# Ultrasound Guided Intravenous Access by Nursing versus Resident Staff in a Community Based Teaching Hospital: A "Noninferiority" Trial

**Thomas Carter,[1] Chris Conrad,[1] J. Link Wilson,[1] and Godwin Dogbey[2]**

[1] *Emergency Department, Southern Ohio Medical Center, Portsmouth, OH 45662, USA*
[2] *CORE Research Office, Ohio University Heritage College of Osteopathic Medicine, Athens, OH 45701, USA*

Correspondence should be addressed to Thomas Carter; carterte@somc.org

Academic Editor: Wen-Jone Chen

*Objectives.* Ultrasound (US) guidance is a safe and effective method for peripheral intravenous (IV) catheter placement. However, no studies have directly compared the success rate of emergency medicine (EM) residents and nurses at using this technique especially in community hospital settings. This prospective "noninferiority" study sought to demonstrate that nursing staff are at least as successful as EM residents at placing US guided IVs. *Methods.* A group of 5 EM residents and 11 nurse volunteers with at least two years' experience underwent training sessions in hands-on practice and didactic instruction with prospective follow-up. Two failed attempts on a patient using standard approach by an emergency department (ED) nurse were deemed to be "difficult sticks" and randomly assigned to either a nurse or resident, based on the day they presented. *Results.* A total of 90 attempts, consisting of trials on 90 patients, were recorded with a success rate of 85% and 86% for residents and nurses, respectively. With a $p$ value of .305, there was no statistically significant difference in the success rate between the residents and nurses. *Conclusion.* Properly trained nursing staff can be as equally successful as EM residents in placing US guided intravenous lines.

## 1. Introduction

The use of ultrasound (US) technology in placing peripheral lines has been shown to reduce the need for central venous catheters—a more painful process with more grave possible complications [1, 2]. Nurses are at the frontline of clinical contact with patients in the emergency department (ED). As a result, there have been repeated calls for training of nurses on the use of US guided IV (USGIV) access in the ED and hospital setting, in general [3]. In response to such calls, programs for nurses have been designed and implemented [4, 5]. When nursing staff in the ED of a hospital are unable to obtain peripheral venous access after multiple attempts, they have the option to forego any venous access, request to place a central venous catheter, or request ultrasound (US) guided IV access by a physician [2, 6]. This is particularly the case in most community teaching hospitals.

Multiple studies [7–10] have demonstrated the efficacy of nurses and ED technicians using US for IV access. This finding has not been widely used and in some institutions a culture of "hands off" for nurses and technicians still exists around ultrasound guidance for some procedures. The emergent issue, therefore, has not been over whether ultrasound is safe and effective but about who should be able to use the machines and for what purpose.

In underserved community hospitals, such as the one under study, low levels of workforce have necessitated that limited available human resources are utilized to the fullest in patient care. Consequently, nurses and residents face the task of performing many procedures including IV placements frequently. Anecdotally, it was observed that fear has led to low levels of comfort among nurses regarding the use of US as a guide for IV access and placement in patients especially those with difficult access, "difficult sticks." The training requirements of emergency residents and physicians have meant that, to a large extent, they are relatively facile with USGIV access and placement [6]. In light of this, it is important within a community hospital environment to

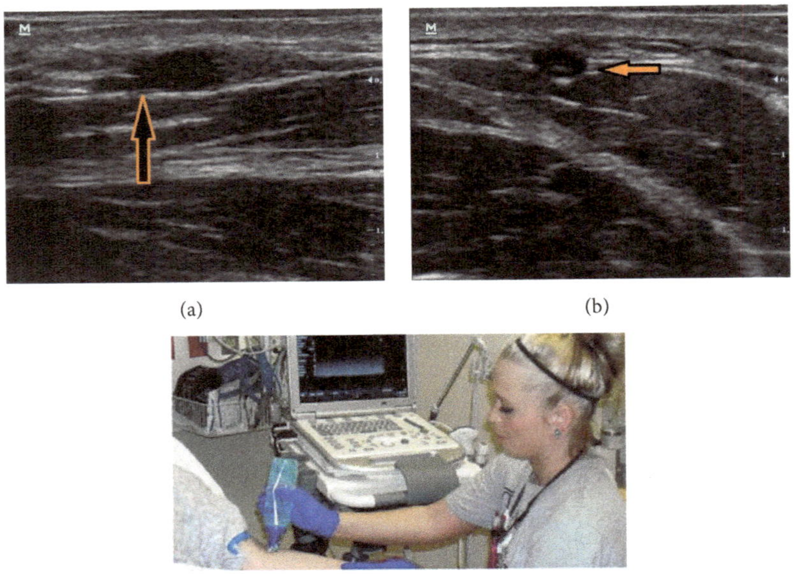

(a) (b) (c)

Figure 1: (a) Catheter tip (hyperechoic or white) shown accessing a vein (hypoechoic or black square) in the oblique access; the catheter is highlighted in by the orange arrow. (b) A catheter tip (hyperechoic or white) shown accessing the peripheral vein (hypoechoic or black circle) circle in the coronal plane delineated by the orange arrow. (c) A nurse preparing to perform US guided IV access notes the location of the ultrasound machine to allow for line of site of both the machine and the patient.

have nurses at par with residents with regard to success in placing USGIVs. However, there are no studies found in the literature comparing the efficacy of ultrasound use by nurses and residents in situations where US guided access to IVs is necessary for the patient.

From the foregoing, therefore, the goal of our study was to directly compare success rate between emergency medicine (EM) residents and emergency room nursing staff at obtaining peripheral venous access under real time ultrasound guidance. We assert that the nursing staff can be, if properly trained, as effective as the emergency medicine residents at this technique.

## 2. Methods

*2.1. Study Design and Setting.* This single center, nonblinded, quasi-randomized, "noninferiority" study was conducted in a 180-bed Midwestern community teaching hospital in the United States. Local Institutional/Ethics Review Board approval was obtained for this study.

*2.2. Population and Sample.* A sample of nurses and residents was self-selected from the population of nurses and emergency medicine (EM) residents in the community teaching hospital. The nursing staff in the emergency department of the community teaching hospital who consented to participate in the study was trained on use of the ultrasound machine through hands-on instruction followed by simulated venous canalization in model gel (see Figures 1(a), 1(b), and 1(c)). After the nurses were introduced to the technique, we determined the extent to which they could effectively use US guidance in the appropriate situations, as directed by a physician, to obtain IV access in situations when it was difficult to access patients.

We began the trial with the self-selected group of 11 highly motivated nurse volunteers who had successfully completed the training sessions. Since nurses in the ED were already quite experienced in IV access, the learning curve was short and only related to visualization on the US screen and the dexterity to insert IV while holding the probe and watching the screen (Figures 1(a) and 1(b)). Setup with the screen at the patients head to allow proper visualization and to maintain orientation with the field was recommended as displayed in Figure 1(c). The group of nurses was pitted against a group of five (5) equally trained and motivated emergency medicine residents who had received one or more years of on-the-job training in ultrasound use for various procedures, including peripheral venous access.

*2.3. Inclusion and Exclusion Criteria.* Inclusion criteria comprised adult patients (18 years or older) who needed peripheral venous access as judged by the treating attending physician. Furthermore, patients should have undergone two unsuccessful attempts at peripheral venous access by anatomic landmarks by any ED nurse, as is the standard procedure at this time. Those excluded from the study were pediatric patients (less than 18 years old), patients with an urgent need for central venous access due to critical status, hemodialysis patients, mastectomy or radiation therapy patients, patients randomly placed in a room to which a participating nurse was not previously assigned, and/or patients who had successful peripheral venous access in two or less attempts using the traditional anatomic landmarks technique. Ultrasound guided anatomy of the upper extremity was the

TABLE 1: Relationship between provider type and success (hit) at ultrasound guided IV access.

| Provider type | Hit | | Total | $p$ value |
|---|---|---|---|---|
| | Yes | No | | |
| Resident | 34 | 6 | **40** | .893 |
| Nurse | 43 | 7 | **50** | |
| Total | 77 | **13** | **90** | |

TABLE 2: Relationship between provider type and complications in the use of ultrasound guided IV access.

| Provider type | Complications | | Total | $p$ value |
|---|---|---|---|---|
| | Yes | No | | |
| Resident | 2 | 38 | **40** | .110 |
| Nurse | 0 | 50 | **50** | |
| Total | **2** | **88** | **90** | |

only decision for access location; no standardized vein was required and only intermediate depth vessels were utilized.

*2.4. Study Protocol and Subject Assignments.* Quasi-randomization was done with patients assigned to rooms based on presentation before peripheral access was ordered. One or more nurses covered the patient room before patient assignment or any order for peripheral venous access was identified. The study nurse assigned to a room continued care after patient consent was obtained and attempts to perform the US guided IV when a nonstudy nurse was unsuccessful using the traditional techniques. Similarly, after patient consent, a resident attempted to perform the ultrasound guided placement. A comparison of the success rates in obtaining a working IV between the nurse and resident groups was made. Success (hit) was defined as the withdrawal of blood from the catheter followed by the ability to freely flush saline without any signs of infiltration.

*2.5. Measurements.* Data was collected simply by measuring either success or lack of success in canalization as defined above. The numbers were compared directly to answer our simple question of whether nurses can be equally efficacious in obtaining peripheral venous access with ultrasound guidance when compared to emergency medicine residents. The chi-squared test of association was used to determine overall relationship between the health professional type (nurses versus residents) and success at the IV placement as well as complications. Furthermore, the nonparametric chi-square test of equality of proportions was used to determine if success rates were different between the two groups. Statistical significance was set at $p < .05$. Data was analyzed using the SPSS version 21 (IBM, Chicago, IL).

## 3. Results

The inclusion criteria were met by 90 patients who consented to participate in the study over the period of interest. The 11 ED nursing staff made 50 attempts while the five EM residents made 40 IV placement attempts. As previously stated, the outcome measures of interest were the number of successes and complications associated with the ultrasound guided IV placement by each member of each of the two groups. There was no statistically significant association between the provider type and success at the IV placement, $p = .893$ (see Table 1).

In all, there were 77 hits out of the 90 attempts yielding an overall success rate of 85.5%. Nurses recorded 43 successes out of the 50 attempts representing a group success rate of 86% while residents scored 34 hits out of 40, a group success rate of 85%. The success rates between nurses and residents were not significantly different statistically, $p = .305$. Regarding complications, similarly no statistically significant relationship was found with provider type, $p = .110$. There were two out of the 90 attempts, a complication rate of 2.2% overall (see Table 2). These two resulted solely from the residents' attempts, a 5% group complication rate.

## 4. Discussion

The success rates of 85% and 86% observed for residents and nurses, respectively, in USGIV placements were consistent with results reported in some studies involving nurses [2, 7]. Those studies reported success rates in the range 53%–85% depending on technique (one-person versus two-person), type of vein (basilic versus brachial), number of attempts (one or multiple), and overall cannulation [11].

Our study observed no statistically significant difference in the success rate between the providers: nurses and EM residents. However, there was a measured difference in complications rate (5% for residents and none for nurses). Further studies involving larger sample size are needed to determine if that result was purely due to chance or a real difference. In this study, no overall association was found between complication and provider type (nurse or resident). Each provider did not work on the same patient more than once and so interoperator reliability (measured by *kappa*) was not relevant and not computed. Moreover, the primary outcome of success as defined was not based on interpreting the sonographic images thereby rendering the issue of reproducibility of images untenable. We did not determine time to success mostly due to the lower acuity of the patient with IV access needs.

## 5. Conclusion

Nurses have used ultrasound to perform peripheral IV insertion in the past but this study has provided further evidence that they are equally adept at this procedure as emergency medicine residents. This was in light of the fact that no significant difference was observed between residents and nurses with regard to the success rate of US guided IV placement. Based on this result, a protocol can be developed for training and routine use of ultrasound for peripheral IV insertion in the ED for nurses. Implementing a program for use of intermediate lines under ultrasound guidance for nurses could expedite care, reduce pain, and decrease possible complications associated with central access.

## Conflict of Interests

The authors declare that there is no conflict of interests regarding the publication of this paper.

## Acknowledgments

The authors would like to acknowledge Southern Ohio Medical Center, Emergency Physicians Medical Group PC, and Ohio University Heritage College of Osteopathic Medicine for technical editing support.

## References

[1] H. Shokoohi, K. Boniface, M. McCarthy et al., "Ultrasound-guided peripheral intravenous access program is associated with a marked reduction in central venous catheter use in noncritically ill emergency department patients," *Annals of Emergency Medicine*, vol. 61, no. 2, pp. 198–203, 2013.

[2] M. Blaivas and M. Lyon, "The effect of ultrasound guidance on the perceived difficulty of emergency nurse-obtained peripheral IV access," *Journal of Emergency Medicine*, vol. 31, no. 4, pp. 407–410, 2006.

[3] N. Mumoli, J. Vitale, M. Cocciolo et al., "Accuracy of nurse-performed compression ultrasonography in the diagnosis of proximal symptomatic deep vein thrombosis: a prospective cohort study," *Journal of Thrombosis and Haemostasis*, vol. 12, no. 4, pp. 430–435, 2014.

[4] C. Moore, "An emergency department nurse-driven ultrasound-guided peripheral intravenous line program," *Journal of the Association for Vascular Access*, vol. 18, no. 1, pp. 45–51, 2013.

[5] G. Miles, A. Salcedo, and D. Spear, "Implementation of a successful registered nurse peripheral ultrasound-guided intravenous catheter program in an emergency department," *Journal of Emergency Nursing*, vol. 38, no. 4, pp. 353–356, 2012.

[6] S. G. Weiner, A. R. Sarff, D. E. Esener et al., "Single-operator ultrasound-guided intravenous line placement by emergency nurses reduces the need for physician intervention in patients with difficult-to-establish intravenous access," *The Journal of Emergency Medicine*, vol. 44, no. 3, pp. 653–660, 2013.

[7] L. Brannam, M. Blaivas, M. Lyon, and M. Flake, "Emergency nurses' utilization of ultrasound guidance for placement of peripheral intravenous lines in difficult-access patients," *Academic Emergency Medicine*, vol. 11, no. 12, pp. 1361–1363, 2004.

[8] E. Schoenfeld, K. Boniface, and H. Shokoohi, "ED technicians can successfully place ultrasound-guided intravenous catheters in patients with poor vascular access," *American Journal of Emergency Medicine*, vol. 29, no. 5, pp. 496–501, 2011.

[9] M. Bauman, D. Braude, and C. Crandall, "Ultrasound-guidance vs. standard technique in difficult vascular access patients by ED technicians," *American Journal of Emergency Medicine*, vol. 27, no. 2, pp. 135–140, 2009.

[10] S. J. Doniger, P. Ishimine, J. C. Fox, and J. T. Kanegaye, "Randomized controlled trial of ultrasound-guided peripheral intravenous catheter placement versus traditional techniques in difficult-access pediatric patients," *Pediatric Emergency Care*, vol. 25, no. 3, pp. 154–159, 2009.

[11] B. Chinnock, S. Thornton, and G. W. Hendey, "Predictors of success in nurse-performed ultrasound-guided cannulation," *Journal of Emergency Medicine*, vol. 33, no. 4, pp. 401–405, 2007.

# 28

# Trauma Simulation Training Increases Confidence Levels in Prehospital Personnel Performing Life-Saving Interventions in Trauma Patients

**Christine M. Van Dillen,[1] Matthew R. Tice,[1] Archita D. Patel,[1] David A. Meurer,[1] Joseph A. Tyndall,[1] Marie Carmelle Elie,[1] and Jonathan J. Shuster[2]**

[1]*Department of Emergency Medicine, University of Florida College of Medicine, Gainesville, FL 32610, USA*
[2]*Department of Health Outcomes and Policy, University of Florida College of Medicine, Gainesville, FL 32610, USA*

Correspondence should be addressed to Christine M. Van Dillen; c.vandillen@ufl.edu

Academic Editor: Selim Suner

*Introduction.* Limited evidence is available on simulation training of prehospital care providers, specifically the use of tourniquets and needle decompression. This study focused on whether the confidence level of prehospital personnel performing these skills improved through simulation training. *Methods.* Prehospital personnel from Alachua County Fire Rescue were enrolled in the study over a 2- to 3-week period based on their availability. Two scenarios were presented to them: a motorcycle crash resulting in a leg amputation requiring a tourniquet and an intoxicated patient with a stab wound, who experienced tension pneumothorax requiring needle decompression. Crews were asked to rate their confidence levels before and after exposure to the scenarios. Timing of the simulation interventions was compared with actual scene times to determine applicability of simulation in measuring the efficiency of prehospital personnel. *Results.* Results were collected from 129 participants. Pre- and postexposure scores increased by a mean of 1.15 (SD 1.32; 95% CI, 0.88–1.42; $P < 0.001$). Comparison of actual scene times with simulated scene times yielded a 1.39-fold difference (95% CI, 1.25–1.55) for Scenario 1 and 1.59 times longer for Scenario 2 (95% CI, 1.43–1.77). *Conclusion.* Simulation training improved prehospital care providers' confidence level in performing two life-saving procedures.

## 1. Introduction

The advancement of patient care is the final goal of all training in medicine. Over the past several decades, significant innovations have been introduced in the educational methodology and tools used to deliver clinical education. With the rapid advancement in technology in medical education, simulation has been shown to facilitate this type of learning, especially with regard to skills needed in the prehospital environment [1]. Simulation provides an optimal environment for learning and can refresh personnel on infrequently performed procedures and patient scenarios [1, 2]. It also allows high-risk scenarios to be repeated for multiple providers to focus on specific management skills and techniques as well as assessment by supervisors and medical directors in critical patient scenarios [1, 3]. In the prehospital setting, personnel in the field operate from medical care protocols. A medical director is often limited to chart review to assess performance of critical thinking, patient interaction, procedural performance, and overall quality of care provided. This method of review is extremely limited by self-reporting and documentation. As a result of these limitations, simulation has become a very useful learning and assessment tool for emergency medical services (EMS) agencies.

Recent meta-analyses focusing on medical simulation in general concluded that the presence of medical simulation in the medical education strategy greatly enhanced skills and knowledge compared with curricula that excluded simulation [4, 5]. Evidence focusing on simulated scenarios for prehospital personnel is still somewhat limited [1]. The literature involving the use of simulation with prehospital care providers broadly covers topics that include intubation,

TABLE 1: Alachua county fire rescue paramedics' descriptive statistics.

| Characteristics | Total # of paramedics (155) |
|---|---|
| Average age | 40.1 |
| Avg. years in service | 12.4 |
| Percent male | 95% |
| Race | |
| White (not Hispanic) | 93% |
| Hispanic/Latino (any race) | 3% |
| Black/African American | 4% |

ventilation, trauma care, cardiopulmonary resuscitation, and resuscitation [1, 6]. In trauma simulation articles, specific assessment skills, triage management, and procedural performance are the topics often discussed. Specific procedural skills such as tourniquet application and chest decompression have received little attention in the medical literature [1]. This study described in this paper evaluated the effect of introducing prehospital personnel to simulated critical trauma patients requiring the emergent use of tourniquets and needle decompression on their confidence levels in performing these procedures. The purpose of this study is to evaluate if the confidence of prehospital personnel can be improved through simulation training.

Previous studies in the prehospital setting have used visual analog scales (VASs) to assess confidence in procedures [7]. Assessment of the efficiency with which paramedics recognized the need for emergent life-saving interventions (specifically needle decompression for pneumothorax and tourniquet placement for amputation) and recognized patients meeting Florida trauma alert criteria was also documented. This study also compared simulated scenario times with actual trauma scene times with regard to the timing of patient evaluation, interventions, and transport, which are key features that EMS medical directors review as part of their assessment of the provision of care to critical trauma patients.

## 2. Methods

Alachua County Fire Rescue (ACFR) provides EMS transport and first responder services in the county and staffs 12 full-time advanced life support (ALS) ambulances that cover 969 square miles and serve a general population of 246,336. Paramedics at ACFR are mostly male with an average of 12 years of service in the agency (Table 1). ACFR responds to approximately 36,000 calls annually. From June 2013 to June 2014, trauma was the primary reason for 2,209 of these calls, and an additional 216 were considered trauma alerts after field assessment. Care provided by crews is guided by medical protocols written and approved by the medical director. Quality assurance and improvement are done through a combination of online medical control (done via the radio), chart review, and a small amount of physician field response. Local system trauma alert criteria at the time of the study can be found in Table 2.

In this retrospective observational study, paramedic and emergency medical technician (EMT-basic) teams were presented with two scenarios. Scenario 1 was a motorcycle crash that caused the amputation of driver's right leg, requiring the life-saving intervention of placing a tourniquet on the limb. Scenario 2 involved an intoxicated patient who had sustained an occult stab wound in a bar fight and who later developed a tension pneumothorax requiring needle decompression. The crew members' perceived confidence levels in the treatment of these critically injured patients were evaluated via a self-assessment standard survey form before and after the presentation of the simulated scenarios. After each scenario, crew members received a debriefing about their performance and were trained to review both tourniquet placement and needle decompression as well as the associated indications, contraindications, and important treatment points. In previous studies, students who had experienced a posttraining debriefing felt that weaknesses and strengths discussed by observers enhanced their knowledge and clinical performance [6]. In our debriefing, clinical weaknesses and strengths as well as on-scene time utilization were discussed.

EMT-basic and paramedic crews came to the training facility during their shifts over a 2- to 3-week period based on the availability of the training teams. A total of 129 prehospital personnel participated in the training. The simulation sessions were presented in place of ACFR's quarterly training along with surveys and evaluations that were completed to assess the quality of the training model. In actual response scenarios, a minimum of an engine crew (one paramedic and two EMTs-basic) as well as a rescue crew (one paramedic and one EMT-basic) would usually be dispatched to the scene of a critical traumatic injury when adequate information is given at the time of dispatch. Therefore, each training group consisted of two to five crew members, depending on their availability. EMT-basic and paramedics participated in the simulation together; however data was only collected on the paramedics as they would normally perform the procedures and make the clinical decisions. We excluded those who were not available for training or did not complete the survey.

Prior to the training, crews completed a survey that asked them to rate their confidence level when evaluating and treating critically injured patients, using a VAS of 1 to 9 (Figure 1). Identifying information was collected and used initially to correlate their pre- and posttraining survey results. Soon after the data were collected, identifying information was removed prior to analysis.

Training was initiated with crew members receiving a simulated call from dispatch for the initial case, along with a brief summary of the setting for their simulation. The simulator mannequin was then revealed to them so that they could start their assessment. Paramedic training officers from ACFR acted as evaluators to record the times of each intervention and to document whether critical actions were completed by crew members, the timing of these interventions, the timing of trauma alert notification, and the time spent on scene on a standard evaluation sheet. An emergency physician or emergency medicine resident was present to lead the scenario and answer questions regarding the patient's

TABLE 2: 64J-2.004 adult trauma scorecard methodology.

*Adult trauma triage criteria and methodology*

The EMT or paramedic will assess the condition of those injured persons with anatomical and physiological characteristics of a person sixteen (16) years of age or older for the presence of at least one of the following four (4) criteria to determine whether to transport as a trauma alert. These four criteria are to be applied in the order listed, and once any one criterion is met that identifies the patient as a trauma alert, no further assessment is required to determine the transport destination.

*Criteria*

(1) Meets color-coded triage system (see below)

(2) GCS ≤ 12 (patient must be evaluated via GCS if not identified as a trauma alert after application of criterion 1)

(3) Meets local criteria (specify)

(4) Patient does not meet any of the trauma criteria listed above but, in the judgment of the EMT or paramedic, should be transported as a trauma alert (document)

| Component | Blue criteria (B) | Red criteria (R) |
|---|---|---|
| Airway[1] | ± sustained RR ≥ 30 | ± active airway assistance[2] |
| Circulation | ± sustained HR > 120 | ± lack of radial pulse with sustained fast heart rate (>120) or<br>± BP <90 |
| Best motor response | ± BMR = 5 | ± BMR of ≤4 or<br>± paralysis or<br>± suspected spinal cord injury |
| Cutaneous | ± tissue loss[3] or<br>± GSW to extremities | ± amputation[4] or<br>± $2^0/3^0$ burns to >15% TBSA or<br>± any penetrating injury to head, neck, or torso[5] |
| Longbone fracture | ± single FX site due to MVA or<br>± fall > 10′ | ± multiple FX sites |
| Age | ± ≥55 | |
| Mechanism of injury | ± ejection from vehicle or<br>± deformed steering wheel[6] | |

(i) R: any *one (1)*-transport as a trauma alert
(ii) B: any *two (2)*-transport as a trauma alert
[1]Airway evaluation is designed to reflect the intervention required for effective care. [2]Not just oxygen. [3]Degloving injuries, major flap avulsions (>5 in). [4]Amputations proximal to the wrist or ankle. [5]Excluding superficial wounds in which the depth of the wound can be easily determined. [6]Only applies to driver of vehicle m: JR/PATTC/6/26/97.

Name________________ Date ________ Crew________

How comfortable do you feel caring for a critically ill trauma patient?

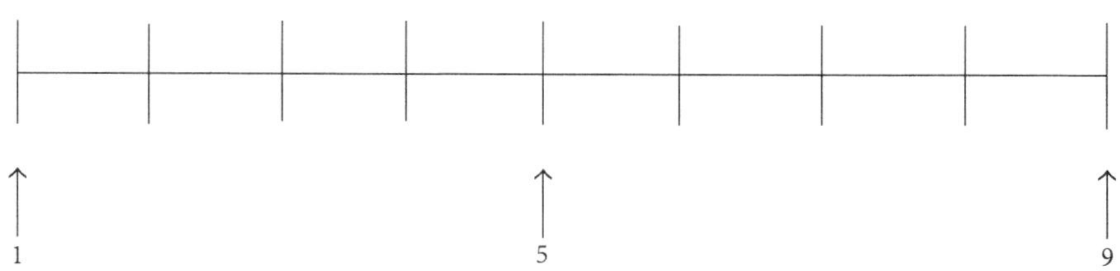


FIGURE 1: Visual analog scale (1–9).

presentation. All physician and training captain team members received training on each scenario and evaluation sheet prior to the simulation to ensure that each group would be exposed to a standard scenario and evaluation process.

The simulation ended when the crew stated that they were leaving the scene to transport the patient or after 15 minutes had passed. The physician simulation leader and the evaluator then led a debriefing session with the crew members to discuss their performance. At this time, each crew received training on the clinical presentation of life-threatening hemorrhage in a trauma patient along with the indications and contraindications for placement of a tourniquet.

After completing the first scenario, the same crew was presented with the second scenario, undergoing active evaluation followed by a debriefing from the physician simulation leader and evaluator. This crew then received training on the identification of tension pneumothorax as well as the indications and contraindications for needle decompression. The postsimulation survey was then filled out by each individual crew member to indicate his or her postsimulation confidence level (a new copy of the same VAS was provided and completed by participants). They also recorded their subjective opinions about the simulation experience.

The primary outcome of interest was whether simulation scenarios increase confidence levels in prehospital care providers performing life-saving interventions on critically injured patients. A secondary outcome of interest was whether medical directors can use simulation as an accurate assessment tool to measure efficiency (the timing of interventions and the time spent on scene) of prehospital personnel at providing care for and transporting critically injured patients.

The evaluation sheet served as our data collection form during the simulation process. In addition, standard pre- and postsurvey sheets were provided to all crew members. These data were entered into Excel spreadsheets and deidentified manually. Analysis was performed using SAS 9.3 (Statistical Analysis Systems, Cary, NC). For timed variables, we used logs to estimate the typical fold changes once converted back to the original units by antilogs. This approach minimizes the adverse impact of outliers. All data collected were used to evaluate the training, not for personnel evaluations or corrective actions.

The data points collected are listed as follows:

(i) Did subjects enjoy the training?

(ii) Did they want to participate in more simulation training?

(iii) Total time spent on motorcycle crash scenario.

(iv) Time on scene for motorcycle crash case.

(v) Total time spent on tension pneumothorax scenario.

(vi) Time on scene for pneumothorax case.

(vii) How comfortable do you feel when caring for a critically injured patient? (Confidence level before the scenario.)

(viii) How comfortable do you feel when caring for a critically injured patient? (Confidence level after the scenario.)

## 3. Results

The providers' confidence levels were recorded in a survey via a VAS before and after participation in the training and then compared directly. When comparing each individual provider's scores, the score increased by a mean of 1.15 (SD = 1.32), with a 95% confidence interval of 1.15 ± 0.27, or from 0.88 to 1.42 for the mean change. This mean change is significant at $P < 0.001$ by a one-sample $t$-test on this paired difference. When asking participants whether they enjoyed the training, 99.0% reported positively and 98.0% reported that they would prefer more simulation training than the previous style of training.

To obtain a real-life comparison, scene times in trauma alert patients were calculated by looking at time of ambulance arrival on scene and ending with ambulance transport, using computer-assisted dispatch records over a 1-year period. When we compared true trauma alert scene times with our two simulated scenarios (Table 3), we found that actual scene times were significantly longer than times in the simulated scenarios. When comparing actual times with Scenario 1 simulated times, we found the point estimate and 95% confidence interval in the log scale is 0.3298 (0.2244, 0.4351). Upon taking antilogs, this converts to a 1.39-fold (1.25, 1.55) difference, with real scenarios being higher. In Scenario 2, we found the point estimate and 95% confidence interval in the log scale is 0.4646 (0.3593, 0.5699). Upon taking antilogs, this converts to 1.59-fold (1.43, 1.77) longer for the real scenario.

Table 3: Scene time ranges for trauma alert patients.

| | |
|---|---|
| *Scenario 1* | |
| Arrival on scene to trauma alert | 0.25–9.96 min |
| Time to initiation of tourniquet placement | 0.4–3.16 min |
| Total time on scene | 5.33–9.96 min |
| *Scenario 2* | |
| Arrival on scene to trauma alert | 1–8.03 min |
| Time to initiation of needle compression | 2.2–5.76 min |
| Total time on scene | 5.2–8.75 min |

## 4. Discussion

Quality prehospital care is a critical function in the continuum of emergency care. In many scenarios, the prehospital phase of care is the health care system's earliest opportunity to improve patient outcomes during episodic care. The importance of creating effective models to develop expertise in prehospital care cannot be understated.

Prehospital personnel must be capable of providing life-saving interventions at a moment's notice. EMT-basic training is between 120 and 150 hours and EMT-paramedic between 1200 and 1800 hours in length, compared with the 2 to 4 years of training that nurses receive and the 11 to 13 years that physicians receive prior to being expected to evaluate and treat patients. Treatment decisions for time-sensitive emergency conditions must be made quickly and correctly; therefore, prehospital care providers must be well trained and have a high degree of confidence in initiating procedures under adverse circumstances. It can be inferred that higher provider confidence should lead to a decrease in time spent on scene because of the greater efficiency with procedures and decreased time to make a decision due to exposure to various scenarios from simulation. Our findings suggest that exposure to a critical trauma scenario requiring a life-saving intervention improves a prehospital care provider's confidence level in performing this procedure. Similar findings have been noted in other simulation studies, although not focusing specifically on tourniquet placement and needle decompression.

Overall, our results suggest that introducing simulation into EMS training can enhance the educational experience of prehospital care providers, allowing them to develop important experiential knowledge about procedures while gaining essential confidence in procedure performance. Previous evidence has suggested that education using clinical simulation can shorten the time it takes for trained personnel to become proficient in critical clinical procedures [6].

Our limitations include that the pre- and posttraining survey were a simple tool that was subjective in the assessment of confidence in performing procedures without specific evidence of outcomes or proficiency. In addition, the scene times documented in the simulation were much shorter than those in real trauma scenes in Alachua County. A clear limitation of the simulation environment is the inability to reliably create the chaos, distractions, and other stressors (e.g., interactions with other agencies and the public, extrication, and environmental factors) that are typically associated with real world situations. While this limitation is to some extent insurmountable and can clearly affect the ability of a simulation environment to precisely evaluate outcomes such as the true time spent on trauma calls, it does not preclude accurate measure of the prehospital care providers' assessments, decision-making, and action times, which directly impact actual scene times.

Future studies should focus on actual patient care outcomes as a result of such education interventions, which could be particularly helpful to rural EMS agencies and other municipalities with fewer scene calls.

In conclusion, this study demonstrates that the introduction of simulation into training can improve prehospital care providers' confidence in performing tourniquet placement and needle decompression in critically injured patients. These scenarios were chosen to test the prehospital personnel in their ability to make critical decisions and perform advanced procedures when necessary. Additional simulations could be done to assess other skills as well. These findings suggest that the integration of more simulation into prehospital care training may be useful, especially for rarely performed time critical life-saving skills.

## Disclosure

The content is solely the responsibility of the authors and does not necessarily represent the official views of the National Institutes of Health.

## Competing Interests

The authors declare that they have no competing interests.

## Acknowledgments

The research reported in this publication was supported by the National Center for Advancing Translational Sciences of the National Institutes of Health under Award no. UL1TR001427. The paper was copyedited by Linda J. Kesselring, M.S., ELS.

## References

[1] A. Abelsson, I. Rystedt, B.-O. Suserud, and L. Lindwall, "Mapping the use of simulation in prehospital care—a literature review," *Scandinavian Journal of Trauma, Resuscitation and Emergency Medicine*, vol. 22, article 22, 2014.

[2] R. L. Lammers, M. Davenport, F. Korley et al., "Teaching and assessing procedural skills using simulation: metrics and methodology," *Academic Emergency Medicine*, vol. 15, no. 11, pp. 1079–1087, 2008.

[3] P. Bradley, "The history of simulation in medical education and possible future directions," *Medical Education*, vol. 40, no. 3, pp. 254–262, 2006.

[4] J. S. Ilgen, J. Sherbino, and D. A. Cook, "Technology-enhanced simulation in emergency medicine: a systematic review and meta-analysis," *Academic Emergency Medicine*, vol. 20, no. 2, pp. 117–127, 2013.

[5] W. F. Bond, M. Kostenbader, and J. F. McCarthy, "Prehospital and hospital-based health care providers' experienced with a human patient simulator," *Prehospital Emergency Care*, vol. 5, no. 3, pp. 284–287, 2001.

[6] A. Abelsson, I. Rystedt, B.-O. Suserud, and L. Lindwall, "Learning by simulation in prehospital emergency care—an integrative literature review," *Scandinavian Journal of Caring Sciences*, vol. 30, no. 2, pp. 234–240, 2015.

[7] D. P. Davis, C. Buono, J. Ford, L. Paulson, W. Koenig, and D. Carrison, "The effectiveness of a novel, algorithm-based difficult airway curriculum for air medical crews using human patient simulators," *Prehospital Emergency Care*, vol. 11, no. 1, pp. 72–79, 2007.

# Children's Mental Health Visits to the Emergency Department: Factors Affecting Wait Times and Length of Stay

**Amanda S. Newton,[1] Sachin Rathee,[2] Simran Grewal,[3]
Nadia Dow,[4] and Rhonda J. Rosychuk[5]**

[1] *Faculty of Medicine & Dentistry, University of Alberta, Edmonton Clinic Health Academy (ECHA), 11405-87 Avenue, Room 3-526, Edmonton, AB, Canada T6G 1C9*
[2] *Faculty of Medicine & Dentistry, University of Alberta, WC Mackenzie Health Sciences Centre, Edmonton, AB, Canada T6G 2R7*
[3] *Faculty of Medicine & Dentistry, University of Alberta, Edmonton Clinic Health Academy (ECHA), 11405-87 Avenue, Room 3-582B, Edmonton, AB, Canada T6G 1C9*
[4] *Faculty of Medicine & Dentistry, University of Alberta, Edmonton Clinic Health Academy (ECHA), 11405-87 Avenue, Room 3-582, Edmonton, AB, Canada T6G 1C9*
[5] *Faculty of Medicine & Dentistry, University of Alberta, Edmonton Clinic Health Academy (ECHA), 11405-87 Avenue, Room 3-524, Edmonton, AB, Canada T6G 1C9*

Correspondence should be addressed to Amanda S. Newton; mandi.newton@ualberta.ca

Academic Editor: Chak W. Kam

*Objective*. This study explores the association of patient and emergency department (ED) mental health visit characteristics with wait time and length of stay (LOS). *Methods*. We examined data from 580 ED mental health visits made to two urban EDs by children aged ≤18 years from April 1, 2004, to March 31, 2006. Logistic regressions identified characteristics associated with wait time and LOS using hazard ratios (HR) with 95% confidence intervals (CIs). *Results*. Sex (male: HR = 1.48, 95% CI = 1.20–1.84), ED type (pediatric ED: HR = 5.91, 95% CI = 4.16–8.39), and triage level (Canadian Triage and Acuity Scale (CTAS) 2: HR = 3.62, 95% CI = 2.24–5.85) were statistically significant predictors of wait time. ED type (pediatric ED: HR = 1.71, 95% CI = 1.18–2.46), triage level (CTAS 5: HR = 2.00, 95% CI = 1.15–3.48), number of consultations (HR = 0.46, 95% CI = 0.31–0.69), and number of laboratory investigations (HR = 0.75, 95% CI = 0.66–0.85) predicted LOS. *Conclusions*. Based on our results, quality improvement initiatives to reduce ED waits and LOS for pediatric mental health visits may consider monitoring triage processes and the availability, access, and/or time to receipt of specialty consultations.

## 1. Introduction

In recent years, there has been considerable documentation of increases in visits by children to the emergency department (ED) for crisis mental health care [1–9]. Studies show that more parents are seeking care for their children in hospital EDs to treat acute emergencies [2, 4–6, 10, 11], request guidance for at-home child management [12], and gain access to health care resources [12]. The current health care system, however, does not meet the needs of families in the emergency care setting [3, 4, 13]. Many children do not receive comprehensive treatment for pediatric mental health visits and are discharged without adequate recommendations for follow-up care [14]. There is also increasing evidence for long waits for care and lengths of ED stay (LOS) [6, 8, 9, 15–19].

A stance among a number of studies is that wait times and LOS are important measures of treatment timeliness and patient safety [20–25]. A number of organizational and patient characteristics have been linked to wait time and LOS and serve to highlight the multifactorial nature of improving ED performance. Longer ED wait times for patients of all ages have been associated with a higher triage level (which denotes a lower level of urgency for the presenting complaint), an increased patient census (ED occupancy), urban-based EDs, day of arrival (Sunday, Monday, or Wednesday), and arrival by "walk-in" (versus ambulance) [26–31]. ED wait times have also been associated with race, ethnicity, and sex [30–35]—sociodemographic disparities that raise issues of access to timely care in terms of issues of bias/discrimination, language barriers, and ED cultural competence. A longer LOS for pediatric visits has also been associated with night shift and early morning arrivals, admitted patients, presentation during the winter season, higher triage acuity, and treatment that includes diagnostic testing and subspecialty consultations [34, 36]. Intentional self-injury, age 6–13 years, use of laboratory testing, hospital location, and patient transfer have also been associated with extended ED stays for pediatric mental health visits [17], while limited staff availability for psychiatric assessments, clinical instability, and limited bed availability have been associated with longer ED LOS for adult mental health visits [37]. In total, this body of literature raises important questions for pediatric emergency mental health care including how to ensure treatment timeliness and quality of care. We analyzed data from a sample of pediatric mental health visits to a general and a pediatric ED over a two-year period to explore organizational and patient characteristics associated with longer wait times and LOS.

## 2. Materials and Methods

*2.1. Study Population Variables of Interest.* We examined data from a previously conducted medical record and administrative database review of a representative sample of pediatric (≤18 years) mental health visits to a general and a pediatric ED, both academic tertiary care centers. Using a proportional allocation stratified random sampling design, 580 ED visits were reviewed from the 2 sites ($n = 164$ for pediatric ED; $n = 416$ for general ED). The site samples ensured that data were representative of mental health emergency visits at each ED location. Characteristics of the EDs and the study protocol are detailed elsewhere [14, 38]. ED visits by children were made between April 1, 2004, and March 31, 2006, for mental illness, substance abuse, or intentional self-harm (International Statistical Classification of Diseases (ICD) codes) [39].

Clinical data included in this study were health care visit and demographic variables of interest. Health care visit data included the type of ED visited (general versus pediatric), the presenting complaint (to indicate primary reason for mental health visit), and ED accompaniment and mode of arrival. Other ED visit information included the time of week (Tuesday to Thursday, Friday to Monday) and season (spring, summer, autumn, or winter) for the visit. We also included triage level data coded according to the Canadian Triage and Acuity Scale (CTAS; CTAS 1 = Resuscitation, CTAS 2 = Emergent, CTAS 3 = Urgent, CTAS 4 = Semi-Urgent, CTAS 5 = Non-Urgent) [40, 41]. This triage level is assigned at ED presentation to establish treatment priority based on the severity of the child's condition. We were also interested in whether a child received a mental health consultation, the number of consults and diagnostic tests (investigations) documented for the ED visit, and the recorded disposition for the visit. Documented ED registration, triage, assessment (physician and nurse), and discharge dates and times were also reviewed to calculate the wait time and LOS for each ED visit. Demographic data included age, sex, the presence of medical or psychiatric comorbidities (yes/no), and socioeconomicstatus (SES) based on median household income [42]. This study was approved by the Health Research Ethics Board of the University of Alberta (Edmonton, Alberta).

*2.2. Outcome Variables.* Two time-to-event outcome variables defined two patient subsets. For patients who had a disposition other than "left without being seen" (admitted, discharged, transferred, or unknown), the ED wait time for the visit was defined as the time of triage to the first time assessed by a health care provider (nurse or physician, whichever time came first). LOS for the visit was defined as the time of triage to the time of discharge from the ED for the subset of patients who were discharged or admitted to hospital.

*2.3. Statistical Analysis.* Data were summarized by frequencies and percentages or median and interquartile range (IQR). If the triage time was missing for the ED visit, the registration time was used in the calculation of the outcome variables. Missing, negative, or implausible wait times were replaced with median times for the respective triage level and censored. The median wait time for triage level 3 was used as the censoring time for patients with missing triage. For LOS, missing, negative, or implausible LOS times were replaced with median times for the respective diagnosis and censored [23].

Kaplan-Meier curves display outcome variables and separate bivariable and multivariable Cox proportional hazards (PH) models (with a random effect for patients) were developed to investigate predictors for each outcome variable. Based on previous studies, variables hypothesized to predict longer ED wait times for pediatric mental health visits were those that occurred over the weekend/early week (Friday to Monday) and had less urgent triage levels and were made by patients with a lower SES and who arrived by "walk-in" (versus ambulance) [26–34]. We also hypothesized that lower SES would predict a longer ED wait time based on bias/discrimination findings from other studies [30–35] and that youth who were not accompanied by a guardian or parent (e.g., arrival alone or with friends) waited longer because of the absence of adult advocacy and communication limitations. Variables hypothesized to predict a longer ED LOS were those visits that occurred over the weekend/early week (Friday to Monday), had more urgent triage levels, involved mental health consultations and other consultations/laboratory investigations, and resulted in the patient being admitted [17, 34, 36]. We also hypothesized that those visits made to the general ED would result in a longer LOS [37] as this hospital had in-house psychiatric service compared to the pediatric ED and would likely involve more assessment/care [14]. An interaction term (ED type and number of investigations) was added to the LOS model to account for known practice variation between EDs [14].

Models were examined for the PH assumption [43]. Hazard ratios (HR) and 95% confidence intervals (CIs) are reported. Statistical software (S-PLUS Version 8.1.1 for Linux, TIBCO Software Inc., Palo Alto, CA, 2008) was used for data analysis; $P < 0.05$ was considered statistically significant.

## 3. Results

Of the 580 mental health ED presentations in this study, visits were made by 551 distinct children and youth. The majority of ED visits were made by females ($n = 326$, 56.2%) and youth aged 13–18 years ($n = 494$, 85.2%) and children aged 6–12 years ($n = 81$, 14.0%). ED visits were represented across all SES groups; however, the majority of visits involved children and youth from median annual family incomes of $50,000–$69,999 ($n = 322$, 55.5%) and $30,000–$49,999 ($n = 91$, 15.7%). Only 2.6% of visits were made by children and youth from a median family income <$30,000 ($n = 15$). Visits were made equitably across seasons (spring: 25.5%, summer: 22.1%, autumn: 25.5%; winter: 26.9%).

Children and youth were most often accompanied by a parent or guardian ($n = 316$, 54.4%) with "walk-in" ($n = 268$, 46.2%) as the most common method of arrival (Table 1). The majority of presentations were assigned a triage level of CTAS 3 ($n = 271$, 46.7%) and CTAS 4 ($n = 215$, 37.1%) at presentation. Mental and behavioural disorders secondary to substance abuse ($n = 161$, 27.8%) and behavioural/emotional disorders and syndromes ($n = 122$, 21.0%) were the most frequent main ambulatory diagnoses. Comorbidities were documented for 249 children and youth (42.9%). Most children and youth did not receive a mental health consultation ($n = 399$, 68.8%). The majority of children and youth presenting for a mental health crisis did not receive any other specialty/subspecialty consultation ($n = 365$, 62.9%) during their ED visit and laboratory investigations were often not ordered ($n = 411$, 70.9%). Most ED presentations for mental health by children and youth ended in discharge ($n = 426$, 73.4%) (Table 1).

We analyzed 558 ED visits (by 531 distinct patients) for modeling predictors of longer wait times. Of these visits, all had a disposition other than "left without being seen" and 1 visit had an unknown triage time. In the medical records for these visits, 3 records did not have recorded sex, 24 records did not have patient accompaniment documented, 23 records did not have mode of ED arrival documented, and 33 records did not have the necessary forward sortation data available to calculate SES. The median wait time for these visits was 1 hour and 5 minutes (IQR: 32 minutes, 1 hour and 50 minutes). When predictor variables were examined separately (Table 2; bivariable model), triage level, ED type, mode of ED arrival, and diagnosis were statistically significant predictors of wait time. When adjusted for other predictors in the multivariable model, sex became statistically significant and only ED type and triage level remained statistically significant (Table 2; multivariable model). As seen in Figure 1, when compared with those children and youth triaged as CTAS 3, children and youth triaged as CTAS 2 had shorter wait times (HR = 3.62, 95% CI = 2.24–5.85). The relatively large CIs reflect small

Table 1: Visit characteristics ($n = 580$), $n$ (%).

| | |
|---|---|
| ED type | |
| General | 416 (71.7) |
| Pediatric | 164 (28.3) |
| Mode of arrival | |
| Medical transport | 267 (46.0) |
| Police | 15 (2.6) |
| Walk-in | 268 (46.2) |
| Unknown | 30 (5.2) |
| Patient accompaniment | |
| Alone | 9 (1.6) |
| Emergency Medical Services (EMS) worker | 213 (36.7) |
| Parent/guardian | 316 (54.4) |
| Friend | 11 (1.9) |
| Unknown | 31 (5.3) |
| Triage level | |
| CTAS 1 | 2 (0.3) |
| CTAS 2 | 76 (13.1) |
| CTAS 3 | 271 (46.7) |
| CTAS 4 | 215 (37.1) |
| CTAS 5 | 15 (2.6) |
| Unknown | 1 (0.2) |
| Main ambulatory diagnosis | |
| Anxiety or stress-related disorder | 112 (19.3) |
| Behavioural or emotional disorder/syndrome | 122 (21.0) |
| Intentional self-harm | 62 (10.7) |
| Mental and behavioural disorder secondary to substance abuse | 161 (27.8) |
| Mood disorder | 100 (17.2) |
| Schizophrenia or other psychotic disorder | 23 (4.0) |
| Comorbidity | |
| None documented | 331 (57.1) |
| Mental health consultation | |
| No | 399 (68.8) |
| Yes | 181 (31.2) |
| Number of consultations | |
| 0 | 365 (62.9) |
| 1 | 206 (35.5) |
| 2 | 9 (1.6) |
| Number of investigations | |
| 0 | 411 (70.9) |
| 1 | 40 (6.9) |
| 2 | 76 (13.1) |
| 3 | 45 (7.8) |
| 4 | 8 (1.4) |
| Disposition | |
| Admitted | 75 (12.9) |
| Discharged | 426 (73.4) |
| Left without being seen/left against medical advice | 22 (3.8) |
| Transferred | 21 (3.6) |
| Unknown | 36 (6.2) |

TABLE 2: Exploratory models of ED wait time predictors for pediatric mental health visits ($n$ = 558).

| | $n$ | Bivariable model | | | Multivariable model | | |
|---|---|---|---|---|---|---|---|
| | | Hazard ratio | 95% CI | $P$ value | Hazard ratio | 95% CI | $P$ value |
| Age | 558 | 1.03 | 0.99–1.07 | 0.210 | 1.01 | 0.97–1.06 | 0.521 |
| Sex | | | | | | | |
| Female | 314 | | Reference | | | Reference | |
| Male | 241 | 1.18 | 0.96–1.44 | 0.108 | 1.48 | 1.20–1.84 | <0.001 |
| Unknown | 3 | 1.26 | 0.39–4.05 | 0.699 | 0.46 | 0.15–1.41 | 0.174 |
| Socioeconomic status | | | | | | | |
| <$30,000 | 15 | 0.77 | 0.49–1.22 | 0.269 | 1.05 | 0.62–1.75 | 0.867 |
| $30,000–$49,999 | 89 | 1.04 | 0.77–1.42 | 0.792 | 0.82 | 0.59–1.14 | 0.230 |
| $50,000–$69,999 | 308 | | Reference | | | Reference | |
| $70,000–$89,999 | 68 | 0.91 | 0.65–1.28 | 0.590 | 0.92 | 0.65–1.31 | 0.653 |
| >$90,000 | 45 | 1.09 | 0.73–1.62 | 0.680 | 1.08 | 0.68–1.70 | 0.753 |
| Unknown | 33 | 1.54 | 0.97–2.45 | 0.068 | 1.07 | 0.71–1.64 | 0.737 |
| Day of the week | | | | | | | |
| Tuesday to Thursday | 265 | | Reference | | | Reference | |
| Friday to Monday | 293 | 1.19 | 0.97–1.45 | 0.098 | 0.98 | 0.79–1.23 | 0.846 |
| Patient accompaniment | | | | | | | |
| Parent/guardian or unknown | 331 | | Reference | | | Reference | |
| EMS, alone, or with friends | 227 | 1.02 | 0.84–1.25 | 0.836 | 1.36 | 0.95–1.95 | 0.094 |
| Mode of arrival | | | | | | | |
| Medical transport/police or unknown | 298 | | Reference | | | Reference | |
| Walk-in | 260 | 0.59 | 0.48–0.72 | <0.001 | 0.86 | 0.57–1.28 | 0.455 |
| ED type | | | | | | | |
| General | 398 | | Reference | | | Reference | |
| Pediatric | 160 | 5.39 | 3.78–7.69 | <0.001 | 5.91 | 4.16–8.39 | <0.001 |
| Triage level | | | | | | | |
| CTAS 1 | 2 | 9.47 | 5.75–15.58 | <0.001 | 2.32 | 0.90–6.01 | 0.082 |
| CTAS 2 | 76 | 7.08 | 4.95–10.12 | <0.001 | 3.62 | 2.24–5.85 | <0.001 |
| CTAS 3 or unknown | 264 | | Reference | | | Reference | |
| CTAS 4 | 201 | 0.89 | 0.71–1.11 | 0.310 | 0.97 | 0.74–1.26 | 0.799 |
| CTAS 5 | 15 | 1.64 | 0.95–2.82 | 0.076 | 1.02 | 0.60–1.72 | 0.952 |
| Diagnosis | | | | | | | |
| Mental/behavioural disorder secondary to substance abuse | 152 | | Reference | | | Reference | |
| Anxiety/stress-related disorder | 109 | 0.42 | 0.31–0.58 | <0.001 | 0.82 | 0.50–1.32 | 0.405 |
| Intentional self-harm | 61 | 0.50 | 0.34–0.75 | <0.001 | 1.15 | 0.73–1.79 | 0.550 |
| Mood disorder | 97 | 0.39 | 0.27–0.56 | <0.001 | 0.97 | 0.64–1.47 | 0.889 |
| Schizophrenia or other psychotic disorder | 20 | 0.42 | 0.25–0.69 | <0.001 | 0.84 | 0.52–1.34 | 0.456 |
| Behavioural or emotional disorder/syndrome | 119 | 0.40 | 0.29–0.56 | <0.001 | 0.97 | 0.63–1.49 | 0.898 |

counts for CTAS 1 ($n$ = 2). Children and youth who visited a pediatric ED were much more likely to wait less time to see a health care provider (HR = 5.91, 95% CI = 4.16–8.39; Figure 2) than those children and youth who visited a general ED. Shorter wait times were associated with male sex (HR = 1.48, 95% CI = 1.20–1.84; Figure 3). The multivariable model showed some deviation from the assumption of proportional hazards for some of the variables including ED type, CTAS, and diagnosis.

We analyzed 501 ED visits with a disposition of either admitted or discharged (by 477 distinct patients) for modeling predictors of longer LOS. Of these visits, 1 visit had an unknown triage time. In the 501 medical records, 2 records were missing sex, 10 did not have patient accompaniment documented, 10 records did not have mode of ED arrival documented, and 27 records did not have the necessary forward sortation data available to calculate SES. The median ED LOS was 3 hours and 53 minutes (IQR: 2 hours and 26 minutes, 6 hours and 24 minutes). When predictor variables were examined separately (Table 3; bivariable model), age, triage level, mental health consultation, disposition, number of consultations, number of laboratory investigations, and diagnosis were statistically significant predictors of LOS For the multivariable model, an interaction term of ED type by

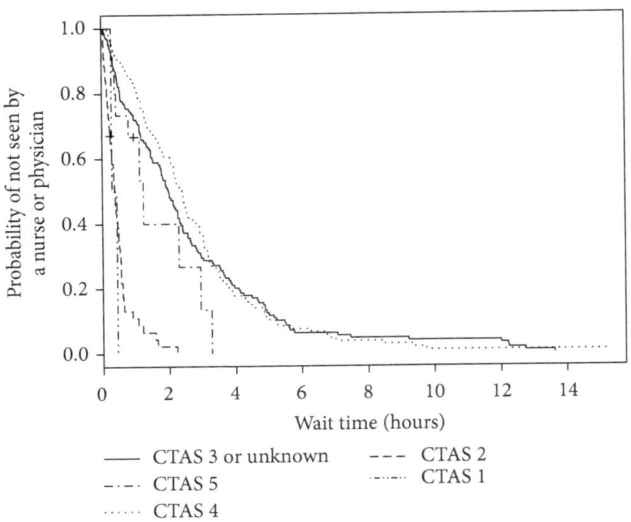


FIGURE 1: Kaplan-Meier estimates of ED wait time by triage level.

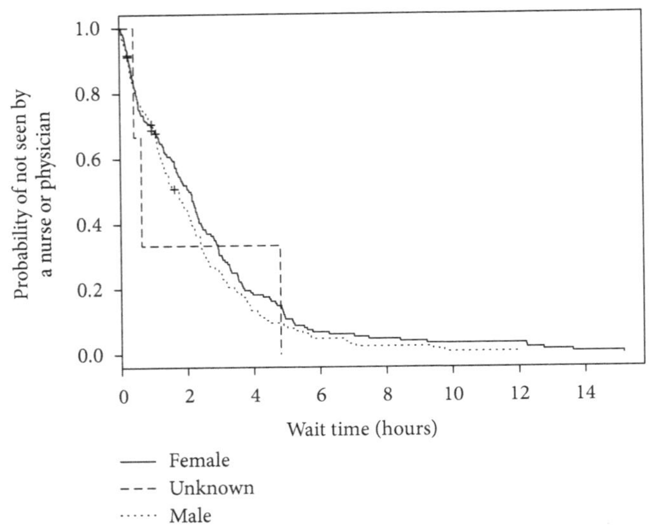


FIGURE 3: Kaplan-Meier estimates of ED wait time by sex.

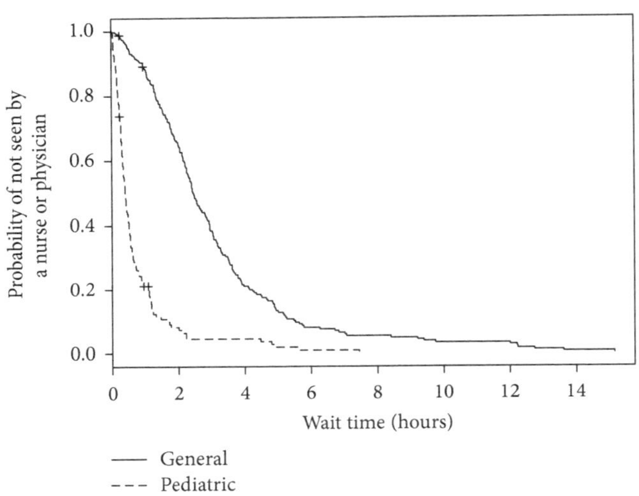


FIGURE 2: Kaplan-Meier estimates of ED wait time by ED type.

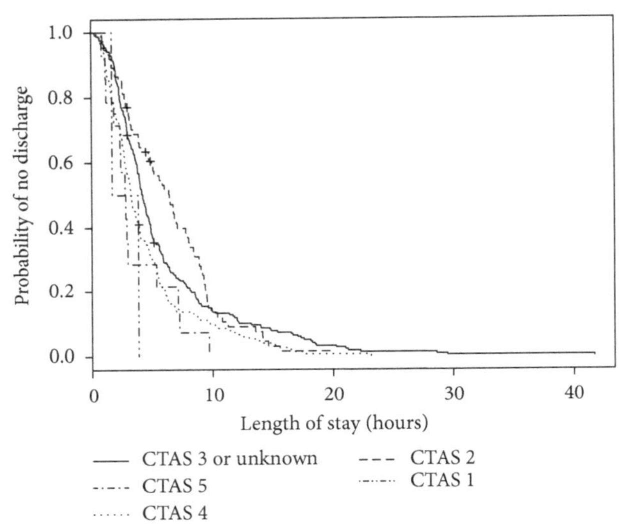


FIGURE 4: Kaplan-Meier estimates of ED LOS by triage level.

number of laboratory investigations was added to account for known practice variation between EDs. When adjusted for other predictors in the multivariable model, ED type became statistically significant. Triage level, number of consultations, and number of laboratory investigations remained statistically significant (Table 3; multivariable model). When compared with those children and youth triaged as CTAS 3, children and youth triaged as CTAS 5 had a shorter LOS (HR = 2.00, 95% CI = 1.15–3.48; Figure 4). The relatively large CIs reflect small counts for CTAS 1 ($n$ = 2). Children and youth who visited a pediatric ED (HR = 1.71, 95% CI = 1.18–2.46; Figure 5) were more likely to experience a shorter LOS than those who visited a general ED. A longer ED LOS for pediatric mental health visits was also associated with the number of consultations (HR = 0.46, 95% CI = 0.31–0.69; Figure 6) and number of laboratory investigations (HR = 0.75, 95% CI = 0.66–0.85; Figure 7) that occurred during the visit. The multivariable model showed some deviation from the assumption of proportional hazards for some of the variables: ED type, number of consults, and number of investigations.

## 4. Discussion

In this study, we explored the association of patient and ED visit characteristics with wait time and LOS for pediatric mental health visits. In our multivariable model, shorter ED wait times were associated with visits to a pediatric ED, children and youth triaged as CTAS 2, and being male, while shorter LOS was associated with visits to a pediatric ED, children and youth triaged as CTAS 5, and fewer consultations and laboratory investigations that occurred during the visit. Based on these results, candidate characteristics for quality

TABLE 3: Exploratory models of ED LOS predictors for pediatric mental health visits ($n$ = 501).

| | $n$ | Bivariable model | | | Multivariable model | | |
|---|---|---|---|---|---|---|---|
| | | Hazard ratio | 95% CI | $P$ value | Hazard ratio | 95% CI | $P$ value |
| Age | 501 | 0.93 | 0.90–0.97 | <0.001 | 0.96 | 0.92–1.01 | 0.079 |
| Sex | | | | | | | |
| Female | 278 | | Reference | | | Reference | |
| Male | 221 | 0.93 | 0.77–1.11 | 0.412 | 0.88 | 0.72–1.07 | 0.210 |
| Unknown | 2 | 1.35 | 0.50–3.60 | 0.554 | 1.77 | 1.23–2.55 | 0.002 |
| Day of the week | | | | | | | |
| Tuesday to Thursday | 245 | | Reference | | | Reference | |
| Friday to Monday | 256 | 1.02 | 0.86–1.22 | 0.825 | 1.05 | 0.87–1.27 | 0.624 |
| ED type | | | | | | | |
| General | 366 | | Reference | | | Reference | |
| Pediatric | 135 | 1.06 | 0.88–1.28 | 0.551 | 1.71 | 1.18–2.46 | 0.004 |
| Triage level | | | | | | | |
| CTAS 1 | 2 | 2.87 | 1.14–7.21 | 0.025 | 4.96 | 1.57–15.68 | 0.006 |
| CTAS 2 | 74 | 0.86 | 0.69–1.07 | 0.181 | 1.13 | 0.82–1.56 | 0.441 |
| CTAS 3 or unknown | 238 | | Reference | | | Reference | |
| CTAS 4 | 173 | 1.40 | 1.13–1.73 | 0.002 | 1.24 | 0.99–1.56 | 0.061 |
| CTAS 5 | 14 | 1.81 | 1.04–3.16 | 0.037 | 2.00 | 1.15–3.48 | 0.015 |
| Mental health consultation | | | | | | | |
| No consultation | 332 | | Reference | | | Reference | |
| Consultation | 169 | 0.48 | 0.40–0.59 | <0.001 | 0.93 | 0.60–1.42 | 0.722 |
| Disposition | | | | | | | |
| Discharged | 426 | | Reference | | | Reference | |
| Admitted | 75 | 0.67 | 0.53–0.84 | <0.001 | 0.99 | 0.77–1.28 | 0.961 |
| Number of consultations | 501 | 0.45 | 0.38–0.54 | <0.001 | 0.46 | 0.31–0.69 | <0.001 |
| Number of laboratory investigations | 501 | 0.75 | 0.70–0.81 | <0.001 | 0.75 | 0.66–0.85 | <0.001 |
| Pediatric ED, number of investigations* | 501 | | | | 0.88 | 0.73–1.07 | 0.197 |
| Diagnosis | | | | | | | |
| Mental/behavioural disorder secondary to substance abuse | 129 | | Reference | | | Reference | |
| Anxiety or stress-related disorder | 102 | 1.66 | 1.27–2.17 | <0.001 | 1.20 | 0.83–1.74 | 0.322 |
| Intentional self-harm | 54 | 0.91 | 0.63–1.31 | 0.599 | 1.04 | 0.70–1.55 | 0.854 |
| Mood disorder | 87 | 1.06 | 0.83–1.35 | 0.637 | 1.10 | 0.77–1.58 | 0.602 |
| Schizophrenia or other psychotic disorder | 17 | 0.83 | 0.59–1.17 | 0.295 | 0.88 | 0.54–1.44 | 0.621 |
| Behavioural or emotional disorder/syndrome | 112 | 1.28 | 0.98–1.66 | 0.068 | 1.13 | 0.79–1.62 | 0.506 |

*Interaction with number of investigations.

improvement initiatives in EDs to reduce waits and LOS for pediatric mental health visits are discussed below.

In this study, it mattered in terms of both wait time and LOS whether a child or youth visited a pediatric or general ED. Consistent with our hypothesis, those visits made to the general ED resulted in a longer LOS. This finding may reflect the psychiatric resources available at the general hospital as previous research has shown that children/youth who visited this ED were more likely to receive mental health consultations and associated care [14]. While a longer LOS due to access to specialized services does not necessarily imply a need for quality improvement, the length of time to accessing such resources in the ED (e.g., wait time for consultations) is of importance and should be tracked by EDs to ensure timely access to assessments and treatment. Other factors that may have affected the longer wait and LOS at the general ED which would be important for addressing treatment timeliness and quality of care, but not assessed in this study, were the mixed patient population (adult and pediatric, emergencies other than mental health) and rates of discharge/admission. These factors have been found to affect health care delivery to children seen in different ED types [25].

Adult, female patients (>18 years) have been found to wait longer for ED assessment and treatment than male patients [31, 36], and it has been proposed for adult patients that differences may be, in part, attributable to a lack of preassessment/treatment testing (e.g., EKG) [31]. The role of sex in influencing ED wait times amongst different ages of children and youth has not been previously documented, and the reasons for this difference seen in our study for pediatric mental health patients remain unclear. Further

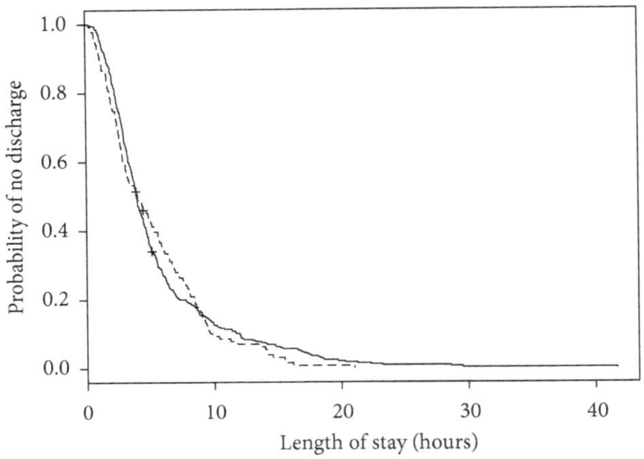


FIGURE 5: Kaplan-Meier estimates of ED LOS by ED type.

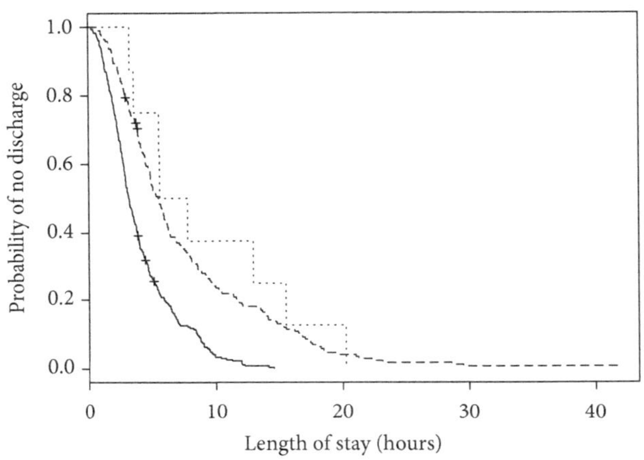


FIGURE 6: Kaplan-Meier estimates of ED LOS by number of consultations.

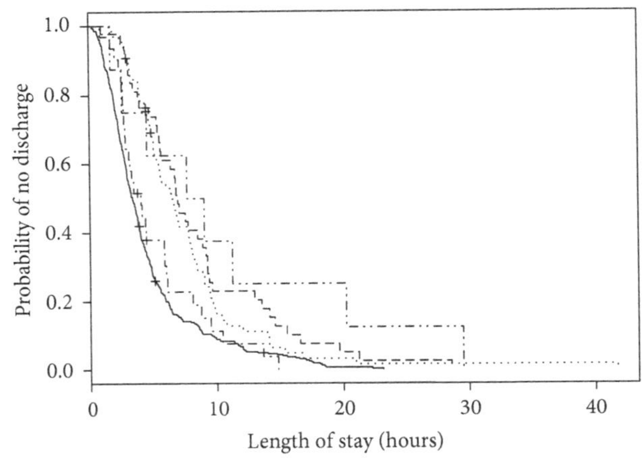


FIGURE 7: Kaplan-Meier estimates of ED LOS by number of investigations.

investigation is important to determine whether a difference in preassessment for these patients is a factor, which may have implications for the utilization of standardized preassessment tools at triage.

While other studies have reported racial and ethnic disparities amongst adult and pediatric ED patients for ED wait time and LOS [30–35], we did not find SES, another type of patient sociodemographic, to be a significant predictor of either time period. In other studies, the influence of insurance status on ED wait times has been mixed with several studies reporting no effect [32, 44] and an Australian study reporting lower SES as a significant predictor of ED wait time [36]. Based on this body of results, it may be that different organizational characteristics (e.g., location of ED, whether mental health services are available in the ED) interact with insurance status and SES to influence ED wait time and LOS. This interaction may be important for future studies interested in developing quality improvement initiatives for ED wait times and LOS.

Day of the week when the ED visit occurred was also not a significant predictor of wait time or LOS as we had hypothesized. While other studies have reported longer times for visits on Sunday, Monday, and Wednesday [27, 28], our findings are similar to Chan et al. [45] who found no difference in day of the week on overall ED LOS. The difference in study patient populations may explain our findings in that adult patients with medical concerns wait until the weekend or those who do not improve over the weekend decide to seek care shortly thereafter, whereas parents caring for a child with mental health needs may be motivated during any day of the week to visit the ED given the caregiving and emotional demands of mental health crises.

In this study, mode of arrival and patient accompaniment were not significant predictors of ED wait time. However, other studies discuss the implications of providing care to an unaccompanied minor [46], and we recommend that those EDs who treat unaccompanied minors in emergency mental health situations use age appropriate language to help elicit information needed to stabilize the crisis, facilitate timely care, and provide a comprehensive referral/discharge plan if needed.

Comparable to other study findings [27, 28, 31, 36], a significant predictor of wait time and LOS in this study was triage level. As expected, mental health visits triaged at the higher acuity CTAS 2 had shorter waits for care. CTAS 1 was also a significant predictor of a shorter LOS, as hypothesized; however, the large confidence interval suggests that further evaluation with a larger sample size would lend confidence to this finding. A longer ED wait time is a known risk factor for a longer LOS [36]. While visits triaged as CTAS 5 in this study had longer recorded wait times, this lower acuity triage level was a significant predictor of a shorter LOS. Less urgent conditions usually require minimal physician/nursing consultation and often only assessment/reassurance, which could lead to more efficient treatment and discharge times [23]. Triage associated initiatives shown to improve timeliness to care that may impact the visits include having a health care provider (i.e., nurse practitioner, physician assistant) in the triage area to perform initial assessments and initiate diagnostic tests [47], general practice clinics adjacent to the ED to divert nonurgent patients [48], and bedside registration/triage which involves the primary care nurse working alongside registration staff at a mobile computer station to log presenting complaints and the initial assessment [49]. These strategies may also improve those mental health visits with a longer LOS (e.g., CTAS 3) by improving time delays caused by waiting for a number of subspecialty consultations and laboratory investigations, which in our study were found to predict a longer LOS.

Of final note, disposition status was not a significant predictor of LOS in our study. Other studies have noted that mental health patients presenting to the ED tend to spend a significant time there for evaluation and disposition due to insufficient psychiatric services and inpatient resources (i.e., available beds for admission) [17, 19]. In some studies, being transferred to another health care facility or being admitted [17, 34] increased the odds of an extended LOS. Variables not evaluated in this study may further explain our finding and be of importance to quality improvement, such as the presence of any quality improvement measures to facilitate discharge and/or the availability of inpatient beds.

## 5. Study Limitations

There are some limitations to this study. The data set was limited by date (March 31, 2006) and thus may not entirely reflect current predictors of ED wait time and LOS.

Other determinants (such as the variable availability of a specialized mental health assessment team or a potential lack of comfort for some physicians in knowing how to manage patients with mental health concerns, thereby preferentially selecting other patients to see first) likely contribute to both ED wait and LOS, but these factors could not be elicited in the medical records we reviewed. Sociodemographic disparities in ED wait and LOS based on race and ethnicity have also been discussed in the literature, but this information was not routinely collected or available in the medical records we reviewed. Further, administrative data such as ED census during the date/time of the mental health visit and the availability of in-patient beds (e.g., boarding time) may also help to explain our findings but were not collected in this study.

## 6. Conclusions

In summary, the results of our multivariable model suggest that, as a first step, quality improvement initiatives in EDs for treatment timeliness and safety for pediatric mental health visits include the monitoring of triage processes, and the availability, access, and/or time to involve specialty consultations. Further work is needed to better understand the role of sex in influencing wait time for pediatric mental health patients as is the influence of ED-wide quality improvement measures to facilitate throughput such as discharge and/or the availability of in-patient beds.

## Conflict of Interests

The authors have no conflict of interests to declare including no direct relation with the commercial identities (statistical software) identified in this paper.

## Acknowledgments

During the execution of this project Mr. Rathee was supported by a Summer Student Research Award from the Health Quality Council of Alberta. Dr. Rosychuk is a Health Scholar with Alberta Innovates-Health Solutions. Dr. Newton holds a Canadian Institutes of Health Research (CIHR) New Investigator Award.

## References

[1] M. R. Sills and S. D. Bland, "Summary statistics for pediatric psychiatric visits to US emergency departments, 1993–1999," *Pediatrics*, vol. 110, no. 4, article e40, 2002.

[2] A. S. Newton, S. Ali, D. W. Johnson et al., "A 4-year review of pediatric mental health emergencies in Alberta," *Canadian Journal of Emergency Medicine*, vol. 11, no. 5, pp. 447–454, 2009.

[3] M. A. Dolan, J. A. Fein, K. N. Shaw et al., "Technical report—pediatric and adolescent mental health emergencies in the emergency medical services system," *Pediatrics*, vol. 127, no. 5, pp. e1356–e1366, 2011.

[4] J. L. Cooper and R. Masi, *Unclaimed Children Revisited (Issue Brief No. 1): Child and Youth Emergency Mental Health Care: A National Problem*, National Center for Children in Poverty, Columbia University, New York, NY, USA, 2007.

[5] S. Reder and L. Quan, "Emergency mental health care for youth in Washington State: qualitative research addressing hospital emergency departments' identification and referral of youth facing mental health issues," *Pediatric Emergency Care*, vol. 20, no. 11, pp. 742–748, 2004.

[6] J. Grupp-Phelan, P. Mahajan, G. L. Foltin et al., "Referral and resource use patterns for psychiatric-related visits to pediatric emergency departments," *Pediatric Emergency Care*, vol. 25, no. 4, pp. 217–220, 2009.

[7] A. Kennedy, P. Cloutier, J. E. Glennie, and C. Gray, "Establishing best practice in pediatric emergency mental health: a prospective study examining clinical characteristics," *Pediatric Emergency Care*, vol. 25, no. 6, pp. 380–386, 2009.

[8] L. I. Santiago, M. G. Tunik, G. L. Foltin, and M. A. Mojica, "Children requiring psychiatric consultation in the pediatric emergency department: epidemiology, resource utilization, and complications," *Pediatric Emergency Care*, vol. 22, no. 2, pp. 85–89, 2006.

[9] A. S. Newton, R. J. Rosychuk, S. Ali et al., "The emergency department compass. Children's mental health," Pediatric mental health emergencies in Alberta, Canada, Emergency department visits by children and youth aged 0 to 17 years, 2002–2008, Edmonton, Canada, 2011.

[10] A. S. Newton, S. Ali, D. W. Johnson et al., "Who comes back? Characteristics and predictors of return to emergency department services for pediatric mental health care," *Academic Emergency Medicine*, vol. 17, no. 2, pp. 177–186, 2010.

[11] E. C. Soto, A. M. Frederickson, H. Trivedi et al., "Frequency and correlates of inappropriate pediatric psychiatric emergency room visits," *Journal of Clinical Psychiatry*, vol. 70, no. 8, pp. 1164–1177, 2009.

[12] P. Cloutier, A. Kennedy, H. Maysenhoelder, E. J. Glennie, M. Cappelli, and C. Gray, "Pediatric mental health concerns in the emergency department: caregiver and youth perceptions and expectations," *Pediatric Emergency Care*, vol. 26, no. 2, pp. 99–106, 2010.

[13] American Academy of Pediatrics, Committee on Pediatric Emergency Medicine, "Pediatric mental health emergencies in the emergency medical services system," *Pediatrics*, vol. 118, no. 4, pp. 1764–1767, 2006.

[14] A. S. Newton, S. Ali, M. P. Hamm et al., "Exploring differences in the clinical management of pediatric mental health in the emergency department," *Pediatric Emergency Care*, vol. 27, no. 4, pp. 275–283, 2011.

[15] J. Meunier-Sham, "Increased volume/length of stay for pediatric mental health patients: one ED's response," *Journal of Emergency Nursing*, vol. 29, no. 3, pp. 229–239, 2003.

[16] K. V. Christodulu, R. Lichenstein, M. D. Weist, M. E. Shafer, and M. Simone, "Psychiatric emergencies in children," *Pediatric Emergency Care*, vol. 18, no. 4, pp. 268–270, 2002.

[17] S. D. Case, B. G. Case, M. Olfson, J. G. Linakis, and E. M. Laska, "Length of stay of pediatric mental health emergency department visits in the United States," *Journal of the American Academy of Child and Adolescent Psychiatry*, vol. 50, no. 11, pp. 1110–1119, 2011.

[18] P. Mahajan, E. R. Alpern, J. Grupp-Phelan et al., "Epidemiology of psychiatric-related visits to emergency departments in a multicenter collaborative research pediatric network," *Pediatric Emergency Care*, vol. 25, no. 11, pp. 715–720, 2009.

[19] M. Waseem, R. Prasankumar, K. Pagan, and M. Leber, "A retrospective look at length of stay for pediatric psychiatric patients in an Urban emergency department," *Pediatric Emergency Care*, vol. 27, no. 3, pp. 170–173, 2011.

[20] D. Ng, G. Vail, S. Thomas, and N. Schmidt, "Applying the lean principles of the Toyota production system to reduce wait times in the emergency department," *Canadian Journal of Emergency Medicine*, vol. 12, no. 1, pp. 50–57, 2010.

[21] S. R. Finamore and S. A. Turris, "Shortening the wait: a strategy to reduce waiting times in the emergency department," *Journal of Emergency Nursing*, vol. 35, no. 6, pp. 509–514, 2009.

[22] B. R. Holroyd, M. J. Bullard, K. Latoszek et al., "Impact of a triage liaison physician on emergency department overcrowding and throughput: a randomized controlled trial," *Academic Emergency Medicine*, vol. 14, no. 8, pp. 702–708, 2007.

[23] M. Soleimani, S. Grewal, R. J. Rosychuk, and A. S. Newton, "wait times and length of stay in Alberta emergency department for children's mental health meeting national benchmarks? Trends from 2002 to 2008," *Paediatrics & Child Health*, vol. 18, no. 6, pp. e26–e31, 2013.

[24] U. Sethuraman, N. Kannikeswaran, X. Chen, and P. V. Mahajan, "Effect of a rapid assessment program on total length of stay in a pediatric emergency department," *Pediatric Emergency Care*, vol. 27, no. 4, pp. 295–300, 2011.

[25] F. T. Bourgeois and M. W. Shannon, "Emergency care for children in pediatric and general emergency departments," *Pediatric Emergency Care*, vol. 23, no. 2, pp. 94–102, 2007.

[26] P. Hutten-Czapski, "Rural-urban differences in emergency department wait times," *Canadian Journal of Rural Medicine*, vol. 15, no. 4, pp. 153–155, 2010.

[27] A. Arkun, W. M. Briggs, S. Patel et al., "Emergency department crowding: factors influencing flow," *Western Journal of Emergency Medicine*, vol. 11, no. 1, pp. 10–15, 2010.

[28] N. Elkum, M. Fahim, M. Shoukri, and A. Al-Madouj, "Which patients wait longer to be seen and when? A waiting time study in the emergency department," *Eastern Mediterranean Health Journal*, vol. 15, no. 2, pp. 416–424, 2009.

[29] M. E. Richards, M. W. Hubble, and C. Crandall, "Influence of ambulance arrival on emergency department time to be seen," *Prehospital Emergency Care*, vol. 10, no. 4, pp. 440–446, 2006.

[30] N. Sonnenfeld, S. R. Pitts, S. M. Schappert, and S. L. Decker, "Emergency department volume and racial and ethnic differences in waiting times in the United States," *Medical Care*, vol. 50, no. 4, pp. 335–341, 2012.

[31] A. P. Wilper, S. Woolhandler, K. E. Lasser et al., "Trends: waits to see an emergency department physician: U.S. trends and predictors, 1997–2004," *Health Affairs*, vol. 27, no. 2, pp. w84–w95, 2008.

[32] C. Y. Park, M. A. Lee, and A. J. Epstein, "Variation in emergency department wait times for children by raceethnicity and payment source: children's care and coverage," *Health Services Research*, vol. 44, no. 6, pp. 2022–2039, 2009.

[33] C. A. James, F. T. Bourgeois, and M. W. Shannon, "Association of race/ethnicity with emergency department wait times," *Pediatrics*, vol. 115, no. 3, pp. e310–e315, 2005.

[34] A. Bekmezian, P. J. Chung, M. D. Cabana, J. H. Maselli, J. F. Hilton, and A. L. Hersh, "Factors associated with prolonged emergency department length of stay for admitted children," *Pediatric Emergency Care*, vol. 27, no. 2, pp. 110–115, 2011.

[35] M. Mohsin, A. Bauman, and S. Ieraci, "Is there equity in emergency medical care? Waiting times and walk-outs in South Western Sydney hospital emergency departments," *Australian Health Review*, vol. 21, no. 3, pp. 133–149, 1998.

[36] K. A. Nelson, S. E. Boslaugh, and D. Hodge, "Risk factors for extremely long length-of-stay among pediatric emergency patients," *Pediatric Emergency Care*, vol. 25, no. 12, pp. 835–840, 2009.

[37] G. Chang, A. P. Weiss, E. J. Orav et al., "Bottlenecks in the emergency department: the psychiatric clinicians' perspective," *General Hospital Psychiatry*, vol. 34, no. 4, pp. 403–409, 2012.

[38] A. Y. Yu, N. Ata, K. Dong, and A. S. Newton, "A description of emergency care received by children and youth with mental health presentations for alcohol and other drug use in two Alberta emergency departments," *Journal of the Canadian Academy of Child and Adolescent Psychiatry*, vol. 19, no. 4, pp. 290–296, 2010.

[39] World Health Organization, International Statistical Classification of Diseases and Related Health Problems (10th Revision), http://www.who.int.login.ezproxy.library.ualberta.ca/classifications/icd/en/.

[40] J. Gravel, S. Manzano, and M. Arsenault, "Validity of the Canadian paediatric triage and acuity scale in a tertiary care hospital," *Canadian Journal of Emergency Medicine*, vol. 11, no. 1, pp. 23–28, 2009.

[41] D. W. Warren, A. Jarvis, L. LeBlanc, and J. Gravel, "Revisions to the Canadian triage and acuity scale paediatric guidelines (PaedCTAS)," *Canadian Journal of Emergency Medicine*, vol. 10, no. 3, pp. 224–243, 2008.

[42] Statistics Canada, Profile for Canada, Provinces, Territories, and Forward Sortation Areas, 2006 Census, http://www.statcan.gc.ca/bsolc/olc-cel/olc-cel?catno=94-581-X2006003&lang=eng.

[43] P. M. Grambsch and T. M. Therneau, "Proportional hazards tests and diagnostics based on weighted residuals," *Biometrika*, vol. 81, no. 3, pp. 515–526, 1994.

[44] L. I. Horwitz and E. H. Bradley, "Percentage of US emergency department patients seen within the recommended triage time: 1997 to 2006," *Archives of Internal Medicine*, vol. 169, no. 20, pp. 1857–1865, 2009.

[45] L. Chan, K. M. Reilly, and R. F. Salluzzo, "Variables that affect patient throughput times in an academic emergency department," *The American Journal of Medical Quality*, vol. 12, no. 4, pp. 183–186, 1997.

[46] J. Urkin, N. Bilenko, Y. Bar-David, E. Gazala, N. Barak, and J. Merrick, "Who accompanies a child to the office of the physician?" *International Journal of Adolescent Medicine and Health*, vol. 20, no. 4, pp. 513–518, 2008.

[47] R. A. Love, J. A. Murphy, T. E. Lietz, and K. S. Jordan, "The effectiveness of a provider in triage in the emergency department: a quality improvement initiative to improve patient flow," *Advanced Emergency Nursing Journal*, vol. 34, no. 1, pp. 65–74, 2012.

[48] A. Sharma and B. Inder, "Impact of co-located general practitioner (GP) clinics and patient choice on duration of wait in the emergency department," *Emergency Medicine Journal*, vol. 28, no. 8, pp. 658–661, 2011.

[49] D. Handel, S. Epstein, R. Khare et al., "Interventions to improve the timeliness of emergency care," *Academic Emergency Medicine*, vol. 18, no. 12, pp. 1295–1302, 2011.

# Management of Fever in Postpneumococcal Vaccine Era: Comparison of Management Practices by Pediatric Emergency Medicine and General Emergency Medicine Physicians

**Hnin Khine,[1,2] David L. Goldman,[2,3] and Jeffrey R. Avner[1,2]**

[1] *Division of Pediatric Emergency Medicine, Children's Hospital at Montefiore, 3415 Bainbridge Avenue, Bronx, NY 10467, USA*
[2] *Department of Pediatrics, Albert Einstein College of Medicine, Bronx, NY 10467, USA*
[3] *Division of Pediatric Infectious Diseases, Children's Hospital at Montefiore, Bronx, NY 10467, USA*

Correspondence should be addressed to Hnin Khine; hkhine@montefiore.org

Academic Editor: Chee-Fah Chong

*Background.* The primary objective of this study was to compare management practices of general emergency physicians (GEMPs) and pediatric emergency medicine physicians (PEMPs) for well-appearing young febrile children. *Methods.* We retrospectively reviewed the charts of well-appearing febrile children aged 3–36 months who presented to a large urban children's hospital (PED), staffed by PEMPs, or a large urban general emergency department (GED), staffed by GEMPs. Demographics, immunization status, laboratory tests ordered, antibiotic usage, and final diagnoses were collected. *Results.* 224 cases from the PED and 237 cases from the GED were reviewed. Children seen by PEMPs had significantly less CXRs (23 (10.3%) versus 51 (21.5%), $P = 0.001$) and more rapid viral testing done (102 (45%) versus 40 (17%), $P < 0.0001$). A diagnosis of a viral infection was more common in the PED, while a diagnosis of bacterial infection (including otitis media) was more common in the GED. More GED patients were prescribed antibiotics (41% versus 27%, $P = 0.002$), while more PED patients were treated with oseltamivir (6.7% versus 0.4%, $P < 0.001$). *Conclusions.* Our findings identify important differences in the care of the young, well-appearing febrile child by PEMPs and GEMPs and highlight the need for standardization of care.

## 1. Introduction

Physicians with varying amounts of pediatric clinical experience manage children seeking emergency care. Because of differences in training and work exposures, the management of ill and injured pediatric patients in the emergency department can vary greatly between pediatric emergency physicians (PEMPs) and general emergency medicine physicians (GEMPs). Prior studies have shown important differences in the management of pediatric patients by GEMPs and PEMPs in a variety of clinical situations including, resuscitation, fracture management, and resource utilization [1–4].

Fever is one of the most common chief complaints of children presenting to the emergency department. This includes otherwise well-appearing children aged 3–36 months, who are at risk for occult bacteremia. In the 1980s and early 1990s, the standard of care for these children included laboratory testing (complete blood count and blood culture) and empiric antibiotic treatment. Practice guidelines from 1993 recommended that children of 3 to 36 months of age with fever of 39.0°C or higher and whose WBC count was 15,000/mm$^3$ or more should have a blood culture performed and be treated with antibiotics pending culture results [5]. With the advent improved conjugated pneumococcal and *Haemophilus* vaccines, the incidence of occult bacteremia in vaccinated, well-appearing febrile children has dramatically decreased and is now estimated to be 0.25–0.7% [6]. Consequently, the risk and cost of routine testing and treating young febrile children for bacteremia likely exceed their potential benefits. A recent review suggests that the only laboratory tests necessary in the evaluation of fever >39.0°C in young children are a urinalysis and urine culture (for circumcised males <6 months of age and uncircumcised males and females <24 months of age) [7].

There have been no recent comparisons of PEMPs with GEMPs in their evaluation and management of well-appearing young children with fever in the postpneumococcal vaccine era. A questionnaire performed by Maldonado et al. found that while PEMPs and GEMPs agreed on level of triage for most pediatric scenarios, GEMPs triaged children with fever at a significantly higher level of triage than PEMPs [8]. Despite the availability of specialized care for children in designated children's centers, the majority of children are cared for in general emergency departments. Differences in care among these sites can have important medical and economic implications. We hypothesized that GEMPs are likely to perform more tests and more likely to prescribe antibiotics when compared with PEMPs.

## 2. Methods

We performed a chart review of cases of well-appearing febrile children aged 3–36 months who presented to either a large urban children's hospital emergency department (PED) or a large urban general emergency department (GED) from September 1, 2009, to December 31, 2009. The children's hospital was located in the urban setting with an annual census of 60,000 per year. The GED was located 5 miles east of the children's hospital and has an annual census of 72,000 per year, 18% of whom are children. The children's hospital is a teaching hospital with residency and fellowship program while the general ED is staffed by general emergency medicine attending physicians and physician assistants. Pediatric patients from both hospitals were admitted to the children's hospital.

Charts were identified through the ED charting system, which is used by both hospitals. Charts were reviewed if the patient was between 3 and 36 months with the triage chief complaint of fever. The investigators manually reviewed all the eligible patients' records from the electronically scanned charts. Patients were excluded if they were admitted or had underlying conditions that predispose to infection, including an indwelling catheter (venous, bladder, or ventriculoperitoneal shunt), sickle cell disease, immunocompromising condition, cancer, or other chronic illness.

Demographic data were extracted from the ED charts of eligible patients using a standardized data collection sheet. In addition, the following information was collected: maximal height of fever (both historical and triage values), immunization status, number and types of laboratory tests ordered, use of antibiotics (type of antibiotic and route of administration), procedures performed, and final diagnosis. Final diagnoses were classified into either viral or bacterial based on the diagnosis and the use of antibiotics.

### 2.1. Statistics

*2.1.1. Power Calculations.* The primary outcome variable was the number of children receiving blood tests. Secondary outcomes included the number of tests performed, the use of empiric antibiotics, and the route of administration of antibiotics. We estimated that about 2.5% of eligible patients at PED received blood testing. In order to detect a 3-fold increase in number of eligible patients receiving blood tests in GED with an alpha error of 0.5 and a statistical power of 0.8, a sample size of 234 in each group was required. During the study period, an average of 81 children aged 3–36 months with fever were seen in the GED monthly, while 411 were seen in the PED monthly. In order to collect patients over the same 4-month interval, we reviewed every 6th patient in the PED group. The investigators manually reviewed every 6th chart of patients, aged 3–36 months with fever. If a patient met the exclusion criteria, the chart of the patient that preceded the eligible patient was reviewed. However, if the preceding patient also met the exclusion criteria, then the patient was counted as excluded.

*2.2. Data Analysis.* Categorical data such as sex and testing status were compared using chi-square or Fisher's exact test. Quantitative data was tested for normality using the Shapiro-Wilk normality test. Nonnormally distributed data was compared using the Mann-Whitney $U$ test. Normally distributed data was compared using the Student's $t$-test. $P$ values <0.05 were considered significant. All statistics were done with GraphPad InStat software (San Diego, CA). This study was approved by the hospital's committee on clinical investigations.

## 3. Results

For 2009, the annual census for the PED was 59,640 patients. In contrast, the annual census for the GED was 72,224 patients of which 12,794 (18%) were pediatric patients. The PED was staffed by 32 providers, while the GED was staffed by 36 providers. During the study period, from the PED, 1644 visits of patients aged 3–36 months with a chief complaint of fever or febrile seizure were identified, of which every 6th chart (274) was reviewed. Fifty of these cases were excluded based on criteria, as outlined above. From the GED, 324 charts were identified and 87 excluded based on criteria. A total of 461 charts (224 from PED and 237 from GED) were reviewed for this study (Figure 1). Demographic data are shown in Table 1. The two groups were similar in terms of age, sex, and insurance status; however, the patients in PED group had a higher temperature, both by history and by triage. Documentation of immunization status by either nurse or physician was more common in PED cases (222/224, 98%) than in GED cases (200/237, 84%, $P < 0.001$).

The frequency of laboratory testing by PEMPs and GEMPs is shown in Table 2. Both PEMPs and GEMPs infrequently obtained complete blood counts and blood cultures. Furthermore, both PEMPs and GEMPs ordered similar numbers of urine cultures. However, GEMPs ordered more chest radiographs while PEMPs ordered more viral testing. The discharge diagnoses of the study patients are listed in Table 3. Overall, the most common diagnosis made by both PEMPs and GEMPs was viral illness/viral syndrome. However, more patients treated by GEMPs received a diagnosis with a bacterial cause compared to those patients treated by PEMPs. GEMPs diagnosed more acute otitis media as

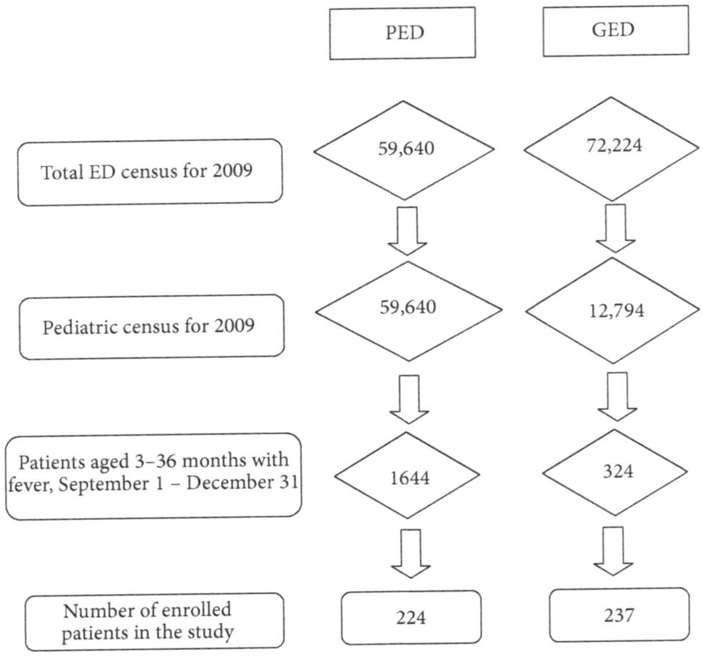


FIGURE 1: Hospital ED census and enrollment numbers are given for the study period, September 1, 2009, to December 31, 2009.

TABLE 1: Demographics.

| | PED | GED | $P$ value |
|---|---|---|---|
| Age (mos) | 16.6 ± 9.1 | 15.2 ± 8.7 | NS |
| Male (%) | 56% | 49% | NS |
| $T_{max}$ by hx (°F) | 102.7 ± 1.4 | 102.2 ± 1.4 | 0.01 |
| Triage temperature (°F) | 101.8 ± 1.9 | 101.3 ± 1.9 | 0.03 |
| Immunization documented (%) | 98% | 84% | <0.001 |
| State assistance insurance/self-pay (%) | 61% | 56% | NS |

TABLE 2: Laboratory test performed.

| | PED ($n$ = 224) | GED ($n$ = 237) | $P$ value |
|---|---|---|---|
| | Diagnostic studies | | |
| CBC (%) | 8 (4) | 9 (4) | NS |
| BCX (%) | 8 (4) | 7 (3) | NS |
| UCX (%) | 20 (9) | 11 (5) | 0.09 |
| CXR (%) | 23 (10) | 51 (22) | 0.001 |
| VIRAL testing (%) | 102 (46) | 40 (17) | <0.001 |

TABLE 3: Discharge diagnoses and prescription patterns.

| | PED ($n$ = 224) | GED ($n$ = 237) | $P$ value |
|---|---|---|---|
| | | Diagnosis | |
| Viral (total) | **163** | **140** | **0.0016** |
| Viral syndrome | 103 | 122 | NS |
| Influenza | 16 | 0 | <0.0001 |
| Bronchiolitis | 15 | 8 | NS |
| AGE* | 13 | 5 | 0.053 |
| Fever | 9 | 1 | 0.0091 |
| Stomatitis/herpangina | 5 | 2 | NS |
| Croup | 2 | 2 | NS |
| Bacterial (total) | **61** | **97** | **0.0017** |
| Otitis media | 50 (22) | 77 (32) | 0.016 |
| UTI/pyelonephritis | 3 | 1 | NS |
| Pneumonia | 3 | 3 | NS |
| Sinusitis | 4 | 1 | NS |
| Pharyngitis | 0 | 10 | 0.0018 |
| Lymphadenitis | 1 | 0 | NS |
| Bronchitis | 0 | 3 | NS |
| Conjunctivitis | 0 | 2 | NS |
| | | Prescriptions | |
| Antibiotics | 61 (27) | 97 (41) | 0.002 |
| Antiviral | 15 (7) | 1 (0) | <0.001 |

*Refers to acute gastroenteritis.

well as pharyngitis than PEMPs (Table 3). Overall, GEMPs prescribed more antibiotics than PEMPs (97/237 (41%) versus 61/224 (27%), $P = 0.002$). Consistent with more viral testing, PEMPs prescribed more antivirals (primarily oseltamivir) than GEMPs (7% versus 0.4%, $P < 0.001$).

## 4. Discussion

The majority of children who seek emergency care in the United States are treated in hospitals staffed by GEMPs.

Children under the age of 18 comprised 22.1% of all hospital emergency department visits. Nonetheless, the annual number of pediatric patients seen in most general hospital EDs is relatively small. The National Health Statistic Report from 2012 noted that 4000 out of 4800 hospital emergency departments see less than 10,000 pediatric patients per year [9]. The relatively limited exposure to pediatric emergencies during training and practice can make the managing of pediatric emergencies especially challenging for the GEMP.

A survey conducted in 2001 to emergency physicians regarding their management of febrile young children reported a very high rate of invasive testing with 69% of correspondents choosing to perform complete blood count and 46% choosing to perform blood cultures [10]. In contrast, we found that the overall rate of invasive testing was low for both GEMPs and PEMPS. The hypothesis that GEMPs rely more heavily on invasive testing to assess young febrile children of 3–36 months of age was not supported by our findings. This minimalistic approach is consistent with recent recommendations that recommend the elimination of routine invasive testing for well-appearing young febrile children based on very low rates of occult bacteremia (<0.5%) among vaccinated children [11, 12].

However, there were important differences in the care provided in the GED and the PED. Firstly, the documentation of immunization status was significantly greater in the PED when compared with the GED. Immunization status is an important consideration in the evaluation of the febrile infant since unvaccinated infants are at increased risk for pneumococcal bacteremia [13]. In addition, we found significantly higher rates of antibiotic prescription and diagnoses of AOM by GEMPs when compared with PEMPs. These findings are similar to those of Isaacman et al. who found that GEMPs diagnosed more bacterial focal infections, mainly otitis media, and prescribed more antibiotics than PEMPS when caring for children with fever [10]. Overuse of antibiotics has important ramifications including the emergence of resistant organisms, like penicillin resistant pneumococci and highly resistant gram-negative organisms. Overuse of antibiotics is also associated with increased cost and adverse effects including anaphylaxis and *C. difficile* colitis. In attempt to limit antibiotic exposure in the pediatric community, the AAP recommends an initial observation for children over 23 months with acute otitis media [14].

We also found that performance of CXR in the evaluation of young febrile child was greater among GEMPs. Again these findings are consistent with those of Isaacman et al. [10]. Nonetheless, the rate of CXR used by GEMPs was significantly lower than that reported in the Isaacmen study (21% versus 40%). Previous studies have noted a wide variation in the utilization of chest radiography in the evaluation of febrile children in PEDs [15]. Guidelines for the use of chest radiographs in the evaluation of children older than 3 months with fever are not precise. The 2003 ACEP Clinical Policies Committee recommends (level C) that a chest radiograph is usually not indicated in febrile children aged older than 3 months with temperature less than 39°C (<102.2°F) without clinical evidence of acute pulmonary disease [16]. Not surprisingly, high chest radiography rates have been associated with increased antibiotic usage [17].

The high rate of viral testing by PEMPs in this study was likely affected by the timing of this study relative to H1N1 outbreak. Children under 2 years of age were considered to be in the high-risk group for complication from influenza and thus were screened for influenza including H1N1. This pattern of practice was reflected in the higher percent of use of antiviral agents among PEMPs. The cost effectiveness of this practice is yet to be determined.

There were several limitations of the study. This was a retrospective study and therefore we cannot comment on the decision making process of physicians. We believe that the two groups of patients that were included in the study were similar in terms of their health care need since the 2 hospitals are geographically located in close proximity. Children presenting to PED may be sicker since more patients with complex health history will seek the specialized care at children's hospital. However, in this study, we only included healthy, well-appearing children; thus we believe that their exposure to pathogens and external factors should be similar. We relied on the clinician assessment of well-appearing child as an inclusion criterion. This may have minimized the potential difference in the test performing behavior between the 2 groups since we are not able to determine the ability of physician's assessment of a healthy child. A child who may have been admitted to the hospital by GEMPs may not have been considered ill by PEMPs. We also included limited number of hospital sites, which may affect the generalizability of our findings. Nonetheless, we note that our findings are consistent with earlier studies regarding differences in the treatment of children by PEMPs versus GEMPs [1, 10].

## 5. Conclusions

Our studies indicate that the rate of invasive testing for well-appearing young febrile children at risk for occult bacteremia is low in EDs staffed by PEMPs and GEMPS. Nonetheless, the use of antibiotics and X-rays by GEMPs remains high when compared with PEMPs. In contrast, both the diagnosis of influenza and oseltamivir use are significantly more common with PEMPS. These findings are consistent with those of previous studies and highlight the differences in care received by febrile children cared for by PEMPs and GEMPs.

## Conflict of Interests

The authors declare that there is no conflict of interests regarding the publication of this paper.

## References

[1] P. V. Scribano, M. D. Baker, and S. Ludwig, "Factors influencing termination of resuscitative efforts in children: a comparison of pediatric emergency medicine and adult emergency medicine physicians," *Pediatric Emergency Care*, vol. 13, no. 5, pp. 320–324, 1997.

[2] M. Dharmar, J. P. Marcin, P. S. Romano et al., "Quality of care of children in the emergency department: association with

hospital setting and physician training," *Journal of Pediatrics*, vol. 153, no. 6, pp. 783–789, 2008.

[3] S. G. Weiner, R. P. Ruffing, and B. A. Barnewolt, "A comparison of resource utilization between emergency physicians and pediatric emergency physicians," *Pediatric Emergency Care*, vol. 28, no. 9, pp. 869–872, 2012.

[4] L. B. Cimpello, H. Khine, and J. R. Avner, "Practice patterns of pediatric versus general emergency physicians for pain management of fractures in pediatric patients," *Pediatric Emergency Care*, vol. 20, no. 4, pp. 228–232, 2004.

[5] L. J. Baraff, J. W. Bass, G. R. Fleisher et al., "Practice guideline for the management of infants and children 0 to 36 months of age with fever without source," *Annals of Emergency Medicine*, vol. 22, no. 7, pp. 1198–1210, 1993.

[6] E. Waddle and R. Jhaveri, "Outcomes of febrile children without localising signs after pneumococcal conjugate vaccine," *Archives of Disease in Childhood*, vol. 94, no. 2, pp. 144–147, 2009.

[7] L. J. Baraff, "Management of infants and young children with fever without source," *Pediatric Annals*, vol. 37, no. 10, pp. 673–679, 2008.

[8] T. Maldonado and J. R. Avner, "Triage of the pediatric patient in the emergency department: are we all in agreement?" *Pediatrics*, vol. 114, no. 2, pp. 356–360, 2004.

[9] S. M. Schappert and F. Bhuiya, "Availability of pediatric services and equipment in emergency departments: United States, 2006," National Health Statistics Reports 47, 2012.

[10] D. J. Isaacman, K. Kaminer, H. Veligeti, M. Jones, P. Davis, and J. D. Mason, "Comparative practice patterns of emergency medicine physicians and pediatric emergency medicine physicians managing fever in young children," *Pediatrics*, vol. 108, no. 2, pp. 354–358, 2001.

[11] G. M. Lee, G. R. Fleisher, and M. B. Harper, "Management of febrile children in the age of the conjugate pneumococcal vaccine: a cost-effectiveness analysis," *Pediatrics*, vol. 108, no. 4, pp. 835–844, 2001.

[12] M. Wilkinson, B. Bulloch, and M. Smith, "Prevalence of occult bacteremia in children aged 3 to 36 months presenting to the emergency department with fever in the postpneumococcal conjugate vaccine era," *Academic Emergency Medicine*, vol. 16, no. 3, pp. 220–225, 2009.

[13] K. L. Carstairs, D. A. Tanen, A. S. Johnson, S. B. Kailes, and R. H. Riffenburgh, "Pneumococcal bacteremia in febrile infants presenting to the emergency department before and after the introduction of the heptavalent pneumococcal vaccine," *Annals of Emergency Medicine*, vol. 49, no. 6, pp. 772–777, 2007.

[14] A. S. Lieberthal, A. E. Carroll, T. Chonmaitree et al., "The diagnosis and management of acute otitis media," *Pediatrics*, vol. 131, no. 3, pp. e964–e999, 2013.

[15] M. I. Neuman, D. Graham, and R. Bachur, "Variation in the use of chest radiography for pneumonia in pediatric emergency departments," *Pediatric Emergency Care*, vol. 27, no. 7, pp. 606–610, 2011.

[16] American College of Emergency Physicians Clinical Policies Committee and American College of Emergency Physicians Clinical Policies Subcommittee on Pediatric Fever, "Clinical policy for children younger than three years presenting to the emergency department with fever," *Annals of Emergency Medicine*, vol. 42, no. 4, pp. 530–545, 2003.

[17] N. Le Saux, C. Bjornson, and C. Pitters, "Antimicrobial use in febrile children diagnosed with respiratory tract illness in an emergency department," *Pediatric Infectious Disease Journal*, vol. 18, no. 12, pp. 1078–1080, 1999.

# Adherence to Follow-Up Recommendations by Triathlon Competitors Receiving Event Medical Care

**Jeremy D. Joslin,[1] Jarem B. Lloyd,[2] Nikoli Copeli,[3] and Derek R. Cooney[4]**

[1]*Department of Emergency Medicine, State University of New York Upstate Medical University, Syracuse, NY, USA*
[2]*Department of Orthopedics and Sports Medicine, St. Luke's University Health Network, Bethlehem, PA, USA*
[3]*Department of Emergency Medicine, New York Hospital Queens, Flushing, NY, USA*
[4]*Department of Emergency Medicine, 550 East Genesee St., Syracuse, NY 13210, USA*

Correspondence should be addressed to Derek R. Cooney; cooneyd@upstate.edu

Academic Editor: Chak W. Kam

*Introduction.* We sought to investigate triathlete adherence to recommendations for follow-up for participants who received event medical care. *Methods.* Participants of the 2011 Ironman Syracuse 70.3 (Syracuse, NY) who sought evaluation and care at the designated finish line medical tent were contacted by telephone approximately 3 months after the initial encounter to measure adherence with the recommendation to seek follow-up care after event. *Results.* Out of 750 race participants, 35 (4.6%) athletes received event medical care. Of these 35, twenty-eight (28/35; 80%) consented to participate in the study and 17 (61%) were available on telephone follow-up. Of these 17 athletes, 11 (11/17; 65%) of participants reported that they had not followed up with a medical professional since the race. Only 5 (5/17; 29%) confirmed that they had seen a medical provider in some fashion since the race; of these, only 2 (2/17; 12%) sought formal medical follow-up resulting from the recommendation whereas the remaining athletes merely saw their medical providers coincidentally or as part of routine care. *Conclusion.* Only 2 (2/17; 12%) of athletes who received event medical care obtained postrace follow-up within a one-month time period following the race. Event medical care providers must be aware of potential nonadherence to follow-up recommendations.

## 1. Introduction

Participation in triathlons has increased over the past two decades [1, 2]. With this rise in popularity, it is important to consider that triathlons have been associated with illness and injury including dehydration, cardiovascular complications, metabolic abnormalities, heat-related illness, and musculoskeletal injuries [2, 3]. USA Triathlon statistics have shown that the average age of triathlon participants is 38 years old, drawing the majority of participants from the 30–50-year-old age demographic: a group older than expected to participate in long duration, high intensity sports, and a group that may conceivably carry greater susceptibility to injury [1].

Factors such as experience, conditioning, environmental conditions, duration and distance of race events, and underlying athlete health can potentially contribute to inability to continue the race and result in the need for on-site medical evaluation [2, 3]. While some injuries occur during the course of the race, some participants may not become symptomatic until well after the athlete has finished the race and left the postrace area [4]. Over 85% of the triathletes seen in the medical area at the Kona Ironman Triathlon (Kailua-Kona, Hawaii) arrived at the main medical tent after finishing the race [4]. The concern for delayed presentation, or the existence of occult illness and injury, has also been expressed in a number of other published works in this area [5–7].

Similar to an emergency department, encounters at a race medical tent are often brief, and treatment guided towards resolution of acute symptoms. Whereas acute care provided in the emergency department setting may be more easily escalated to hospital admission or clinical referral, acute care in ultradistance medical tents is often limited by minimal supplies, limited infrastructure, with little-to-no established protocols besides hospital transfers by ambulance for true clinical emergencies.

Because medical encounters at race events are often limited and noncomprehensive, it is essential for patients to obtain follow-up care. Review of the current literature revealed no studies investigating how often patients who are evaluated in a race medical tent seek follow-up care when instructed to do so. Because of the importance of this follow-up care, the authors sought to investigate the adherence to recommendations that triathletes seek follow-up care after medical tent evaluation and treatment.

## 2. Methods

As part of a quality assurance review of athlete education on the importance of follow-up, participants of the 2011 Ironman 70.3 Syracuse (Syracuse, NY) who visited the designated finish line medical tent were evaluated by medical staff using a standardized encounter form which requested the athlete's follow-up contact information, as well as a checkbox to indicate their willingness to participate in our telephone follow-up at approximately three months after the event [IRB 294979-2].

The Ironman 70.3 Syracuse consists of three segments: a 1.2-mile swim, a 56-mile bike ride, and a 13.1-mile run. All triathlete participants treated in the medical tent were counseled to follow up with a medical provider for more definitive evaluation and to ensure resolution of symptoms. The participants were not advised of a specific time period to follow up. The medical encounter form used included a carbon copy tear-off sheet which was given to athletes upon medical tent discharge. All encounters were coded on the sheet with standard diagnoses (see the following list) at the time of evaluation. Athletes transferred off course or out of the medical tent by ambulance were excluded.

Standardized diagnoses used were

(i) mild to moderate heat-related illness;

(ii) severe heat illness;

(iii) dehydration or fatigue;

(iv) gastric dysfunction;

(v) orthopedic or soft tissue injury;

(vi) other.

Participants were contacted by telephone approximately 3 months after the initial encounter and asked if they did indeed follow up as instructed at their race medical tent evaluation. In the event that they did not follow up, they were asked to share the reason.

## 3. Results

Out of a total of 750 race participants, 35 (4.6%) athletes received event medical care at the medical tent. Of these 35, twenty-eight (28/35; 80%) consented to participate in the study and 17 (61%) were available to discuss their postevent care by telephone. Of these 17 athletes, 11 (11/17; 65%) of participants reported they had not followed up with a medical professional since the race. Only 5 (5/17; 29%) confirmed they had been seen by a medical provider since the race. Of these 5, only 2 (2/17; 12%) could be considered actual event medical follow-up, whereas the remaining athletes actually saw their medical providers coincidentally or as part of routine care. Athletes' own perception of symptom resolution was the most common reason among those who did not follow up. Results of the telephone interviews are summarized in Table 1.

## 4. Discussion

Endurance events demand sustained and elevated physiologic function under a variety of environmental conditions and therefore may incur a range of different injuries and physiologic insults. Common injury patterns seen at triathlon and other endurance events are well established in the literature [3, 8–11].

There are many examples in which an athlete's condition appears benign, yet requires diligent evaluation and should receive appropriate follow-up. These include, but are not limited to, subtle skeletal injuries that are only detected on radiographic imaging [12], hematuria that should be evaluated with serum biomarkers [10], and chest pain that should be risk stratified by electrocardiogram and serum marker assays due to related risk of cardiac events [13].

Although acute kidney injury (AKI) in this setting is typically self-limiting, an episode of severe AKI may warrant hospitalization and may not be caught until follow-up. McCullough found that 40% of marathon runners in a single event experienced only transient rises in creatinine level seen in AKI but suggests that chronic damage may accumulate in repeat participants [14]. Professional and amateur triathletes with repetitive AKI require the attention of follow-up care beyond the scope of the average event medical tent. Broad use of NSAIDs by athletes during endurance events may potentially increase the risk of AKI and exercise-associated hyponatremia, decreasing the glomerular filtration rate already lowered by exercise [15–17]. One urine dipstick method has been described to help risk stratify athletes with suspected renal injury at a medical tent [7].

Medical tents do not commonly have the capacity to perform radiographic examinations. One case series following stress fracture presentations among athletes found that diagnosis was delayed by an average of 3.5 months [18]. Our data reinforce the importance of follow-up care for orthopedic pain as one athlete reported a fracture found on radiographs at a follow-up visit (Athlete #7).

While there are clear differences between a race medical tent and an emergency department, the brief period of patient contact allowing a potential for complications after discharge is similar. In an emergency department study, leaving the patient to schedule their own follow-up was associated with poor follow-up adherence [19]. On the other hand, patients showed improved adherence among a comparison group where the follow-up appointment was prearranged [19]. Although it could be argued that not all athletes evaluated in a race medical tent require follow-up care, it may be difficult in the moment to stratify those who do and those who do not require that follow-up. In emergency medicine practice, it is common to recommend for these same reasons that

Table 1: Follow-up characteristics of athletes.

| Athlete | Complaint | Medical tent diagnosis | Medical tent intervention | Follow-up timeframe | Comments |
|---|---|---|---|---|---|
| 1 | Leg pain | (1) Orthopedic or soft tissue injury | (1) Comfort measures | 3-4 weeks | Chronic iliotibial band pain |
| 2 | Paresthesias | (1) Other | (1) Comfort measures<br>(2) Supplemental oxygen | None | Symptoms resolved so did not perceive need to follow up |
| 3 | Nausea & headache | (1) Dehydration or fatigue<br>(2) Gastric dysfunction | (1) Comfort measures<br>(2) Oral ondansetron<br>(3) Oral hydration | None | Symptoms resolved so did not perceive need to follow up |
| 4 | Ankle pain | (1) Orthopedic or soft tissue injury | (1) Cold pack applied | 2-3 months | Expected call from race staff to organize follow-up |
| 5 | Knee pain | (1) Orthopedic or soft tissue injury | (1) Cold pack applied | None | Symptoms resolved so did not perceive need to follow up |
| 6 | Nausea & dizziness | (1) Dehydration or fatigue | (1) Comfort measures<br>(2) Oral ondansetron<br>(3) Oral hydration | None | (1) Symptoms resolved so did not perceive need to follow up<br>(2) Did not have PCP for follow-up |
| 7 | Fall with abrasion | (1) Orthopedic or soft tissue injury | (1) Topical antibiotic ointment<br>(2) Cold pack applied<br>(3) Wound dressing | 2-3 weeks | Pain did not improve so sought follow-up care<br>Diagnosed with fracture |
| 8 | Leg pain | (1) Orthopedic or soft tissue injury | (1) Cold pack applied | None | Symptoms resolved so did not perceive need to follow up |
| 9 | Fall with abrasion | (1) Orthopedic or soft tissue injury | (1) Topical antibiotic ointment<br>(2) Cold pack applied<br>(3) Wound dressing | None | Symptoms resolved so did not perceive need to follow up |
| 10 | Foot pain | (1) Orthopedic or soft tissue injury | (1) Comfort measures | 2-3 months | Symptoms resolved so did not perceive need to follow up acutely |
| 11 | Knee pain | (1) Orthopedic or soft tissue injury | (1) Cold pack applied | None | Symptoms resolved so did not perceive need to follow up |
| 12 | Leg pain | (1) Orthopedic or soft tissue injury | (1) Comfort measures<br>(2) Oral hydration | 2-3 days | Symptoms persisted so followed up acutely |
| 13 | Blisters | (1) Orthopedic or soft tissue injury | (1) Topical antibiotic ointment<br>(2) Wound dressing | None | Symptoms resolved so did not perceive need to follow up |
| 14 | Nausea & dizziness | (1) Dehydration or fatigue | (1) Comfort measures | None | Symptoms resolved so did not perceive need to follow up |
| 15 | Weakness & dizziness | (1) Dehydration or fatigue | (1) Comfort measures | None | Symptoms resolved so did not perceive need to follow up |
| 16 | Asthma exacerbation | (1) Other | (1) Inhaled beta agonist treatment | None | Symptoms resolved so did not perceive need to follow up |
| 17 | Itching | (1) Other | (1) Comfort measures | None | Symptoms resolved so did not perceive need to follow up |

all patients discharged from the emergency department be reevaluated in the near term.

Another factor found to improve adherence to recommended follow-up among self-pay and Medicaid patients was to provide a clinical appointment date before discharge [20]. In that subject pool where no appointment was provided, only 13% followed up with a medical provider. By comparison, in Roy Magnusson's study, where a prearranged clinical appointment was offered, approximately half of every comparison group followed up [19].

It may also be helpful to reflect on the "athlete attitude" which may include amplified feelings of health and wellness. Some athletes are likely to question a physician's or other provider's recommendation to obtain follow-up care, especially if the athlete has no prior relationship with the medical tent provider. Athletes may also carry feelings that they are "unbreakable" and too healthy to require medical care. Finally, it is not uncommon for athletes to simply not have a primary care provider if they have been generally healthy or are of a young age.

Considerations for improving follow-up rates include a primary follow-up care provider referral on the race registration form, documentation of participant primary care provider information on registration, or establishment of a designated follow-up provider for participants who visit the medical tent. Primary care sports medicine providers trained in both primary care and sports medicine offer an attractive option to triathletes requiring follow-up care [21]. The triathlete racer demographic possesses a more stable socioeconomic status [1], which presumably entails greater access to both insurance and follow-up medical care.

## 5. Limitations

This study represents a small sample size from a single event. The lack of comparable published literature limits the analysis to some degree as no other data set or expected rates of follow-up are known. Though a larger sample size may have enhanced the level of generalizability of the study, the results are consistent with common sense expectations and require further study. The unique practice environment typically involves care providers of various backgrounds, training, and licensure or certification. Because of this, it is not common practice to detail-oriented diagnoses. Typically general categories of field-expedient diagnoses are utilized, limiting potential subanalysis.

## 6. Conclusions

This study demonstrated that follow-up care recommendations were for the most part dismissed by athletes based on resolution of symptoms despite consistent medical staff advisement of all athletes who were seen in the medical tent to follow up with their healthcare professional. Athletes' perception of symptom resolution was the most common reason cited among those who did not follow up. Event medical care providers must be aware of potential nonadherence to recommendations and should consider potential strategies to improve follow-up compliance, especially in cases where the provider deems clinical follow-up to be important. Further studies are required to verify the causes of noncompliance with medical follow-up and the long-term outcome of subclinical triathlon or endurance sports injuries.

## Competing Interests

The authors declare that they have no competing interests.

## Acknowledgments

The authors warmly thank Anthony Giuffrida for his work on data gathering and Dr. Martin Hoffman for his review and assistance.

## References

[1] TribeGroup, *The Mind of the Triathlete: Executive Summary*, USA Triathlon, 2009.

[2] C. M. Gosling, A. B. Forbes, J. McGivern, and B. J. Gabbe, "A profile of injuries in athletes seeking treatment during a triathlon race series," *The American Journal of Sports Medicine*, vol. 38, no. 5, pp. 1007–1014, 2010.

[3] G. M. Dallam, S. Jonas, and T. K. Miller, "Medical considerations in triathlon competition: recommendations for triathlon organisers, competitors and coaches," *Sports Medicine*, vol. 35, no. 2, pp. 143–161, 2005.

[4] R. H. Laird and D. Johnson, "The medical perspective of the Kona Ironman Triathlon," *Sports Medicine and Arthroscopy Review*, vol. 20, no. 4, p. 239, 2012.

[5] V. Vleck, G. P. Millet, and F. B. Alves, "The impact of triathlon training and racing on Athletes' General Health," *Sports Medicine*, vol. 44, no. 12, pp. 1659–1692, 2014.

[6] B. R. Kupchak, B. M. Volk, L. J. Kunces et al., "Alterations in coagulatory and fibrinolytic systems following an ultramarathon," *European Journal of Applied Physiology*, vol. 113, no. 11, pp. 2705–2712, 2013.

[7] M. D. Hoffman, K. J. Stuempfle, K. Fogard, T. Hew-Butler, J. Winger, and R. H. Weiss, "Urine dipstick analysis for identification of runners susceptible to acute kidney injury following an ultramarathon," *Journal of Sports Sciences*, vol. 31, no. 1, pp. 20–31, 2013.

[8] W. D. B. Hiller, M. L. O'toole, E. E. Fortess, R. H. Laird, P. C. Imbert, and T. D. Sisk, "Medical and physiological considerations in triathlons," *The American Journal of Sports Medicine*, vol. 15, no. 2, pp. 164–167, 1987.

[9] S. Migliorini, "The triathlon: acute and overuse injuries," *Journal of Sports Traumatology*, vol. 22, no. 4, pp. 186–195, 2000.

[10] P. K. Korkia, D. S. Tunstall-Pedoe, and N. Maffulli, "An epidemiological investigation of training and injury patterns in British triathletes," *British Journal of Sports Medicine*, vol. 28, no. 3, pp. 191–196, 1994.

[11] R. H. Laird, "Medical complications during the Ironman Triathlon World Championship 1981–1984," *Annals of Sports Medicine*, vol. 3, no. 2, pp. 113–116, 1987.

[12] A. M. Spiker, S. Dixit, and A. J. Cosgarea, "Triathlon: running injuries," *Sports Medicine and Arthroscopy Review*, vol. 20, no. 4, pp. 206–213, 2012.

[13] J. H. Kim, R. Malhotra, G. Chiampas et al., "Cardiac arrest during long-distance running races," *The New England Journal of Medicine*, vol. 366, no. 2, pp. 130–140, 2012.

[14] P. A. McCullough, K. M. Chinnaiyan, M. J. Gallagher et al., "Changes in renal markers and acute kidney injury after marathon running," *Nephrology*, vol. 16, no. 2, pp. 194–199, 2011.

[15] S. J. Warden, "Prophylactic use of NSAIDs by athletes: a risk/benefit assessment," *Physician and Sportsmedicine*, vol. 38, no. 1, pp. 132–138, 2010.

[16] J. Baker, J. D. Cotter, D. F. Gerrard, M. L. Bell, and R. J. Walker, "Effects of indomethacin and celecoxib on renal function in athletes," *Medicine and Science in Sports and Exercise*, vol. 37, no. 5, pp. 712–717, 2005.

[17] J. Joslin, J. Lloyd, T. Kotlyar, and S. Wojcik, "NSAID and other analgesic use by endurance runners during training, competition and recovery," *South African Journal of Sports Medicine*, vol. 25, no. 4, pp. 101–104, 2013.

[18] S. Orava and A. Hulkko, "Delayed unions and nonunions of stress fractures in athletes," *The American Journal of Sports Medicine*, vol. 16, no. 4, pp. 378–382, 1988.

[19] A. Roy Magnusson, J. R. Hedges, M. Vanko, K. McCarten, and J. C. Moorhead, "Follow-up compliance after emergency department evaluation," *Annals of Emergency Medicine*, vol. 22, no. 3, pp. 560–567, 1993.

[20] D. Barlas, C. S. Homan, J. Rakowski, M. Houck, and H. C. Thode Jr., "How well do patients obtain short-term follow-up after discharge from the emergency department?" *Annals of Emergency Medicine*, vol. 34, no. 5, pp. 610–614, 1999.

[21] "American Medical Society for Sports Medicine. In: What is a Sports Medicine Specialist?" 2014 http://www.amssm.org/Content/pdf%20files/WhatisSMSpec-Patient-broch.pdf.

# 32

# Emergency Ultrasound Predicting the Need for Therapeutic Laparotomy among Blunt Abdominal Trauma Patients in a Sub-Saharan African Hospital

**P. C. M. Musiitwa,[1] M. Galukande,[1] S. Bugeza,[2] H. Wanzira,[3] and R. Wangoda[1]**

[1] *Department of Surgery, College of Health Sciences, Makerere University, Kampala, Uganda*
[2] *Department of Radiology, College of Health Sciences, Makerere University, Kampala, Uganda*
[3] *Infectious Diseases Research Collaboration, Makerere University, Kampala, Uganda*

Correspondence should be addressed to M. Galukande; mosesg@img.co.ug

Academic Editor: Rade B. Vukmir

*Background.* The trauma burden globally accounts for high levels of mortality and morbidity. Blunt abdominal trauma (BAT) contributes significantly to this burden. Patient's evaluation for BAT remains a diagnostic challenge for emergency physicians. SSORTT gives a score that can predict the need for laparotomy. The objective of this study was to assess the accuracy of SSORTT score in predicting the need for a therapeutic laparotomy after BAT. *Method.* A prospective observational study. Eligible patients were evaluated for shock and the presence of haemoperitoneum using a portable ultrasound machine. Further evaluation of patients following the standard of care (SOC) protocol was done. The accuracy of SSORTT score in predicting therapeutic laparotomy was compared to SOC. *Results.* In total, 195 patients were evaluated; M : F ratio was 6 : 1. The commonest injuries were to the head 80 (42%) and the abdomen 54 (28%). A SSORTT score of >2 appropriately identified patients that needed a therapeutic laparotomy (with sensitivity 90%, specificity 90%, PPV 53%, and NPV 98%). The overall mortality rate was 17%. *Conclusion.* Patients with a SSORTT score of 2 and above had a high likelihood of requiring a therapeutic laparotomy. SSORTT scoring should be adopted for routine practice in low technology settings.

## 1. Introduction

Trauma burden globally is on the increase accounting for high levels of mortality and morbidity. It is the second largest single cause of disease accounting for 16%, only second to parasitic and infectious diseases at 23%. WHO also estimates that, by the year 2020, trauma will be the first or second leading cause of "years of productive life lost" for the entire world population in both developed and developing world [1].

Blunt abdominal trauma (BAT) is injury to intra-abdominal or retroperitoneal viscera as a result of a non-penetrating force. It is commonly due to rapid deceleration or acceleration in combination with shearing and rotational forces [2, 3]. Common manifestations are hemorrhage and visceral perforation, either intraperitoneal or retroperitoneal; morbidity and mortality are associated with delay in diagnosis and treatment of BAT [4–6].

Common causes include road traffic crushes (RTC), industrial accidents, falls from heights, sporting, and farm accidents (in rural areas) and sometimes the cause of BAT is unknown, for example, with child abuse and domestic violence [7, 8].

Evaluation of patients with BAT is often a diagnostic challenge for emergency physicians and trauma surgeons [9, 10]. Uncontrolled hemorrhage is responsible for over 50% of trauma related deaths [11–13].

Other times overly aggressive management can lead to nontherapeutic laparotomy. The negative laparotomy rate is 16% and negative laparotomy carries the risk of incisional hernia and small bowel obstruction over time. Emergent sonography in form of Focused Abdominal Sonography for Trauma (FAST) has emerged and been embraced as a rapid, noninvasive, and accurate method of evaluating blunt abdominal trauma that can be easily used by emergency room clinicians and trauma surgeons [14–17]. FAST is a rapid, four-view ultrasound examination carried out during the primary survey that assesses for haemoperitoneum, haemothorax, and haemopericardium.

A newer dimension of emergency sonography is the Sonographic Scoring for Operating Room Triage in Trauma (SSORTT score) which was developed in a trauma center in the United States of America with the aim of enabling emergency room clinicians to quickly and reliably predict which patients require an emergent laparotomy. It has three components: (1) FAST findings, (2) systolic blood pressure and, (3) pulse rate which together give a score that can predict whether patient would most likely not require a therapeutic laparotomy.

The objective of this study therefore was to determine whether specific SSORTT scores are good predictors of a need for a therapeutic laparotomy among blunt abdominal trauma patients in a low resource settings.

## 2. Methods

*2.1. Study Design.* A prospective observational cohort study carried out from December 2012 to April 2013.

*2.2. Study Setting.* The study was conducted in the 24/7 A and E department of Mulago National referral hospital situated in Kampala, Uganda. This is a fully fledged unit with a medical and surgical emergency wing, two operating rooms, an X-ray facility, ultrasound facility, resuscitation room with 3 beds, and a 26-bed holding emergency ward; adjacent to it are the blood bank, hematology, microbiology, and chemistry laboratories.

It receives about 1500 trauma patients per month, 300 with suspected torso injuries and 20 with actual torso injuries [18].

*2.3. Study Procedure.* Upon arrival in the A&E unit patients with suspected BAT were screened.

BAT was defined as injury to intra-abdominal viscera or retroperitoneal as a result of a nonpenetrating object or force indicated by presence of torso abrasions and bruises, abdominal tenderness among multiply injured patients with long bone fractures, fracture pelvis, and spine injuries.

Patients meeting these eligibility criteria were recruited and subsequently informed written consent was obtained. All patients were adequately resuscitated and investigated as per the standard of care protocol. Patients with subcutaneous emphysema over the abdomen in whom abdominal assessment with sonography would be difficult to interpret were excluded.

Assessment was done using ATLS protocol. History and physical examination findings were recorded on pre-coded questionnaires. Patients suspected to be having BAT were positioned in supine position and underwent FAST using SonoSite TITAN portable ultrasound machine with a transducer frequency ranging from 3.5 to 5 MHz. A cumulative sum of the three parameters ultrasound score, systolic blood pressure, and pulse rate were determined and used as the SSORTT score.

Patient then underwent secondary survey, which was followed by other routine investigations and management according to the hospital guidelines. As and when appropriate patients were sent to the emergency radiology room for a full ultrasound scan and abdominal X-ray. All admitted patients were followed up for three days to determine whether they had laparotomy or not.

*2.4. Study Variables.* These included the SSORTT score, age, sex, and mechanism of injury, for example, RTC. In addition and therapeutic laparotomy, nontherapeutic laparotomy, and outcomes of nonoperative management (lived/died).

*2.5. Data Collection, Management, and Analysis.* Data were collected using pretested questionnaires and double entered, coded, and cleaned using Epi data version 5.3.2 software. Stored data were exported to Stata version 12 for analysis. Accuracy of the SSORTT score in predicting patients that would need therapeutic laparotomy was determined by calculating sensitivity, specificity, PPV, NPV, and ROC curve of SSORTT score. ROC curve was used to determine diagnostic accuracy of SSORTT score for predicting the need for therapeutic laparotomy.

*2.6. Quality Control.* The investigator(s) underwent didactic tutorials on FAST also performed at least 30 ultrasound scans to determine presence of haemoperitoneum prior to starting the study.

The ultrasound machine was maintained and calibrated by hospital staff from the department of radiology. We stored the examinations images (sonographs) and had them reread (validated) by a consultant radiologist.

*2.7. Ethical Considerations.* Written informed consent for patients above 18 years and assent for those less than 18 years were obtained from the participants. Ethical approval was obtained from the Research and Ethics Committee of the College of Health Sciences of Makerere University.

## 3. Results

A total of 195 trauma patients clinically suspected to have sustained BAT were subjected to emergency ultrasound scanning and were SSORTT scored at the A&E unit of Mulago Hospital from December 2012 to April 2013. The study profile is shown in Figure 1. The patients' characteristics and laparotomy findings are outlined in Table 1.

The male : female ratio was 6 : 1. Age group between 20 and 40 years comprised majority of patients 153 (79%). Road traffic crashes (RTC) were the leading cause of injury in this study accounting for 59%.Others causes included assault 32%, falls 7%, and others 2% as shown in Table 1.

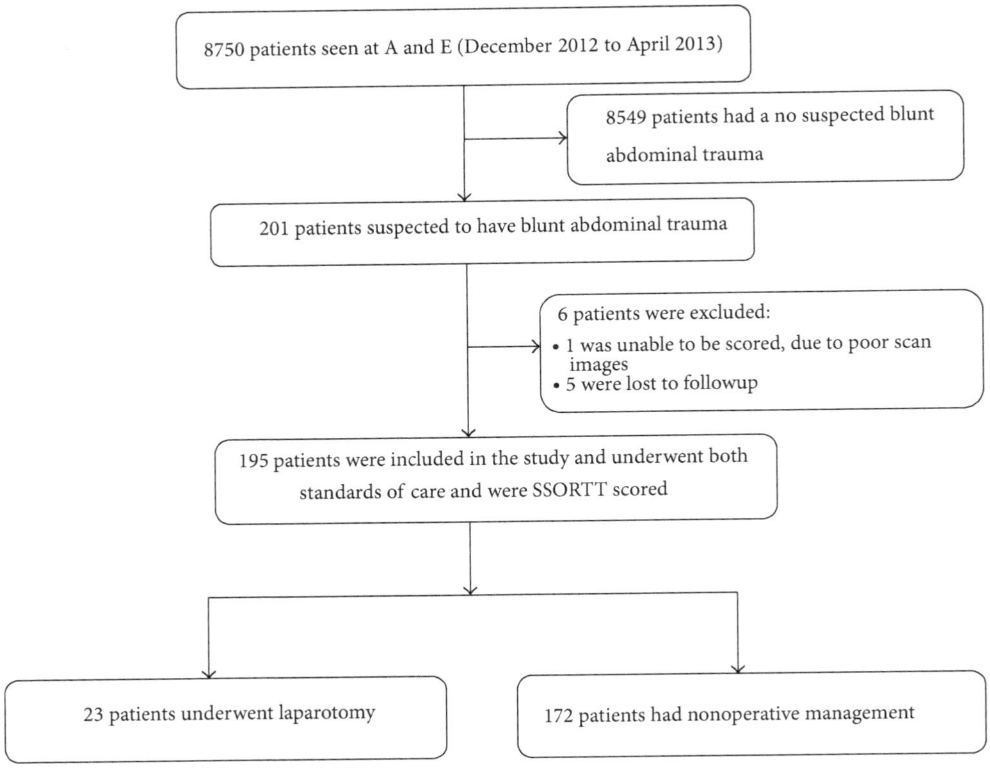


FIGURE 1: Study profile.

Most of patients with BAT had clinically suffered injuries to the head, abdomen, or limbs.

Table 1 shows the distribution of SSORTT scores by intervention. 20/23 (86%) patients who had therapeutic laparotomy had a SSORTT score of ≥3. 156/173 (90%); patients who had nonoperative management had a SSORTT score of ≤2.

Table 2 shows the laparotomy predictions at selected cut offs.

Table 3 shows that the majority of patients who had a laparotomy had high Glasgow coma scores. A small proportion had Glasgow coma score < 13.

More than 80% of the patients with abdominal tell-tale signs and head injury were subjected to a laparotomy.

Majority of the patients with head injury were subjected to nonoperative management.

Among therapeutic laparotomy patients, massive haemoperitoneum was the commonest finding (47%), followed by solid organ injury at 35% and gut perforation at 6%.

Among nontherapeutic laparotomy retroperitoneal hematoma and <grade3 solid organs injury were findings.

The general trend for sensitivity at the various cut-off levels of the SSORTT score was that it reduced with an increasing score; see Table 3.

Values of specificity gradually increase as

at SSORTT score 0, sensitivity = 91% and specificity = 82%;

at SSORTT score 6, sensitivity = 0% and specificity = 100%;

at SSORTT score 0, PPV = 39% and NPV = 99%;

at SSORTT score 6, PPV = 0% and NPV = 89%.

*3.1. Accuracy* . For Accuracy of the Test, the following ranking was considered:

.90–1 = excellent (A);

.80–.90 = good (B);

.70–.80 = fair (C);

.60–.70 = poor (D);

.50–.60 = fail (F).

The area under the ROC curve measured accuracy; see Figure 2.

The closer the curve follows the left-hand border and then the top borders of the ROC space, the more accurate the test is. The area under ROC curve measured 0.91 a high value for accuracy.

The presence of signs which included bruises, abrasions, lacerations, and cuts did not predict staying alive or dying. The patients who had a laparotomy were less likely to die OR 1.64 though it was not statistically significant $P = 0.370$.

Of 23 patients that had laparotomy 21 patients had therapeutic laparotomy and 2 being nontherapeutic, one had a moderately large retroperitoneal haematoma and the other

TABLE 1: Distribution of baseline characteristics and laparotomy findings for the 195 participants.

| Characteristics | Participants | |
|---|---|---|
| | Number | Percentage |
| Age groups | | |
| <20 | 22 | 11 |
| 20–40 | 153 | 79 |
| 41–60 | 18 | 9 |
| >60 | 2 | 1 |
| Gender | | |
| Male | 168 | 86 |
| Female | 27 | 14 |
| Time since injury in hours* | | |
| <1 | 20 | 10 |
| 1-2 | 84 | 43 |
| >2 | 73 | 37 |
| Unknown | 18 | 10 |
| Mechanism of injury* | | |
| Road traffic crash | 116 | 59 |
| Assault | 62 | 32 |
| Fall | 13 | 6 |
| Others | 4 | 2 |
| Therapeutic laparotomy | | |
| Massive haemoperitoneum | 16 | 47 |
| Grade 4/5 solid organs injury | 12 | 35 |
| Gut perforation | 2 | 6 |
| Mesenteric tears | 1 | 3 |
| Bladder injury | 1 | 3 |
| Nontherapeutic laparotomy | | |
| Retroperitoneal haematoma | 1 | 3 |
| Grade 3 solid organs injury | 1 | 3 |
| SSORTT score | Laparotomy $N = 23$ | No laparotomy $N = 172$ |
| | Number (%) | Number (%) |
| 0 | 2 (9) | 142 (83) |
| 1 | 0 | 13 (8) |
| 2 | 1 (4) | 1 (1) |
| 3 | 5 (22)* | 12 (7) |
| 4 | 6 (26) | 3 (2) |
| 5 | 3 (13) | 1 (1) |
| 6 | 6 (26)* | 1 (0) |

*Two participants had nontherapeutic laparotomy with scores of 3 and 6.

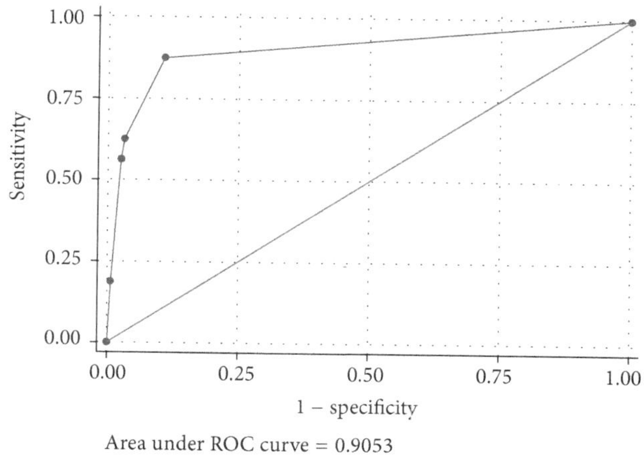


FIGURE 2: ROC curve for SSORTT score.

had a grade two splenic laceration with a haemoperitoneum of about 500 cc. Of the 172 patients that did not undergo laparotomy 28 patients passed away and the rest were either discharged or still admitted by day three. Of the 28 patients, 18 patients were multiply injured with severe extra-abdominal injuries. This can be shown in Table 3 where majority of patient; that is; 18 patients that died; had SSORTT 0 and 23 patients had Glasgow coma score less than 8 indicating presence of severe extra-abdominal injuries.

16 patients did not have a postmortem done because the relatives declined. Haemoperitoneum was found in 3 patients and 7 patients had blunt force trauma with extra-abdominal injury.

Majority of patients that died had a SSORTT score of 0 (55%).

Majority of deaths were in the severely deranged GCS range, that is, 3–8.

Seven patients with intra-abdominal fluid died.

All patients that passed away with intra-abdominal fluid had scores of >2.

## 4. Discussion

We set out to determine the diagnostic accuracy of emergency ultrasound scanning using the SSORTT score in predicting the need for a therapeutic laparotomy for blunt abdominal trauma patients. The SSORTT score was defined as a sum of the ultrasound haemoperitoneum score, systolic blood pressure, and pulse rate [19, 20]. Patients with a SSORTT score of 2 and above had a high likelihood of requiring a therapeutic laparotomy and those below that were unlikely to need one.

SSORTT scoring had excellent diagnostic accuracy for identifying patients that needed or did not need a therapeutic laparotomy with sensitivity of 91% and specificity of 90%.

The findings of this study are comparable to findings by Manka et al. where patients with score of less than 1 were less likely to require a laparotomy [21].

The youths were mostly affected because they fall in the most active age bracket exposed to most injury risks [8, 22, 23].

Motorcycle accidents accounted for most (62%) of the injuries; the use of motorcycles a cheap means of transportation is on the increase in many countries in Africa and are a leading cause of blunt abdominal trauma [22–28].

TABLE 2: Laparotomy predictions at selected cutoffs.

| SSORTT score | Standard of care | | Sensitivity | Specificity | PPV (%) | NPV (%) |
|---|---|---|---|---|---|---|
| | Laparotomy | No laparotomy | | | | |
| *Score cutoffs* | | | | | | |
| At 0 | | | | | | |
| Laparotomy | 19 | 30 | | | | |
| No laparotomy | 2 | 142 | 91 | 82 | 39 | 99 |
| ≥1 | | | | | | |
| Laparotomy | 19 | 17 | | | | |
| No laparotomy | 2 | 155 | 90 | 90 | 53 | 99 |
| ≥2 | | | | | | |
| Laparotomy | 18 | 16 | | | | |
| No laparotomy | 3 | 156 | 86 | 91 | 53 | 98 |
| ≥3 | | | | | | |
| Laparotomy | 14 | 4 | | | | |
| No laparotomy | 8 | 168 | 67 | 98 | 78 | 96 |
| ≥4 | | | | | | |
| Laparotomy | 8 | 1 | | | | |
| No laparotomy | 14 | 171 | 38 | 99 | 89 | 93 |
| ≥5 | | | | | | |
| Laparotomy | 5 | 0 | | | | |
| No laparotomy | 17 | 172 | 24 | 100 | 100 | 91 |
| At 6 | | | | | | |
| Laparotomy | 0 | 0 | | | | |
| No laparotomy | 22 | 172 | 0 | 100 | 0 | 87 |

TABLE 3: Comparison of the fatalities and survivors.

| Injuries | Patient status | | OR (95% CI) | *P* value |
|---|---|---|---|---|
| | Alive Number (%) | Died Number (%) | | |
| Bruises | 66 (47) | 21 (66) | 0.5 (0.2–1.0) | 0.063 |
| Abrasions | 30 (21) | 8 (25) | 0.8 (0.3–2.0) | 0.661 |
| Lacerations | 79 (56) | 18 (56) | 1.0 (0.5–2.2) | 0.985 |
| Cuts | 10 (7) | 3 (9) | 0.7 (0.2–2.9) | 0.667 |
| Burns | 2 (1) | 1 (3) | 0.5 (0.1–5.1) | 0.519 |
| Abdominal | 43 (30) | 7 (22) | 1.6 (0.6–3.9) | 0.334 |
| Chest | 16 (11) | 6 (19) | 0.6 (0.2–1.6) | 0.262 |
| Others | 120 (86) | 23 (74) | 2.2 (0.9–5.6) | 0.100 |
| Standard of care laparotomy | 17 (11) | 6 (18) | 1.6 (0.6–4.9) | 0.370 |
| SSORTT score | | | | |
| 0 | 123 | 18 | — | — |
| 1 | 10 | 3 | — | — |
| 2 | 2 | 0 | — | — |
| 3 | 11 | 6 | — | — |
| 4 | 8 | 1 | — | — |
| 5 | 3 | 1 | — | — |
| 6 | 2 | 4 | — | — |
| Glasgow coma score | | | | |
| Severe | 13 | 21 | — | — |
| Moderate | 21 | 9 | — | — |
| Mild | 125 | 3 | — | — |

Many studies have demonstrated that physical examinations are unreliable in assessing trauma patient especially those with neurological injury (brain or spinal cord), and in those with painful distracting injuries such as long bone or pelvic fractures, or in those with alcohol or other intoxicants in their systems [29, 30].

Eighty patients suffered head injuries (42%) and 50 (26%) had potentially distracting limb extremity injuries. In the absence of diagnostic aids a proportion of the severely injured would be vulnerable to delays in diagnosis of major intra-abdominal visceral injuries. We contend that proper use of ultrasound in the emergency room in early identification of life threatening injuries like intra-abdominal hemorrhage, haemothorax, or haemoperitoneum may save lives in low technology settings. The additional advantage of sonographers is that it is noninvasive compared to techniques like peritoneal lavage which we many times use in the absence of sonography [22].

We found that 23 patients (12%) received laparotomy and of these 21 were therapeutic, that is, surgically correctable lesions. Massive haemoperitoneum with solid organ injury was the commonest finding at laparotomy with ruptured spleen being the commonest solid organ injured followed by liver lacerations. There were two cases of gut perforations, one urinary bladder rupture and one with mesenteric tears.

This pattern of injuries is consistent with many other studies done in the country and the region [6, 22–26, 31, 32].

Five patients of the 23 that had laparotomy passed away, due to anesthesia related complications and aneamia or coagulopathy due to shortage of blood. The laparotomy rate in this study was 11% and the overall mortality rate was 17%, comparable to previous studies [22, 23] which reported a mortality rate between 10 and 30%.

*4.1. Study Limitations.* This study was not without limitations; the sensitivity and specificity of emergency US scanning could have been affected by possible sonography operator differences; however some studies show that FAST can be done reliably by both radiologist and nonradiologists [15, 33, 34].

In the calculation of the SSORTT score, ideally blood pressure and pulse rate should be obtained at the beginning of resuscitation. However, often blood pressure and pulse rates would be taken after fluid infusions that were started to resuscitate patients; this could be assumed to influence the SSORTT score leading to an under estimation of severity of injury. Postmortem to determine cause of death were not done for various reasons like attendants declining.

## 5. Conclusion

SSORTT score is a noninvasive, reproducible test that can be performed easily and reliably predicts the need for a therapeutic laparotomy among blunt abdominal trauma patients. It should be adopted for routine use in low technology settings.

## Abbreviations

| | |
|---|---|
| AE: | Accident and emergency |
| BAT: | Blunt abdominal trauma |
| FAST: | Focused abdominal sonography for trauma |
| RTC: | Road traffic crashes |
| SSORTT: | sum of ultrasound score, systolic blood pressure, and pulse rate. |

## Conflict of Interests

The authors declare that there is no conflict of interests regarding the publication of the paper.

## Authors' Contribution

P. C. M. Musiitwa, M. Galukande, and R. Wangoda redesigned the experiment. P. C. M. Musiitwa collected data. M. Galukande wrote the first draft. All authors performed critical reviews for intellectual input. All authors approved the final draft.

## Acknowledgment

The authors would like to thank the staff in AE unit of Mulago and Department of Surgery, College of Health Sciences, Makerere University.

## References

[1] C. N. Mock, G. J. Jurkovich, D. Nii-Amon-Kotei, C. Arreola-Risa, and R. V. Maier, "Trauma mortality patterns in three nations at different economic levels: implications for global trauma system development," *The Journal of Trauma*, vol. 44, no. 5, pp. 804–814, 1998.

[2] J. J. Davis, I. Cohn Jr., and F. C. Nance, "Diagnosis and management of blunt abdominal trauma," *Annals of Surgery*, vol. 183, no. 6, pp. 672–678, 1976.

[3] W. C. Wilson, C. M. Grande, and D. B. Hoyt, *Trauma: Critical Care*, vol. 1, Informa Healthcare, New York, NY, USA, 1st edition, 2007.

[4] I. Matovu, *Abdominal injuries in paediatrics as seen in Mulago hospital [M.S. thesis]*, Makerere University, Kampala, Uganda, 1978.

[5] J. A. Moylan, D. E. Detmer, J. Rose, and R. Schulz, "Evaluation of the quality of hospital care for major trauma," *The Journal of Trauma*, vol. 16, no. 7, pp. 517–523, 1976.

[6] D. Birabwa-Male, *Abdominal injuries in Mulago hospital [M.S. thesis]*, Makerere University, Kampala, Uganda, 1989.

[7] W. Odero, P. Garner, and A. Zwi, "Road traffic injuries in developing countries: a comprehensive review of epidemiological studies," *Tropical Medicine and International Health*, vol. 2, no. 5, pp. 445–460, 1997.

[8] M. M. Ajiko, *Outcome of blunt abdominal trauma in Mulago hospital [M.S. thesis]*, Makerere University, Kampala, Uganda, 2006.

[9] B. F. K. Odimba, "Plea for use of peritoneal lavage in management of blunt abdominal trauma victims in developing

countries," *East and Central African Journal of Surgery*, vol. 3, no. 2, pp. 49–52, 1997.

[10] T. Kirschning, F. Brenner, M. Stier, C. F. Weber, and F. Walcher, "Pre-hospital emergency sonography of trauma patients," *Anaesthesist*, vol. 58, no. 1, pp. 51–60, 2009.

[11] K. Brohi, M. J. Cohen, M. T. Ganter, M. A. Matthay, R. C. MacKersie, and J.-F. Pittet, "Acute traumatic coagulopathy," *The Journal of Trauma*, vol. 54, no. 6, pp. 1127–1130, 2003.

[12] J. B. A. MacLeod, M. Lynn, M. G. McKenney, S. M. Cohn, and M. Murtha, "Early coagulopathy predicts mortality in trauma," *The Journal of Trauma*, vol. 55, no. 1, pp. 39–44, 2003.

[13] M. Maegele, R. Lefering, N. Yucel et al., "Early coagulopathy in multiple injury: an analysis from the German trauma registry on 8724 patients," *Injury*, vol. 38, no. 3, pp. 298–304, 2007.

[14] C. Tunuka, *Extended focused assessment with sonography for trauma among blunt torso injury patients at Mulago hospital injury patients at Mulago hospital [M.S. thesis]*, Makerere University, Kampala, Uganda, 2012.

[15] G. S. Rozycki, M. G. Ochsner, J. H. Jaffin et al., "Prospective evaluation of surgeons' use of ultrasound in the evaluation of trauma patients," *The Journal of Trauma*, vol. 34, no. 4, pp. 516–526, 1993.

[16] V. H. Thourani, B. J. Pettitt, J. A. Schmidt, W. A. Cooper, and G. S. Rozycki, "Validation of surgeon-performed emergency abdominal ultrasonography in pediatric trauma patients," *Journal of Pediatric Surgery*, vol. 33, no. 2, pp. 322–328, 1998.

[17] S. R. Shackford, F. B. Rogers, T. M. Osler, M. E. Trabulsy, D. W. Clauss, and D. W. Vane, "Focused abdominal sonogram for trauma: the learning curve of nonradiologist clinicians in detecting hemoperitoneum," *The Journal of Trauma*, vol. 46, no. 4, pp. 553–564, 1999.

[18] "Accident and emergency mulago hospital trauma registry," unpublished.

[19] O. J. Ma, M. P. Kefer, K. F. Stevison, and J. R. Mateer, "Operative versus nonoperative management of blunt abdominal trauma: role of ultrasound-measured intraperitoneal fluid levels," *The American Journal of Emergency Medicine*, vol. 19, no. 4, pp. 284–286, 2001.

[20] K. L. McKenney, M. G. McKenney, S. M. Cohn et al., "Hemoperitoneum score helps determine need for therapeutic laparotomy," *The Journal of Trauma*, vol. 50, no. 4, pp. 650–656, 2001.

[21] M. Manka, R. Moscati, K. Raghavendran, and A. Priya, "Sonographic scoring for operating room triage in trauma," *The Western Journal of Emergency Medicine*, vol. 11, no. 2, pp. 138–143, 2010.

[22] R. Wangoda, A. L. Upoki, and F. N. Owori, "Use of urethral catheters for diagnostic peritoneal lavage in blunt abdominal trauma," *East and Central African Journal of Surgery*, vol. 7, no. 1, pp. 63–66, 2002.

[23] O. Kobusingye, D. Guwatudde, and R. Lett, "Injury patterns in rural and urban Uganda," *Injury Prevention*, vol. 7, no. 1, pp. 46–50, 2001.

[24] S. Bugeza, *The pattern of sonographic findings in blunt abdominal trauma at Mulago hospital [M.S. thesis]*, Medical School Library, Makerere University, 2006.

[25] G. Ruhinda, P. Kyamanywa, D. Kitya, and F. Bajunirwe, "Abdominal injury at mbarara regional referral hospital, Uganda," *East and Central African Journal of Surgery*, vol. 13, no. 2, pp. 29–36, 2008.

[26] P. Chalya, J. B. Mabula, R. M. Dass et al., "Injury characteristics and outcome of road traffic crash victims at Bugando Medical Centre in Northwestern Tanzania," *Journal of Trauma Management & Outcomes*, vol. 6, no. 1, atricle 1, 2012.

[27] M. Galukande, J. Jombwe, J. Fualal, and A. Gakwaya, "A boda-boda injuries a health problem and a burden of disease in Uganda: a tertiary hospital survey," *East and Central African Journal of Surgery*, vol. 14, no. 2, pp. 33–37, 2009.

[28] C. N. Andrews, O. C. Kobusingye, and R. Lett, "Road traffic accident injuries in Kampala," *East African Medical Journal*, vol. 76, no. 4, pp. 189–194, 1999.

[29] S. S. Lingawi and A. R. Buckley, "Focused abdominal US in patients with trauma," *Radiology*, vol. 217, no. 2, pp. 426–429, 2000.

[30] M. Blaivas, P. Sierzenski, and D. Theodoro, "Significant hemoperitoneum in blunt trauma victims with normal vital signs and clinical examination," *The American Journal of Emergency Medicine*, vol. 20, no. 3, pp. 218–221, 2002.

[31] S. Bugeza, E. Kiguli-Malwadde, and Z. Muyinda, "Evaluation of ultrasonography for solid organ injury in blunt abdominal trauma: experience at Mulago hospital Makerere University Uganda," in *Proceedings of the 12th World Congress of the World Federation for Ultrasound in Medicine and Biology (WFUMB '09)*, Sydney Convention & Exhibition Centre, Sydney, Australia, September 2009.

[32] F. Kirya, S. Kijjambu, and I. Ezati, "Outcome of major trauma at Mulago hospital in Uganda: assessment using the TRISS methodology," *East and Central African Journal of Surgery*, vol. 7, no. 1, pp. 59–62, 2002.

[33] G. R. Buzzas, S. J. Kern, R. S. Smith, P. B. Harrison, S. D. Helmer, and J. A. Reed, "A comparison of sonographic examinations for trauma performed by surgeons and radiologists," *The Journal of Trauma*, vol. 44, no. 4, pp. 604–608, 1998.

[34] S. W. Branney, E. E. Moore, S. V. Cantrill, J. M. Burch, and S. J. Terry, "Ultrasound based key clinical pathway reduces the use of hospital resources for the evaluation of blunt abdominal trauma," *The Journal of Trauma*, vol. 42, no. 6, pp. 1086–1090, 1997.

# Qualitative Inquiry into Challenges Experienced by Registered General Nurses in the Emergency Department: A Study of Selected Hospitals in the Volta Region of Ghana

**Confidence Alorse Atakro,[1] Jerry Paul Ninnoni,[2] Peter Adatara,[3] Janet Gross,[4,5] and Michael Agbavor[6]**

[1] *University of Cape Coast, Cape Coast, Ghana*
[2] *Faculty of Nursing and Midwifery School, University of Cape Coast, Cape Coast, Ghana*
[3] *The School of Nursing and Midwifery, University of Health and Allied Sciences, Ho, Ghana*
[4] *Morehead State University, Morehead, KY, USA*
[5] *Global Health Services Partnership, US Peace Corps, Washington, DC, USA*
[6] *Volta Regional Hospital, Ho, Ghana*

Correspondence should be addressed to Confidence Alorse Atakro; confidenceatakro@gmail.com

Academic Editor: Seiji Morita

Registered General Nurses (RGNs) play crucial roles in emergency departments (EDs). EDs in Ghana are primarily staffed by RGNs who have had no additional formal education in emergency care. Additionally, basic, master's, or doctoral level nursing education programs provide limited content on the complexities of emergency nursing. Nurses in EDs are affected by many challenges such as growing patient population, financial pressures, physical violence, verbal abuse, operational inefficiencies, overcrowding, and work overload. There is a paucity of research on challenges experienced by RGNs in EDs in the Volta Region of Ghana. In this qualitative study, twenty RGNs in EDs from three selected hospitals in the Volta Region of Ghana were interviewed. All recorded interviews were transcribed, reviewed several times by researchers and supervisors, and analyzed using content analysis. Five thematic categories were identified. These thematic categories of challenges were lack of preparation for ED role, verbal abuse from patients relatives, lack of resources in ED, stressful and time consuming nature of ED, and overcrowding in ED. Formal education of RGNs in the advanced role of emergency care, adequate supply of resources, increased hospital management support, and motivations for RGNs working in ED are necessary to improve the practice of emergency care.

## 1. Introduction

Emergency care is care that must be rendered without delay [1]. The task of emergency departments (EDs) is to provide safe emergency health care to all who need it while adopting a caring, cost-effective approach [2, 3]. Nurses are frontline workers in EDs [4] and experience challenges of overcrowding, growing admission volumes, inadequate resources, and operational inefficiencies in ED [5, 6]. The actual situation in an ED is that when the number of ED patients increases or patients with more severe conditions are admitted to an ED, individual demands for direct nursing care increases; therefore, patients' needs often cannot be met by the same number of nursing staff members [7]. Nursing staff are forced to reduce contact time with patients [7]. Reducing contact time with patients poses threats to the provision of quality nursing care to clients in EDs [7]. Challenges experienced by RGNs working in ED are aggravated by leadership issues and inadequate preparations for ED roles [8]. The scope of practice for emergency nurses in Africa is limited with no clearly defined advanced nurse practitioner roles [9]. Despite the fact that care provided by nurse practitioners practicing in ED requires a body of knowledge relating to acute illness and injury [9], there are few institutions that offer emergency nurse training in Africa and, therefore, few emergency nurses are available to provide care in EDs [10]. While emergency medicine training programs for physicians are on the rise, there are few established training programs for emergency nurses [11]. Caring for emergency patients in Africa is particularly challenging because nurses must often treat severely injured patients who have coexisting conditions, such as Human Immunodeficiency Virus (HIV), Acquired Immunodeficiency Syndrome (AIDS), or Tuberculosis (TB) [10]. The presence of HIV, AIDS, and TB complicates client care and has health implications for staff themselves [10]. Nurses working in EDs in Africa also work with limited resources [10]. Most emergency departments in Africa are staffed by RGNs with no additional formal education in emergency nursing [10]. In Ghana, as in other developing and middle-income countries, little consideration has traditionally been given to optimising the training of nursing staff for the care of acutely ill or injured patients [12]. Additionally, existing emergency care systems in Ghana are rudimentary in comparison to those in developed countries [12] aggravating an already bad situation of overcrowding and inadequate preparations of nurses in emergency care [13]. Though RGNs in EDs are challenged in the provision of safe, quality care to clients, ED nurses' experiences of challenges within accident and emergency units are seldom investigated [14]. Knowledge of challenges experienced by RGNs in ED is necessary to address challenges in EDs. The purpose of this study was to explore challenges experienced by RGNs working in EDs in selected hospitals of the Volta Region of Ghana.

## 2. Materials and Methods

A qualitative phenomenology study design was used in carrying out this study. Phenomenology, rooted in a philosophical tradition, is an approach to explore people's everyday life experiences [15]. The qualitative study design was chosen to explore challenges experienced by RGNs in emergency departments in selected hospitals of the Volta Region of Ghana.

*2.1. Setting.* The settings for data collection were three public hospitals in the Volta Region of Ghana that had emergency departments. These hospitals were Volta Regional Hospital, Keta Municipal Hospital, and Ho Municipal Hospital.

*2.2. Study Population.* The target population for this study was RGNs working at the ED in the Volta Regional Hospital (VRH), Keta Municipal Hospital (KMH), and Ho Municipal Hospital (HMH) in the Volta Region of Ghana.

*2.3. Data Collection and Analysis.* Participants for data collection were selected through purposive sampling technique. Data were collected in January 2015, within a three-week period. A list of all RGNs in EDs was requested from Nurse Managers of EDs. Inclusion criteria were RGNs with professional identification numbers (PINs) who had worked for one year or more and were willing to give written consent. The eligible sample size was estimated to be 20 participants, large enough for data saturation. Saturation was reached after interviewing 20 participants, when new data confirmed previous data without adding new insights [16]. The mobile phone numbers of selected participants were requested. Participants were called on phone to arrange a convenient time and place for interviews. As no validated interview guide relevant to the topic of interest was available, the themes of the interview and the questions were developed by the research group, based on previous scientific literature. EDs were visited prior to data collection to present the study and inform the staff about the study. Staff had opportunity to ask questions and receive answers concerning the study. One semistructured interview was conducted with each participant. Interviews took place at places convenient for participants. Interviews were audio-recorded and recordings were transcribed verbatim. Participants told their stories with minimal interruption. The interviews ranged from 30 to 60 minutes. Transcribed interviews were stored in electronic folders that were created and labeled appropriately for easy identification. These folders were kept on a pen drive solely meant for the purpose of the study and kept under lock and key. Transcribed data were analyzed using conventional qualitative content analysis. Each transcribed interview was read several times and the primary codes were extracted. Then, the related codes were put in groups. Categories were developed based on similarity and content of codes. To ensure trustworthiness of data, continuous investigation of the data (transcription of the data and investigating until the main themes were obtained), peer check and member check were performed. Moreover, the objectivity of the data was determined through continuous, accurate, and proper treatment of all stages of the research study and clarity of the research method. Also, using a team approach in data analysis (i.e., reviewing the data analysis by the research team), the reliability of the results was confirmed. Themes developed were (a) lack of preparation for ED role, (b) verbal abuse from patients' relatives, (c) lack of resources in ED, (d) stressful and time consuming nature of ED, and (e) overcrowding in ED.

*2.4. Ethical Considerations.* The research proposal was submitted to and approved by the University of Cape Coast Institutional Review Board (UCCIRB). Additionally, study received approval from each hospital where research was conducted. Adherence to all principles of research ethics was strictly observed. Participants were briefed about the study aim and procedures before written informed consent was obtained from them. Participants were informed about their rights to refuse to participate in the study or to leave at any time without giving any reason. Also, participants were informed that their refusal to participate in the study would not be used against them in any form. Confidentiality of participants was enforced, and they were assured that the data would be used only for research purposes. The study process did not entail any harmful effects on participants.

## 3. Results and Discussions

*3.1. Results.* In this study, 75% of respondents were between 25 to 29 years of age. A majority of RGNs working at the emergency department (90%) studied general nursing at the Nurses' Training College (NTC). Only 5% of RGNs had additional knowledge of critical care nursing (an advanced diploma course in critical care nursing) to practice emergency care in ED. None of the respondents studied emergency nursing as a degree program. Seventy percent (70%) of participants had worked for two years or less in ED. As many as 75% of participants indicated that there was only one professional nurse in a shift in ED. Five thematic categories were extracted after data analysis. The categories of challenges experienced by RGNs working in ED in selected hospitals in the Volta Region of Ghana were lack of preparation for ED role, verbal abuse from patient relatives, lack of resources in ED, stressful and time consuming nature of ED, and overcrowding in ED.

*3.1.1. Lack of Preparation for ED Role.* Almost all RGNs interviewed considered lack of preparation for ED role as a challenge in ED. One participant likened ED to a battle ground.

> *Nurses are just brought into the emergency unit to battle like soldiers who don't even know how to shoot guns. You have to push yourself to learn because there is no emergency nurse role models to learn from. [participant 7]*

The majority of participants described how the unavailability of emergency nurses and physicians in ED affected their learning experiences. A participant described this in the following statement:

> *ED exposes you to so many conditions but there are no emergency nurses or emergency physicians in ED. I have to force myself to learn. Sometimes I try something to see whether it will work. It's like lotto which is not good enough. [Participant 2]*

Many participants reported that there were many deaths in ED which could have been prevented by the presence of well-educated emergency nurses and physicians. This was evident in the words of a participant.

> *Working in ED is emotional because patients die easily. I think if there were trained emergency nurses and physicians, we could prevent some of the deaths. I feel sad when people die like that.*

Many participants wished that, in the absence of formal education in ED practice, they could be taken through some emergency care workshops before placement in the emergency care unit. A participant explains this in the following statement:

> *We are all RGNs and have no specialist education in emergency care. At least before one is placed in ED, He or she should be taken through some training in the form of a workshop so that he or she will be ready for ED nursing. [participant 14]*

*3.1.2. Verbal Abuse from Relatives toward ED Nurses.* Most of the participants in this study considered verbal abuse from relatives toward ED nurses as another challenge in ED. In this regard a participant stated the following:

> *Relatives here sometimes are ungrateful. Some relatives insult and talk to you very rudely. [participant 10]*

Another participant also said the following:

> *There is stress in ED and patient relatives don't appreciate. Sometimes you are exhausted and the patient and relative coming in don't know and always want immediate attention. If they don't get it, they insult you. [participant 4]*

Another participant explained his/her frustration with patient relatives:

> *Here, relatives want to tell us what emergency care should be. They always put pressure on you to take care of their relative even if it's not an emergency. They verbally abuse you when they feel you are not taking care of them the way they want. [participant 6]*

*3.1.3. Lack of Resources in ED.* Another category of challenges extracted from interviews was lack of resources in ED. In this regard a participant stated:

> *"The supply of essential materials is not the best. Sometimes supply of materials delay and you are embarrassed when clients come and you cannot care for them as a result of lack of materials. We also need more doctors and nurses in ED [participant 19]".*

Moreover, one other participant stated the following:

> *The problem is about staffing. At least staff strength should be increased. Nurses are really sacrificing in ED. We do not have items too and patients come and it looks like we are not prepared for them. [participant 7]*

*3.1.4. Stress and Time Consumption Nature of ED.* Stress and time consuming nature of ED was the fourth challenge in ED that participants described. The majority of respondents indicated that ED was stressful and time consuming. A participant described this in the following statements:

> *I do extra hours on duty but am not motivated in any way. I do not partake in church activities as I used to do. Sometimes friends call me but I am not able to call back because of tiredness. [participant 7]*

Yet one other participant stated the following:

> *Sometimes you don't have time for yourself or even your family, because of the staff situation. Social life is affected. You can't go for occasions. [participant 1]*

A participant also described the stress in ED in the following statement:

> *It's like going to work and never sitting your ass down, working, going up and down. Sometimes you leave work late because you have to assist colleagues who have come to work. [participant 2]*

*3.1.5. Overcrowding in ED.* Participants said that lack of space was a major challenge experienced in ED. In this regard one of the study participants said the following:

> *Accident and Emergency unit is always hectic. We always add extra stretchers. The place is always messy. [participant 1]*

One other participant believed that there was always pressure on nurses in ED as a result of ED overcrowding. This is described in the following statement:

> *There is so much pressure over here and we are not organised. And if you are not careful, you may give the wrong medication to a client. Sometimes we misplace clients medications as well. The lack of space and disorganisation makes the pressure worse. [participant 12]*

One participant explains reasons for overcrowding in the ED in the following statement:

> *This place is choked with clients because the place is too small and also other wards do not want to accept stabilised cases. They will always tell you they don't have beds meanwhile when you go there you will see so many empty beds. [participant 19]*

## 4. Discussion

The findings of this study showed a clear picture of challenges experienced by RGNs in ED. The study participants stated their experiences in ED through five thematic categories.

Almost all nurses taking part in this study mentioned lack of formal education in emergency care as a challenge in emergency care and believed formal education in emergency care will help prevent unnecessary deaths in ED. Additionally, sociodemographic results show that only 5% of participants had specialist education to practice emergency nursing [17] Graneheim and Lundman showed that while emergency medicine training programs for physicians are on the rise, there are few established training programs for emergency nurses [16]. Little time is spent in teaching or learning the content of emergency nursing during the basic, master's, or doctoral level nursing education programs [8]. Caring for the acutely ill or injured patient requires multiple disciplines and specialists working seamlessly together; this care is a team-based continuum and does not end with the Emergency Physician [12]. In spite of the importance of formal education in emergency care, little consideration has been given to optimising the education of nursing staff for the care of acutely ill or injured patients in Ghana [12]. It has been estimated that persons with life-threatening but salvageable injuries were six times more likely to die in Ghana than in the United States of America [12]. Mishandling of severely injured patients by untrained persons, inadequately trained staff, and inadequate equipment were reported as contributory factors to the high mortality rates of ED clients in Ghana [12]. Emergency nursing as a profession is very new to Africa and therefore the availability of guidelines and standards is also limited [17]. Improvements in training such as developing an education curriculum for staff in all areas of the emergency care, holding in-service training on protocols for triage, and emergency care could improve nursing care in ED [18]. There should be enough protocols to help nurses deal with emergency cases in EDs. Management of health facilities within the Volta Region should also have plans of sponsoring nurses to pursue emergency nursing as a specialist course so that these emergency nursing specialists can return to provide leadership and mentorship in the EDs. Unit heads of EDs should organise frequent internal workshops on emergency nursing for ED nurses to upgrade their knowledge in emergency care. Resource person such as emergency physicians, critical care nurses, nurse anesthetists, and emergency care nurses should be invited from teaching hospitals to educate nurses at the EDs in a workshop. Orientations in ED in a form of workshop will improve the readiness of nurses to work in EDs. An Emergency Nursing Association could be formed by the few emergency and critical care nurses in Ghana to push the agenda of the education of more emergency care nurses in Ghana.

Another important dimension of challenges experienced by nurses in the emergency department was verbal abuse from relatives. Participants mentioned that patient relatives were sometimes aggressive toward them and verbally abused them. Participants indicated that, most of the time, relatives of clients want to tell nurses what constituted emergencies. These situations make ED a vulnerable setting for workplace violence [19]. Violence against ED nurses is prevalent [19]. A study conducted in the United States of America (USA) to investigate emergency nurses' experiences and perceptions of violence from patients and visitors in EDs found that approximately 25% of respondents experienced physical violence at least 20 times in 3 years [19]. Similarly almost 20% reported experiencing verbal abuse more than 200 times during the same period [19]. The main perceived reasons for violence were overcrowded emergency rooms, long waiting times, and inadequate systems of security [20]. Respondents who experienced frequent physical violence and/or frequent verbal abuse indicated lack of support from hospital administration and ED management in dealing with abuses [19]. A similar study conducted in South Africa by Kennedy and Julie concluded that the absence of policies to deal with ED violence contributed to underreporting [21]. There is need for hospital management support and policies that deal with emergency care abuses by patient relatives. A preventive, risk-management approach that addresses policies, restraint, security arrangements, and legal precedents is particularly important in managing ED violence [22]. Identification of trends and patterns of violence in ED is necessary so that better health care planning and service provision as well as effective preventive and safe strategies for nurses in the ED workplace can be implemented [23]. Management in hospitals in the Volta Region could organise educative programs on local radio stations and in churches or mosques in order to make the public know about challenges and processes in emergency care. This may reduce the verbal attacks on nurses from patient relatives.

Lack of resources in ED was a challenge participants thought must be addressed for the provision of quality emergency nursing care. RGNs working in ED said there were inadequate material and human resources to provide timely care to clients in ED. Nurses usually felt embarrassed when clients reported at the EDs without the necessary available resources to care for them. This is in agreement with Hines et al. [24] who indicated that nurses working in ED face a number of challenges which include decreased reimbursement by insurers and fewer health care resources including medical staff, facilities, adequate financing, and modern technologies [24]. In most emergency units in Ghana, patients presenting are not triaged and most emergency centres are poorly equipped and overcrowded [12]. Existing emergency care systems in Ghana are rudimentary in comparison to those in developed countries [12]. An assessment of an ED at Police Hospital, a second-level hospital in Accra, Ghana, revealed marked deficiencies in many essential items and services [18]. Nurses in Ghana are currently an underdeveloped resource for the provision of high quality emergency care [13]. However, the future of emergency care can be bright with support from hospital management, government, and international partners [12]. EDs should be allocated more material and human resources by hospital managements to be able to deal with the high patient acuity of EDs.

Another important category of challenges in emergency care was stress and time consuming nature of ED. Nurses on emergency wards indicated that they worked overtime without any motivations. Stress and time consuming nature of ED prevented some nurses from participating in social activities such as weddings and funerals. Emergency work is filled with unanticipated situations and is complicated by disturbed rest periods, long working hours, and limitations in staffing levels [25]. These factors tend to affect RGNs in EDs negatively [25]. RGNs in EDs work in a charged atmosphere that is overloaded with sensory stimuli (ringing phones, rushing people, and beeping monitors), all in a framework of urgency [26]. The quietest day in ED may suddenly become extremely hectic [26]. Rapid disposition of patients to other wards may be necessary to make space for patients in more critical condition [26]. Recent studies have shown that occupational stress is much greater for nurses who work within EDs [27]. A study carried out by Adeb-Saeedi, to identify sources of stress for nurses working within the ED of teaching hospitals, identified dealing with patients' pain and suffering, heavy workload, and the presence of the patients' family in the ED as sources of stress reported by RGNs [27]. Other factors identified as stressors were physical working environment and lack of staff [27]. A study was conducted by Ross-Adjie et al. to determine which stress-evoking incidents in Western Australian emergency department nurses perceive as most significant [28]. Violence against staff was the top ranked stressor, with workload as second [28]. Dealing with a mass casualty incident, the death/sexual abuse of a child, and dealing with high acuity patients were all closely ranked as third, fourth, and fifth, respectively [28]. Nurses working in EDs stated that debriefing after stress-evoking incidents in the workplace should be mandatory and should be conducted by professionals with specific debriefing and counseling skills [28]. Nurses also suggested other ways in which occupational stress could be reduced, including employing more staff and providing a "time-out" room [29]. It is suggested that while it may not be possible to decrease the demands of the ED nursing care, improving work conditions and providing greater support by hospital management to nurses may assist in decreasing the stressors associated with working in the EDs [27]. Currently no motivations exist for nurses working in EDs in VRH, KMH, and HMH. Nurses in EDs should be motivated by managements of EDs for overtime work. Motivations could be in the form of extra duty allowances or food for lunch.

Findings from this study also confirmed overcrowding as a challenge RGNs working in EDs experienced in the Volta Region. All participants confirmed the necessity to create enough space at the ED to make it easier to care for clients. Many of the participants see ED as a messy or disorganised environment. In most emergency units in Ghana, patients presenting are not triaged and most emergency centres are poorly equipped and overcrowded [12]. This is consistent with Coughlan and Corry who conducted a study in which participants described the emergency departments as resembling a disaster zone or a hospital scene from a third-world country [30]. Causes of ED overcrowding included hospital bed shortages, high medical acuity of patients, increasing patient volume, limited examination spaces, and shortage of staff nurses [31]. Overcrowding results in death, permanent disability, additional procedures, and increased length of hospitalization in EDs [31]. A study of California EDs found that 90% had overcrowded conditions and that overcrowding was present in both urban and rural areas [31]. The inability to provide timely service results from overcrowded conditions and has been implicated in poor outcomes for patients [31]. Although overcrowding has been the topic of discussion among many emergency health personnel, few scientific studies actually document and analyze the problems [31]. Despite dramatic headlines and photos of congested EDs, overcrowding has been largely ignored by governments and health care policy makers [31]. A survey by Richardson et al. showed that overcrowding is perceived to be a serious problem by emergency department directors [32]. Most of the factors that contribute to overcrowding are beyond the control of emergency departments [32]. ED overcrowding has multiple effects, including prolonged pain and suffering, long patient waits, patient dissatisfaction, decreased nurse and physician productivity, increased frustration in medical staff, and violence [31]. Solving the problem of overcrowding will not only require a major financial commitment from government and local hospitals, but will also require cooperation from management of hospitals [31]. Nurses in other wards should be educated on the challenges of overcrowding in ED so that they will be willing to accept cases transferred to them from EDs in order to create space for more acute cases in EDs.

Unless the problems in EDs are solved in the near future, the general public may no longer be able to rely on EDs for quality and timely emergency care, placing the people of this country at risk [31].

## 5. Conclusion

Though RGNs play crucial roles in EDs, they experience many challenges that are seldom investigated. It is important for stakeholders of EDs such as government, nongovernmental organisations (NGO), hospital managements, corporate organisations, and local authorities to invest attention and resources into EDs to reduce challenges in EDs. Steps that could improve emergency care include sponsoring nurses to pursue emergency nursing care as a specialty and provision of overtime allowances or lunch to nurses in EDs. Currently, there is only one university in Ghana offering emergency care nursing [33]. Emergency nursing should be introduced in other universities in Ghana in order to increase the number of emergency nurses in Ghana. A similar study could be extended to other regions of Ghana in order to compare results.

## Competing Interests

The authors declare that there is no conflict of interests regarding the publication of this paper.

## References


[1] S. C. Smelter, B. G. Bare, J. L. Hinkle, and K. H. Cheever, *Brunner and Suddart's Textbook of Medical-Surgical Nursing*, Lippincott William & Wilkin, Philadelphia, Pa, USA, 11th edition, 2008.

[2] H. Andersson, B. W. Sundström, K. Nilsson, and E. Jakobsson, "Competencies in Swedish emergency departments-the practitioners' and managers' perspective," *International Emergency Nursing*, vol. 22, no. 2, pp. 81–87, 2014.

[3] World Health Organisation, *Emergency Medical Systems in Low and Middle-income Countries: Recommendations for Action*, World Health Organization, Geneva, Switzerland, 2005.

[4] World Health Organisation, *Guideline to Essential Trauma Care*, World Health Organisation, Geneva, Switzerland, 2004.

[5] U. Hwang, M. N. Shah, J. H. Han, C. R. Carpenter, A. L. Siu, and J. G. Adams, "Transforming emergency care for older adults," *Health Affairs*, vol. 32, no. 12, pp. 2116–2121, 2013.

[6] Institute of Medicine, *Hospital-Based Emergency Care: At the Breaking Point*, National Academies Press, Washington, DC, USA, 2006.

[7] C. H. Chang, D. Harnod, and S. Shih, "Research of patient's nursing care demand at Emergency room," *The Journal of Human Resource and Adult Learning*, vol. 6, no. 2, pp. 110–117, 2010.

[8] E. Weiner, "Preparing nurses internationally for emergency planning and response," *Online Journal of Issues in Nursing*, vol. 11, no. 3, pp. 1–6, 2006.

[9] Emergency Nurses Association, *Competencies for Nurse Practitioners in Emergency Care*, Emergency Nurses Association, Des Plaines, Ill, USA, 2008.

[10] P. Brysiewicz, "South Africa's emergency care professionals are learning fast," *Emergency Nurse*, vol. 18, no. 10, p. 7, 2011.

[11] S. A. Bell, R. Oteng, R. Redman et al., "Development of an emergency nursing training curriculum in Ghana," *International Emergency Nursing*, vol. 22, no. 4, pp. 202–207, 2014.

[12] M. Osei-Ampofo, G. Oduro, R. Oteng, A. Zakariah, G. Jacquet, and P. Donkor, "The evolution and current state of emergency care in Ghana," *African Journal of Emergency Medicine*, vol. 3, no. 2, pp. 52–58, 2013.

[13] S. Rominski, S. A. Bell, D. Yeboah, K. Sarna, H. Hartney, and R. Oteng, "Skills and educational needs of accident and emergency nurses in Ghana: an initial needs analysis," *African Journal of Emergency Medicine*, vol. 1, no. 3, pp. 119–125, 2011.

[14] R. Gallagher, M. Fry, L. Chenoweth, P. Gallagher, and J. Stein-Parbury, "Emergency department nurses' perceptions and experiences of providing care for older people," *Nursing and Health Sciences*, vol. 16, no. 4, pp. 449–453, 2014.

[15] D. F. Polit and C. T. Beck, *Essentials of Nursing Research—Apraising Evidence for Nursing Practice*, Lippincott Williams & Wilkins, 2010.

[16] U. H. Graneheim and B. Lundman, "Qualitative content analysis in nursing research: concepts, procedures and measures to achieve trustworthiness," *Nurse Education Today*, vol. 24, no. 2, pp. 105–112, 2004.

[17] L. Wolf, P. Brysiewicz, N. LoBue et al., "Developing a framework for emergency nursing practice in Africa," *African Journal of Emergency Medicine*, vol. 2, no. 4, pp. 174–181, 2012.

[18] K. B. Japiong, G. Asiamah, E. Owusu-Dabo et al., "Availability of resources for emergency care at a second-level hospital in Ghana: a mixed methods assessment," *African Journal of Emergency Medicine*, vol. 6, no. 1, pp. 30–37, 2015.

[19] J. Gacki-Smith, A. M. Juarez, L. Boyett, C. Homeyer, L. Robinson, and S. L. MacLean, "Violence against nurses working in US emergency departments," *Journal of Nursing Administration*, vol. 39, no. 7-8, pp. 340–349, 2009.

[20] K. O. Ogundipe, A. C. Etonyeaku, I. Adigun et al., "Violence in the emergency department: a multicentre survey of nurses' perceptions in Nigeria," *Emergency Medicine Journal*, vol. 30, no. 9, pp. 758–762, 2013.

[21] M. Kennedy and H. Julie, "Nurses' experiences and understanding of workplace violence in a trauma and emergency department in South Africa," *Health SA Gesondheid*, vol. 18, no. 1, pp. 1–9, 2013.

[22] F. W. Lavoie, G. L. Carter, D. F. Danzl, and R. L. Berg, "Emergency department violence in United States teaching hospitals," *Annals of Emergency Medicine*, vol. 17, no. 11, pp. 1227–1233, 1988.

[23] J. Crilly, W. Chaboyer, and D. Creedy, "Violence towards emergency department nurses by patients," *Accident and Emergency Nursing*, vol. 12, no. 2, pp. 67–73, 2004.

[24] A. Hines, T. Fraze, and C. Stocks, *Emergency Department Visits in Rural and Non-Rural Community Hospitals*, Agency for Healthcare Research and Quality, Rockville, Md, USA, 2011.

[25] J. T. Mitchell and A. Dyregrow, *Traumatic Stress in Disaster Workers and Emergency Personnel, International Handbook of Traumatic Stress Syndromes*, Emergency Health Services Department, University of Maryland, Catonsville, Md, USA, 1993.

[26] L. Phipps, "Stress among doctors and nurses in the emergency department of a general hospital," *Canadian Medical Association Journal*, vol. 139, no. 5, pp. 375–376, 1988.

[27] J. Adeb-Saeedi, "Stress amongst emergency nurses," *Australian Emergency Nursing Journal*, vol. 5, no. 2, pp. 19–24, 2002.

[28] G. M. Ross-Adjie, G. Leslie, and L. Gillman, "Occupational stress in the ED: what matters to Nurses?" *Australasian Emergency Nursing Journal*, vol. 10, no. 3, pp. 117–123, 2007.

[29] S. Helps, "Experiences of stress in accident and emergency nurses," *Accident and Emergency Nursing*, vol. 5, no. 1, pp. 48–53, 1997.

[30] M. Coughlan and M. Corry, "The experiences of patients and relatives/significant others of overcrowding in accident and emergency in Ireland: a qualitative descriptive study," *International Emergency Nursing*, vol. 15, no. 4, pp. 201–209, 2007.

[31] R. W. Derlet and J. R. Richards, "Emergency department overcrowding in Florida, New York, and Texas," *Southern Medical Journal*, vol. 95, no. 8, pp. 846–849, 2002.

[32] S. Richardson, M. Casey, and P. Hider, "Following the patient journey: older persons' experiences of emergency departments and discharge," *Accident and Emergency Nursing*, vol. 15, no. 3, pp. 134–140, 2007.

[33] Kwame Nkrumah University of Science and Technology, *Emergency Nursing Course Outline*, Kwame Nkrumah University of Science and Technology, Kumasi, Ghana, 2010.

# Paramedic Recognition of Sepsis in the Prehospital Setting

**Robert S. Green,[1,2] Andrew H. Travers,[3,4] Edward Cain,[3] Samuel G. Campbell,[3] Jan L. Jensen,[3,4] David A. Petrie,[3] Mete Erdogan,[2] Gredi Patrick,[5] and Ward Patrick[1]**

[1] *Department of Critical Care, Dalhousie University, Suite 377, Bethune Building, 1276 South Park Street, Halifax, NS, Canada B3H 2Y9*
[2] *Trauma Nova Scotia, Room 1-026B, Centennial Building, 1276 South Park Street, Halifax, NS, Canada B3H 2Y9*
[3] *Department of Emergency Medicine, Dalhousie University, Division of EMS, 1796 Summer Street, Halifax Infirmary, Suite 355, Halifax, NS, Canada B3H 3A7*
[4] *Emergency Health Service, 239 Brownlow Avenue, Suite 300, Dartmouth, NS, Canada B3B 2B2*
[5] *Performance Excellence, Nova Scotia Health Authority, Halifax, NS, Canada B3H 4R2*

Correspondence should be addressed to Robert S. Green; greenrs@dal.ca

Academic Editor: Rade B. Vukmir

*Background.* Patients with sepsis benefit from early diagnosis and treatment. Accurate paramedic recognition of sepsis is important to initiate care promptly for patients who arrive by Emergency Medical Services. *Methods.* Prospective observational study of adult patients (age ≥ 16 years) transported by paramedics to the emergency department (ED) of a Canadian tertiary hospital. Paramedic identification of sepsis was assessed using a novel prehospital sepsis screening tool developed by the study team and compared to blind, independent documentation of ED diagnoses by attending emergency physicians (EPs). Specificity, sensitivity, accuracy, positive and negative predictive value, and likelihood ratios were calculated with 95% confidence intervals. *Results.* Overall, 629 patients were included in the analysis. Sepsis was identified by paramedics in 170 (27.0%) patients and by EPs in 71 (11.3%) patients. Sensitivity of paramedic sepsis identification compared to EP diagnosis was 73.2% (95% CI 61.4–83.0), while specificity was 78.8% (95% CI 75.2–82.2). The accuracy of paramedic identification of sepsis was 78.2% (492/629, 52 true positive, 440 true negative). Positive and negative predictive values were 30.6% (95% CI 23.8–38.1) and 95.9% (95% CI 93.6–97.5), respectively. *Conclusion.* Using a novel prehospital sepsis screening tool, paramedic recognition of sepsis had greater specificity than sensitivity with reasonable accuracy.

## 1. Introduction

Despite numerous clinical trials of specific treatments, sepsis remains a leading cause of morbidity and mortality in patients arriving at the emergency department (ED) or staying in hospital [1, 2]. Early detection and protocol-based care (PBC) of sepsis with resuscitation, antibiotics, and source control are considered the optimal management strategy [3–6]. Of patients seen in the ED with sepsis, approximately half are transported there by Emergency Medical Services (EMS) [7]. Previous studies have demonstrated that septic patients who arrive by EMS receive treatment rapidly compared to ambulatory patients [8, 9], as with other time sensitive conditions such as myocardial infarction [10, 11].

Paramedic recognition of sepsis is important for the appropriate triage and initiation of early treatment for septic patients transported by EMS. However, identification of sepsis can be challenging for paramedics since they cannot access the laboratory and imaging adjuncts available to physicians in the ED. There is limited information available on how well paramedics are able to identify sepsis compared to emergency physicians (EPs) [12–14], and few screening tools have been developed to assist with prehospital recognition of sepsis [14–17].

Most previous screening tools have focused on detection of patients with severe sepsis, and only one of these tools has been validated to date [15]. Importantly, these screening tools incorporate limited information regarding recent findings of infection in patients and criteria of organ dysfunction remote from the site of infection. To address these limitations, the study team developed a novel prehospital tool to screen for patients with any degree of sepsis. The goal of this study was to evaluate use of this tool by EMS personnel and to compare paramedic detection of septic patients with EP diagnoses.

## 2. Methods

This prospective observational study was of a convenience sample of adult patients (age ≥ 16 years) transported by paramedics to a Canadian tertiary ED. Patients were enrolled into the study by paramedics if they were dispatched as follows: having abdominal pain, having breathing problems, being sick, having unknown problems, being unconscious/fainting, having chest pain, or any case in which paramedics considered sepsis a possible diagnosis. A novel paper-based prehospital sepsis screening tool was developed by the study team. Relevant data points were determined through literature searches related to diagnosis of sepsis, in addition to consensus or guideline statements. The prehospital sepsis screening tool is available in Supplementary Material available online at http://dx.doi.org/10.1155/2016/6717261.

The content of the tool relied heavily upon sepsis criteria definitions developed by the 2001 SCCM/ESICM/ACCP/ATS/SIS sepsis definitions conference [18]. Possible data elements were vetted through use of a Delphi approach with provincial leaders in paramedicine, emergency medicine, and critical care medicine. The tool was evaluated by a focus group of 40 EMS paramedics to obtain feedback and ensure that data elements could be obtained in the prehospital environment without delaying the implementation of the current standard of care to patients. Prior to study initiation, paramedics attended a 3-hour training session and received instruction on sepsis including definitions, epidemiology, basic pathophysiology, identification, and optimal management of septic patients.

In this Canadian provincial ground ambulance system, most paramedics are primary care paramedics (PCPs) or advanced care paramedics (ACPs) (http://novascotia.ca/dhw/ehs/international-applicants/levels-of-paramedics.asp). PCP training is one to two years in length. PCPs can provide basic level emergency care, including performing semiautomated external defibrillation, oxygen administration, intravenous therapy, cardiac monitoring, and administration of select medications. ACP training is 18 to 36 months in length. ACPs are able to provide advanced level emergency care, including a broad array of emergency medications, advanced airway management, and invasive interventions. Training requirements follow the National Occupational Competency Profile (http://www.paramedic.ca/site/nocp?nav=02).

Immediately following transport to hospital and transfer of care to the ED, paramedics were prompted by the EMS dispatch center to complete the prehospital sepsis screening tool. The tool was used to collect data on patient history, vital signs, recent findings (within past 10 days), signs and symptoms, criteria for organ dysfunction remote from the site of infection, and presence of fever. The determination of whether a patient had a fever was based on self-reporting by the patient or the presence of symptoms such as abnormally warm forehead/neck, flushed face, lethargy, and body aches; thermometers were not routinely used by EMS personnel at the time of this study. Based on data collected using the tool, paramedics made a determination of whether or not the patient had any degree of sepsis which was compared to blind, independent documentation of diagnoses by attending EPs.

The EPs used a study ED screening tool to indicate if patients were septic, which served as the gold standard for this study. If the EP did not mark whether or not the patient had sepsis, the final EP diagnosis recorded on the patients' medical record was obtained through retrospective review of the electronic ED database and study investigators determined if the final diagnosis indicated that the patient had sepsis. Data was entered into a dedicated study database (Microsoft® Access, Redmond WA). Analysis was conducted in IBM SPSS Statistics Version 21 (IBM, Armonk NY) [19]. Simple descriptive statistics were used to describe characteristics of paramedics and the patient cohort. Specificity, sensitivity, accuracy, positive and negative predictive value, and likelihood ratios were calculated with 95% confidence intervals. This study was approved by the Institutional Review Board.

Table 1: Paramedic certification level.

| | Frequency |
|---|---|
| Advanced care paramedic | 257 (43.8) |
| Primary care paramedic | 219 (37.4) |
| Intermediate care paramedic | 97 (16.6) |
| Critical care paramedic | 13 (2.2) |

Parentheses denote percentage.
$n$ = 586 responses.

## 3. Results

Overall, 956 patients were enrolled by paramedics during the study period. A flow diagram outlining the selection of study participants and recognition of sepsis by paramedics and EPs is shown in Figure 1. We excluded 327 cases with no paramedic diagnosis recorded ($n = 249$), no EP diagnosis available ($n = 73$), or if the patient left the ED without being seen or before the EP diagnosis was made ($n = 5$). The remaining 629 (65.8%) cases were included in the final analysis.

The certification level of paramedics who participated in the study is shown in Table 1. In most cases, the EMS personnel were an ACP (43.8%) or a PCP (37.4%). Characteristics of the patients seen by paramedics are described in Table 2. Patients commonly presented with fever (27.9%) and with a recent infection within the prior 10 days (25.2%). Paramedics identified 170/629 (27.0%) patients as septic, while EPs identified sepsis in 71/629 (11.3%) patients. Disagreement in the diagnosis of sepsis often occurred in patients ultimately diagnosed with pneumonia, cellulitis, urinary tract infection, peritonitis, and renal failure.

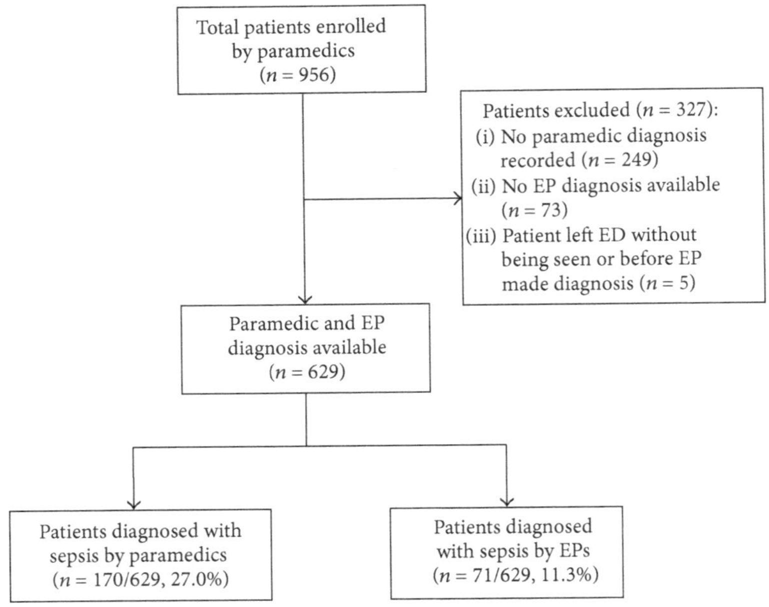


FIGURE 1: Selection of study participants and identification of sepsis by paramedics and EPs. ED, emergency department; EP, emergency physician.

Table 3 shows paramedic identification of sepsis and EP diagnosis of sepsis as a contingency table. The sensitivity and specificity of paramedic diagnoses of sepsis compared to EP diagnoses were 73.2% (95% CI 61.4–83.0) and 78.8% (95% CI 75.2–82.2), respectively. Accuracy was 78.2% (492/629, 52 true positive, 440 true negative). The positive predictive value was 30.6% (95% CI 23.8–38.1), and the negative predictive value was 95.9% (95% CI 93.6–97.5). The positive likelihood ratio was 3.46 (95% CI 2.80–4.29), and negative likelihood ratio was 0.34 (95% CI: 0.23–0.50).

## 4. Discussion

This prospective study assessed the ability of paramedics to recognize septic patients using a novel prehospital sepsis screening tool. Compared with the EPs' diagnosis, we observed that paramedics were able to identify septic patients with 73.2% sensitivity, 78.8% specificity, and 78.2% accuracy using this tool. This study provides evidence that paramedics can identify sepsis with reasonable accuracy in the EMS setting. Increasing paramedic awareness of the importance of early recognition through directed training is critical to reducing the burden of sepsis-related morbidity and mortality.

Few previous studies have examined the ability of prehospital personnel to recognize sepsis in adult patients. Using presence of both an ED report of acute infection and patient admission as their reference standard, one prospective study employed a questionnaire to examine the ability of EMS providers to identify serious infection and reported a sensitivity of 31% (95% CI 17–50) and specificity of 93% (95% CI 87–96) [20]. Other studies have found the sensitivity of sepsis identification by prehospital personnel to be 70% or higher [21, 22], similar to the results of our study.

There are limited reports of validated screening tools for recognition of sepsis in the prehospital setting. One tool recently developed and validated is the prehospital severe sepsis (PRESS) screening tool which involves a score calculated from EMS data on 6 risk factors [15]. Using the PRESS tool in the setting of an urban public hospital, prehospital recognition of severe sepsis by EMS staff had a sensitivity of 86% and a specificity of 47% [15]. The Sepsis Alert Protocol is another screening tool for EMS providers and was found to accurately identify severe sepsis in 47.8% of cases in a pilot study [14]. Unlike these tools, our prehospital screening tool was designed to identify patients with any degree of sepsis, not only those with severe sepsis. Comparing the accuracy of our tool with these other tools is difficult due to variations in study designs, institutional settings, EMS services, and populations served. Additional validation is required before these tools can be recommended for widespread clinical use.

Our study evaluated the ability of paramedics to identify sepsis using a prehospital screening tool and found promising levels of accuracy, sensitivity, and specificity (>70%). These findings are significant in order to capitalize on early alerts to further reduce the time window to treatment initiation [23]. Additional areas for future research may involve integrating the use of biomarkers and evaluating the impact of moving ED treatments earlier into the EMS phase of care. Another opportunity that is yet unexplored is the identification of patients who may have sepsis by EMS dispatchers [24]. There is tremendous potential to reduce the morbidity and mortality associated with sepsis by developing and validating new tools for early recognition and management of the septic patient.

TABLE 2: Patient characteristics.

| | Frequency |
|---|---|
| Patient history[1] | |
| Diabetes mellitus | 117 (21.1) |
| Oral steroids or chemotherapy in last 6 weeks | 38 (6.8) |
| Chronic renal failure | 23 (4.1) |
| Organ/tissue transplant | 5 (0.9) |
| Human immunodeficiency virus | 1 (0.2) |
| None of the above | 394 (71.0) |
| Vital signs, mean [SD] | |
| Respiratory rate | 21.6 [8.3] |
| Heart rate | 90.9 [22.6] |
| Systolic blood pressure[2] | 132.3 [29.5] |
| Diastolic blood pressure[3] | 72.8 [14.8] |
| Blood sugar[4] | 8.1 [3.3] |
| Fever at present[5] | |
| Yes | 163 (27.9) |
| Recent finding of any infection[6] | |
| Yes | 155 (25.2) |
| Signs and symptoms of infection[7] | |
| Pulmonary, cough/hypoxia | 170 (27.5) |
| Abdominal tenderness | 81 (13.1) |
| Soft tissue swelling/redness/pain | 62 (10.0) |
| Altered sensorium | 56 (9.0) |
| Urinary, foul/puss | 52 (8.4) |
| Meningitis, stiff neck | 5 (0.8) |
| None of the above | 259 (41.8) |
| Organ dysfunction criteria[8] | |
| Diaphoresis | 47 (7.8) |
| Cool peripheral limbs | 38 (6.3) |
| Systolic blood pressure < 90 mmHg | 36 (6.0) |
| Knee mottling | 1 (0.2) |
| Periumbilical mottling | 0 (0) |
| None of the above | 498 (82.7) |

SD: standard deviation
Brackets denote standard deviation. Parentheses denote percentage.
[1]Paramedics could make more than one selection for patient history, $n = 555$ responses.
[2]$n = 627$ responses.
[3]Diastolic blood pressure unavailable when palpation was required, $n = 554$ responses.
[4]Blood sugar was often unavailable and only collected in nondiabetic patients, $n = 446$ responses.
[5]Paramedic determination of whether patient had a fever at present, $n = 584$ responses.
[6]Paramedic finding of any infection within prior 10 days, $n = 614$ responses.
[7]Any sign or symptom of infection (both present and new). Paramedics could make more than one selection, $n = 619$ responses.
[8]Any criteria of organ dysfunction present and remote from site of infection that were not chronic conditions. Paramedics could make more than one selection, $n = 602$ responses.

This study has the limitations of an observational study including possible selection and information bias. This study was conducted at a single academic tertiary care center (65,000 ED visits per year) with a single EMS service that takes care of urban, suburban, and rural populations; thus, our findings may not be generalizable to other centers. While we did capture paramedic certification level, data on number of years of experience for paramedics and EPs was not collected. While this study is limited because the reference standard was EP diagnosis instead of a more definitive marker, this reference was chosen as EP diagnosis is the sentinel trigger of PBC at our institution. Another limitation of this study is the number of potentially eligible patients that were excluded, mostly because paramedics did not complete the diagnosis on the study form. At the time of the study, this EMS system did not use thermometers or point of care lactate testing, which may limit generalizability to settings that do use these diagnostic tools.

TABLE 3: Contingency table comparing paramedic identification of sepsis with emergency physician diagnosis of sepsis.

| | Emergency physician diagnosis of sepsis | |
|---|---|---|
| | Yes | No |
| Paramedic identification of sepsis | | |
| Yes | 52 | 118 |
| No | 19 | 440 |

## 5. Conclusion

Using a novel screening tool, paramedic identification of sepsis in this limited single center study cohort revealed a greater specificity than sensitivity in comparison to EP diagnosis. Further research is required to validate the use of this sepsis screening tool in the prehospital setting.

## Conflict of Interests

The authors declare that there is no conflict of interests regarding the publication of this paper.

## Acknowledgments

The authors would like to thank John Kasemets (CCP) for his significant contribution to study design, David Urqhart for developing the study database, and Emily Morash, Maureen Sturgeon (ACP), and Zach Dewar (PCP) for their work on data entry and chart reviews.

## References

[1] D. F. Gaieski, J. M. Edwards, M. J. Kallan, and B. G. Carr, "Benchmarking the incidence and mortality of severe sepsis in the united states," *Critical Care Medicine*, vol. 41, no. 5, pp. 1167–1174, 2013.

[2] J. C. Marshall, "Why have clinical trials in sepsis failed?" *Trends in Molecular Medicine*, vol. 20, no. 4, pp. 195–203, 2014.

[3] R. P. Dellinger, M. N. Levy, A. Rhodes et al., "Surviving sepsis campaign: international guidelines for management of severe sepsis and septic shock: 2012," *Critical Care Medicine*, vol. 41, no. 2, pp. 580–637, 2013.

[4] The ProCESS Investigators, "A randomized trial of protocol-based care for early septic shock," *The New England Journal of Medicine*, vol. 370, no. 18, pp. 1683–1693, 2014.

[5] D. M. Yealy, D. T. Huang, A. Delaney et al., "Recognizing and managing sepsis: what needs to be done?" *BioMed Central Medicine*, vol. 27, no. 13, article 98, 2015.

[6] R. L. Gauer, "Early recognition and management of sepsis in adults: the first six hours," *American Family Physician*, vol. 88, no. 1, pp. 44–53, 2013.

[7] C. W. Seymour, T. D. Rea, J. M. Kahn, A. J. Walkey, D. M. Yealy, and D. C. Angus, "Severe sepsis in pre-hospital emergency care: analysis of incidence, care, and outcome," *American Journal of Respiratory and Critical Care Medicine*, vol. 186, no. 12, pp. 1264–1271, 2012.

[8] R. A. Band, D. F. Gaieski, J. H. Hylton, F. S. Shofer, M. Goyal, and Z. F. Meisel, "Arriving by emergency medical services improves time to treatment endpoints for patients with severe sepsis or septic shock," *Academic Emergency Medicine*, vol. 18, no. 9, pp. 934–940, 2011.

[9] J. R. Studnek, M. R. Artho, C. L. Garner Jr., and A. E. Jones, "The impact of emergency medical services on the ED care of severe sepsis," *The American Journal of Emergency Medicine*, vol. 30, no. 1, pp. 51–56, 2012.

[10] T. Camp-Rogers, S. Dante, M. C. Kontos, C. S. Roberts, L. Kreisa, and M. C. Kurz, "The impact of prehospital activation of the cardiac catheterization team on time to treatment for patients presenting with ST-segment-elevation myocardial infarction," *The American Journal of Emergency Medicine*, vol. 29, no. 9, pp. 1117–1124, 2011.

[11] R. A. Ducas, A. W. Wassef, D. S. Jassal et al., "To transmit or not to transmit: how good are emergency medical personnel in detecting STEMI in patients with chest pain?" *The Canadian Journal of Cardiology*, vol. 28, no. 4, pp. 432–437, 2012.

[12] M. Groenewoudt, A. A. Roest, F. M. M. Leijten, and P. M. Stassen, "Septic patients arriving with emergency medical services: a seriously ill population," *The European Journal of Emergency Medicine*, vol. 21, no. 5, pp. 330–335, 2014.

[13] C. W. Seymour, C. R. Cooke, S. R. Heckbert et al., "Prehospital intravenous access and fluid resuscitation in severe sepsis: an observational cohort study," *Critical Care*, vol. 18, no. 5, article 533, 2014.

[14] W. F. Guerra, T. R. Mayfield, M. S. Meyers, A. E. Clouatre, and J. C. Riccio, "Early detection and treatment of patients with severe sepsis by prehospital personnel," *The Journal of Emergency Medicine*, vol. 44, no. 6, pp. 1116–1125, 2013.

[15] C. C. Polito, A. Isakov, A. H. Yancey II et al., "Prehospital recognition of severe sepsis: development and validation of a novel EMS screening tool," *The American Journal of Emergency Medicine*, vol. 33, no. 9, pp. 1119–1125, 2015.

[16] U. M. Wallgren, M. Castrén, A. E. V. Svensson, and L. Kurland, "Identification of adult septic patients in the prehospital setting: a comparison of two screening tools and clinical judgment," *The European Journal of Emergency Medicine*, vol. 21, no. 4, pp. 260–265, 2014.

[17] O. Bayer, D. Schwarzkopf, C. Stumme et al., "An early warning scoring system to identify septic patients in the prehospital setting: the PRESEP score," *Academic Emergency Medicine*, vol. 22, no. 7, pp. 868–871, 2015.

[18] M. M. Levy, M. P. Fink, J. C. Marshall et al., "2001 SCCM/ESICM/ACCP/ATS/SIS international sepsis definitions conference," *Critical Care Medicine*, vol. 31, no. 4, pp. 1250–1256, 2003.

[19] IBM Corp, *IBM SPSS Statistics for Windows, Version 21.0*, IBM Corp, Armonk, NY, USA, 2012.

[20] B. Suffoletto, A. Frisch, A. Prabhu, J. Kristan, F. X. Guyette, and C. W. Callaway, "Prediction of serious infection during prehospital emergency care," *Prehospital Emergency Care*, vol. 15, no. 3, pp. 325–330, 2011.

[21] C. W. Seymour, C. R. Cooke, M. E. Mikkelsen et al., "Out-of-hospital fluid in severe sepsis: effect on early resuscitation in the emergency department," *Prehospital Emergency Care*, vol. 14, no. 2, pp. 145–152, 2010.

[22] K. Clesham, S. Mason, J. Gray, S. Walters, and V. Cooke, "Can emergency medical service staff predict the disposition of patients they are transporting?" *Emergency Medicine Journal*, vol. 25, no. 10, pp. 691–694, 2008.

[23] A. A. Báez, P. Hanudel, M. T. Perez, E. M. Giraldez, and S. R. Wilcox, "Prehospital sepsis project (PSP): knowledge and attitudes of united states advanced out-of-hospital care providers," *Prehospital and Disaster Medicine*, vol. 28, no. 2, pp. 104–106, 2013.

[24] J. Herlitz, A. Bång, B. Wireklint-Sundström et al., "Suspicion and treatment of severe sepsis. An overview of the prehospital chain of care," *Scandinavian Journal of Trauma, Resuscitation and Emergency Medicine*, vol. 20, article 42, 2012.

# Using Fresh Frozen Plasma for Acute Airway Angioedema to Prevent Intubation in the Emergency Department

**Aya Saeb,[1,2,3] Karen H. Hagglund,[1] and Christine T. Cigolle[2,3,4]**

[1]*Department of Internal Medicine, St. John Hospital & Medical Center, 22101 Moross Road, Detroit, MI 48236, USA*
[2]*Geriatric Research Education and Clinical Center (GRECC), VA Ann Arbor Healthcare System, 2215 Fuller Road 11 G, Ann Arbor, MI 48105, USA*
[3]*Department of Internal Medicine, University of Michigan, 3110 Taubman Center, SPC 5368, 1500 East Medical Center Drive, Ann Arbor, MI 48109, USA*
[4]*Department of Family Medicine, University of Michigan, 1150 W. Medical Center Drive, M7300 Med Sci I, SPC 5625, Ann Arbor, MI 48109, USA*

Correspondence should be addressed to Aya Saeb; drayasaeb@gmail.com

Academic Editor: Wen-Jone Chen

*Background.* Angioedema (AE) is a common condition which can be complicated by laryngeal edema, having up to 40% mortality. Although sporadic case reports attest to the benefits of fresh frozen plasma (FFP) in treating severe acute bouts of AE, little evidence-based support for this practice is available at present. *Study Objectives.* To compare the frequency, duration of intubation, and length of intensive care unit (ICU) stay in patients with acute airway AE, with and without the use of FFP. *Methods.* A retrospective cohort study was conducted, investigating adults admitted to large community hospital ICU with a diagnosis of AE during the years of 2007–2012. Altogether, 128 charts were reviewed for demographics, comorbidities, hospital courses, and outcomes. A total of 20 patients received FFP (108 did not). *Results.* Demographics and comorbidities did not differ by treatment group. However, nontreated controls did worse in terms of intubation frequency (60% versus 35%; $p = 0.05$) and ICU stay (3.5 days versus 1.5 days; $p < 0.001$). Group outcomes were otherwise similar. *Conclusion.* In an emergency department setting, the use of FFP should be considered in managing acute airway nonhereditary AE (refractory to steroid, antihistamine, and epinephrine). Larger prospective, better controlled studies are needed to devise appropriate treatment guidelines.

## 1. Introduction

Angioedema (AE), defined as self-limited, localized swelling, can manifest as an acute attack of asymmetric, nonpruritic, nonpitting subcutaneous or submucosal edema [1]. The reported prevalence varies, depending on etiology, population studied, and method of study (self-reported versus medically diagnosed). The World Allergy Organization (WAO) estimates that up to 20% of individuals will experience urticaria or AE at least once in their lifetime [2, 3]. In related studies, 5%–15% of patients with AE developed obstructive laryngeal edema [4], which is the leading cause of death. The latter carries a mortality rate of 25%–40% [1].

For emergency physicians, evaluation and management of patients who present with acute airway AE may be challenging. This disorder can be caused by a wide variety of immunologic and nonimmunologic mechanisms. Not surprisingly, there are a number of classification systems of AE in the medical literature. For the clinician, we found that dividing AE into two broad categories, histamine-mediated (also mast cell-mediated/allergic) and bradykinin-mediated, is the most clinically relevant and practical in guiding the management approach. When assessing acute AE affecting the airway, the emergency physician must rely on the patient's history and physical examination. With the exception of hereditary AE (HAE), laboratory studies such as serum levels

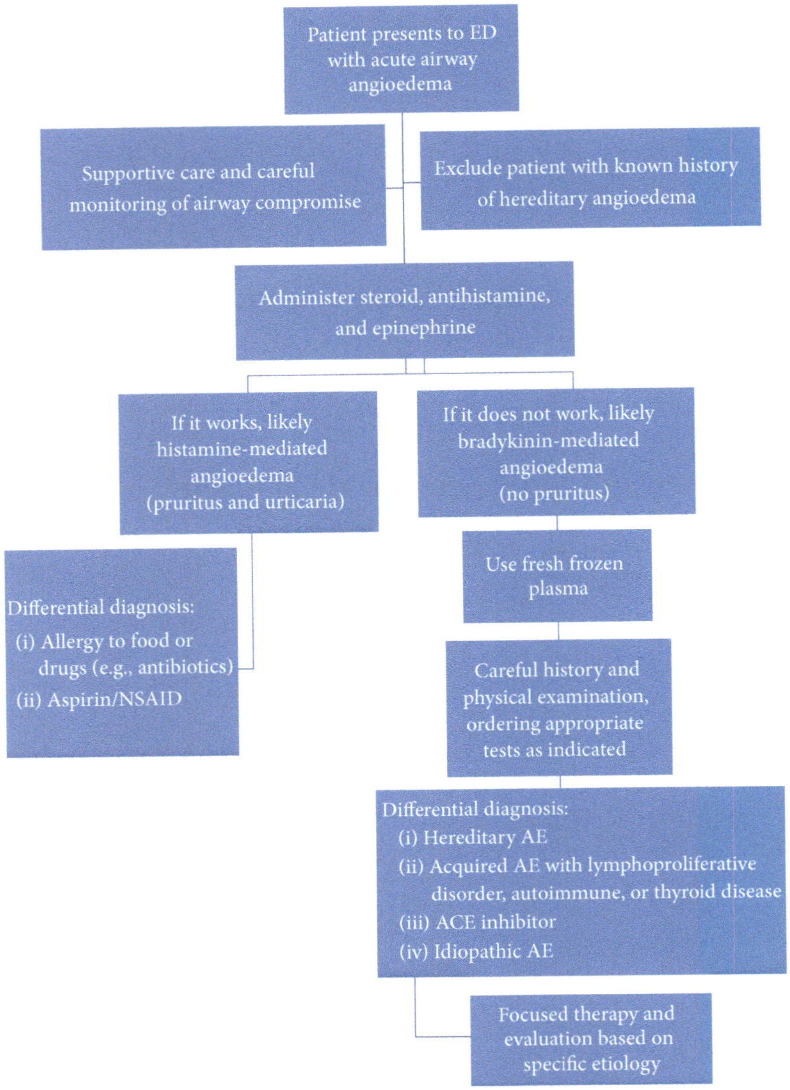


FIGURE 1: Management algorithm.

of Complement 4, tryptase levels, C1 inhibitor protein, and the C1 inhibitor functional activity have been shown to have no utility in the evaluation of acute AE especially in the acute setting [1]. Most common cause of acute AE is thought to be histamine-mediated and is frequently responsive to antihistamine, epinephrine, and steroids; however, refractory cases may be secondary to bradykinin [5].

Fresh frozen plasma (FFP) is one treatment option for acute bradykinin-induced AE with airway compromise. The first report of its successful use was in hereditary AE in 1969 [6]. Subsequent case reports have demonstrated the effectiveness of FFP (given within 45 minutes to 12 hours) for both HAE and non-HAE [7, 8]. However, no randomized clinical trials have investigated the use of FFP for either condition [7]. Likewise, there are no studies that examine the frequency of intubation or the length of stay in intensive care unit (ICU) settings after administration of FFP for airway AE.

Recent literature demonstrates that FFP is effective and can be used if C1 esterase inhibitor (a recently approved treatment for HAE by the US Food and Drug Administration in 2009) is not available (e.g., due to cost) or if initial treatment does not work (i.e., steroid, antihistamine, and epinephrine) (strength of evidence, Level III Grade B) [9]. However, based on a large survey of physicians in the United States in 2011, only 34.9% use FFP in acute episodes of AE [10].

Given the challenge facing emergency physicians managing life-threatening acute AE with airway compromise, we investigated the use of FFP to examine its ability to prevent intubation and shorten the course of airway angioedema and hence ICU stays. After reviewing the comprehensive differential diagnosis for AE acute attacks, we devised our own simplified algorithm to illustrate the decision points for the emergency physician in managing airway angioedema and the place of FFP as an intervention (Figure 1). Proper management includes early recognition and aggressive airway management. For some etiologies, however, both treatment and patient disposition remain controversial [9].

Of note, our investigation focused on patients presenting with idiopathic angioedema. These episodes, those having an unidentified etiology (possibly histamine-mediated, initial attacks of hereditary or acquired angioedema) or those linked with angiotensin-converting enzyme (ACE) inhibitors use, are of interest, given the limited evidence base to guide management and the lack of any treatments approved specifically for these conditions by the US Food and Drug Administration.

We conducted a retrospective cohort study, to determine the frequency of intubation and its duration in patients who presented to our emergency department (ED) with acute AE involving the airway which required ICU admission, comparing patients with airway AE treated with FFP to those not treated with FFP (cases and controls, resp.). We also compared the length of stay in ICU settings for both groups, examining whether FFP administration shortens ICU stays in severe, acute attacks of AE. We hypothesized that using FFP in an acute AE attack with airway compromise can prevent or shorten intubation and lead to shortened ICU stays.

## 2. Methods

*2.1. Design.* A keyword search of PubMed (i.e., angioedema, intensive care unit, fresh frozen plasma, and intubation) identified no studies comparing the frequency of intubation, duration of intubation, or the length of ICU stays in AE cases with airway involvement managed with or without FFP.

We conducted a retrospective cohort study of all adults admitted to the ICU (medical and surgical) in a community teaching hospital in Detroit, MI (772 beds) with a diagnosis of AE during the years of 2007–2012. The scope was confined to chart review; therefore signed patient consent documents were not required. Once St. John Hospital and Medical Center Institutional Review Board approval was granted, all data obtained via electronic medical records and paper charts of ICU/hospital stays were handled in Health Insurance Portability and Accountability Act, compliant manner. The inclusion criteria were as follows:

(1) Age ≥18 years.

(2) Admission to medical or surgical ICU.

(3) Primary diagnosis of AE (indicated by ICD-9 code) and airway involvement (indicated by documented history and physical exam). (The subset of patients taking ACE inhibitors was of particular interest.)

The exclusion criteria included the following:

(1) Food allergy (if specified as a cause of AE).

(2) Intubation unrelated to airway AE.

(3) ICU admission for other indications (not AE primarily).

(4) Known history of HAE. (Patients with histories of HAE were excluded on the grounds that their diagnoses were already established and therefore prophylactic treatments were likely in use, perhaps with the access to other recently FDA-approved targeted therapies.)

*2.2. Study Population and Main Measures.* Paper and electronic medical records/charts were reviewed retrospectively. Dependent variables included intubation frequency, duration (in hours), site of intubation (ED, ICU, or hospital floor), performing physician (emergency physician versus anesthesiologist or otolaryngologist), and route (oral versus nasal), as well as the need for cricothyroidotomy or tracheostomy, ICU stay (in days), and patient outcome/disposition (discharged home, transitioned to extended care facility, or deceased). Important covariates included patient demographics (age, gender, and race), admission and discharge dates, admission source (ED, extended care facility, or direct admission from clinic), comorbidities (diabetes mellitus, hypertension, congestive heart failure, asthma, chronic obstructive pulmonary disease, obstructive sleep apnea, chronic kidney disease, and others), ACE inhibitor use, known specific allergies (food or antibiotics) by history, individual or family history of AE, and history of prior intubation.

We conducted a retrospective cohort study given the anticipated limited use of FFP for airway AE in the ED settings plus our interest in measuring multiple outcomes. The rationale behind the ED or ICU physician's choice of FFP was not always indicated in the medical chart. It is possible that one explanation is a lack of knowledge about the role of FFP as a treatment of airway AE; this lack of knowledge could be a major confounder in our analyses. Data were collected by the primary author from multiple parts of the electronic and paper medical records (e.g., physician progress note, respiratory therapist note, etc.) to ascertain consistency and avoid recall/information bias.

*2.3. Statistical Analysis.* Given that most of the studies evaluating FFP for airway AE are descriptive and that there is a lack of data in prior studies on the frequency of intubation, a reference rate was not available. We conservatively estimated that 90% of patients evaluated in the ED for acute AE with airway compromise and not treated with FFP would require intubation; in contrast, 70% of those treated with FFP would require intubation. Given this effect size, 62 patients were needed for each group (FFP versus no FFP) for 80% power and alpha = 0.05.

By chart review, we had 160 charts but only 128 patients met the inclusion criteria. Twenty patients had received FFP, with the remainder ($n = 108$) serving as controls. Despite being underpowered, statistically significant results were achieved.

The frequencies and other descriptive statistics were calculated, and associations between categorical variables were assessed via the chi-square test. Between-group differences in continuous variables were measured using $t$-tests for independent groups. Standard software was used (SPSS v12.0; SPSS Inc., Chicago, IL, USA), with statistical significance set at $p < 0.05$.

## 3. Results

Out of 160 charts only 128 patients met our inclusion criteria. Mean ± SD patient age was 61 ± 14.8 years. Just over half

Table 1: Patient characteristics.

| Parameter | FFP ($n$ = 20) | No FFP ($n$ = 108) | $p$ value |
|---|---|---|---|
| Age, years, mean (SD) | 62.9 (11.1) | 61.2 (15.4) | 0.64 |
| Male gender, $n$ (%) | 10 (50) | 50 (46) | 0.81 |
| Race, $n$ (%) | | | 1.00 |
| Caucasian | 3 (15) | 18 (17) | |
| African-American | 17 (85) | 89 (83) | |
| Admission type, $n$ (%) | | | — |
| ED | 19 (95) | 98 (90) | |
| ECF | 1 (5) | 5 (5) | |
| Direct | 0 (0) | 5 (5) | |
| Comorbidities, $n$ (%) | | | |
| Diabetes mellitus | 9 (45) | 28 (26) | 0.11 |
| Hypertension | 19 (95) | 97 (90) | 0.69 |
| CHF | 2 (10) | 7 (7) | 0.63 |
| Asthma | 1 (5) | 12 (11) | 0.69 |
| COPD | 6 (30) | 26 (24) | 0.58 |
| OSA | 4 (20) | 8 (7) | 0.09 |
| CKD | 1 (5) | 20 (19) | 0.19 |
| Cancer | 0 (0) | 10 (9) | 0.36 |
| History of allergies, $n$ (%) | 20 (100) | 106 (98) | 1.00 |
| Number of allergies, mean (SD) | 2.0 (1.0) | 2.4 (1.6) | 0.34 |
| History of ACE-I, $n$ (%) | 18 (90) | 92 (85) | 0.74 |
| History of angioedema, $n$ (%) | 6 (30) | 26 (24) | 0.58 |
| History of intubation, $n$ (%) | 3 (15) | 4 (4) | 0.08 |

ACE-I, ACE inhibitor; CHF, congestive heart failure; CKD, chronic kidney disease; COPD, chronic obstructive pulmonary disease; ECF, extended care facility; ED, emergency department; FFP, fresh frozen plasma; OSA, obstructive sleep apnea; SD, standard deviation.

Table 2: Intubation characteristics.

| Parameter | FFP ($n$ = 20) | No FFP ($n$ = 108) | $p$ value |
|---|---|---|---|
| Prevalence, $n$ (%) | 7 (35) | 65 (60) | 0.05 |
| Duration, hours, mean (SD) | 60.3 (38.2) | 97.1 (126.9) | 0.45 |
| Type, $n$ (%) | | | 1.00 |
| PO | 5 (83) | 51 (81) | |
| Nasal | 1 (17) | 12 (19) | |
| Location, $n$ (%) | | | — |
| ED | 3 (43) | 45 (69) | |
| ICU | 1 (14) | 3 (5) | |
| Floor | 0 (0) | 9 (14) | |
| OR | 3 (43) | 8 (12) | |
| Procedure administrator, $n$ (%) | | | 0.59 |
| ED physician | 0 (0) | 9 (14) | |
| Anesthesiologist/ENT | 7 (100) | 56 (86) | |
| Procedures, $n$ (%) | | | |
| Cricothyroidotomy | 1 (14) | 1 (2) | 0.19 |
| Tracheostomy | 1 (14) | 3 (5) | 0.34 |

ED, emergency department; ENT, ear, nose, and throat surgeon; FFP, fresh frozen plasma; ICU, intensive care unit; OR, operating room; PO, per-oral; SD, standard deviation.

of the cohort was female, and 84% were African-American. Demographics, comorbidities, and medical histories did not differ significantly by group ($p > 0.05$) (Table 1).

Hypertension was prevalent in both FFP-treated (95%) and control groups (90%), and ACE inhibitors were frequently used (90% and 85%, resp.). Most patients had documented allergies to two or more medications. Past histories of AE were documented in 30% of FFP-treated patients, compared with 24% of controls. Subanalysis of each comorbidity indicated no measured effect on either primary or secondary outcomes.

Intubation was done in 35% of the FFP-treated patients, compared with 60% of controls ($p = 0.050$). FFP recipients were intubated for 60 hours, as opposed to 97 hours in controls ($p = 0.45$) (Table 2). Surprisingly, most intubations were performed by an anesthesiologist or an otolaryngology surgeon (FFP, 100%; controls, 86%). Cricothyroidotomy or tracheostomy was performed in small numbers of patients of both groups, with no statistically significant difference ($p$ = 0.19 and $p = 0.34$, resp.).

By comparison, FFP-treated patients had shorter ICU stays (1.5 days versus 3.5 days; $p < 0.001$). Although the extent of hospital stay differed by group, this difference was not statistically significant (FFP, 5 days; controls, 7.5 days; $p = 0.23$) (Figures 2 and 3).

There were no differences in discharge dispositions between the groups ($p = 0.76$) (Figure 4). Overall, 78% returned home and 19% were released to an extended care facility (ECF).

## 4. Discussion

The goal of our study was to determine the frequency of intubation and ICU length of stay in patients presenting with acute (nonhereditary) AE and airway compromise who received FFP, comparing these findings with non-FFP-treated patients. To the best of our knowledge, this is the first paper to examine this relationship. Given the retrospective nature of the study, we acknowledge the limitation to ascertain the exact frequency or duration for both outcomes. However we were able to observe a reduction in the ICU length of stay among FFP-treated patients by comparison with non-FFP-treated patients. In addition, there was a reduction in the frequency of intubation that just missed statistical significance ($p = 0.050$).

The various AE syndromes all share the characteristic swelling and subcutaneous/submucosal tissue edema due to the release of vasoactive mediators, including histamine and bradykinin. We selectively studied patients with idiopathic AE (nonhereditary). As explained earlier, well-designed studies and clear management guidelines for this fairly common condition are lacking.

The role of bradykinin and bradykinin type 2 receptors in the development of AE is well documented and has

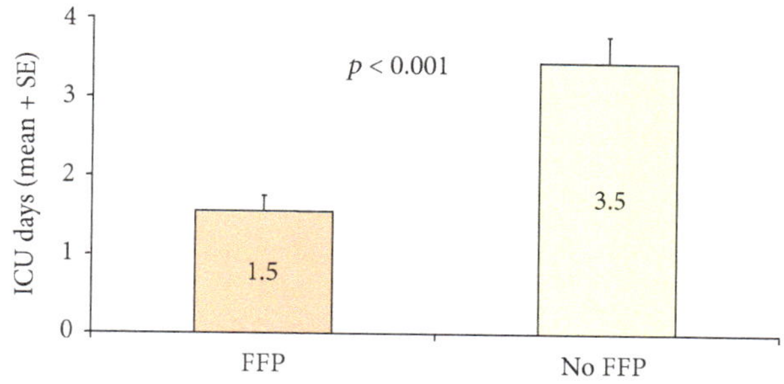


FIGURE 2: ICU stays differed significantly by group. FFP, fresh frozen plasma; ICU, intensive care unit; SE, standard error.

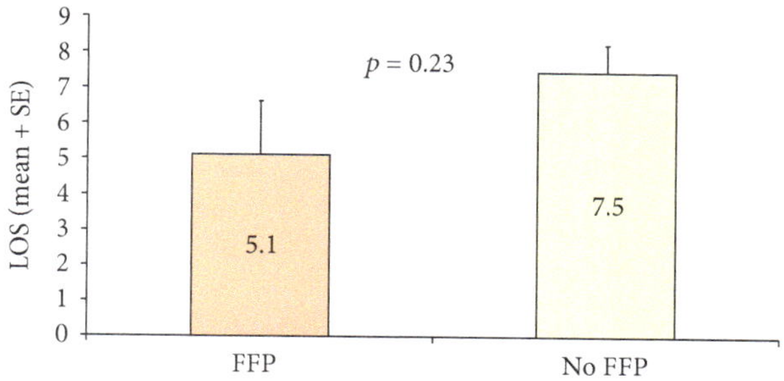


FIGURE 3: Difference in total hospital stays by group. FFP, fresh frozen plasma; LOS, length of stay; SE, standard error.

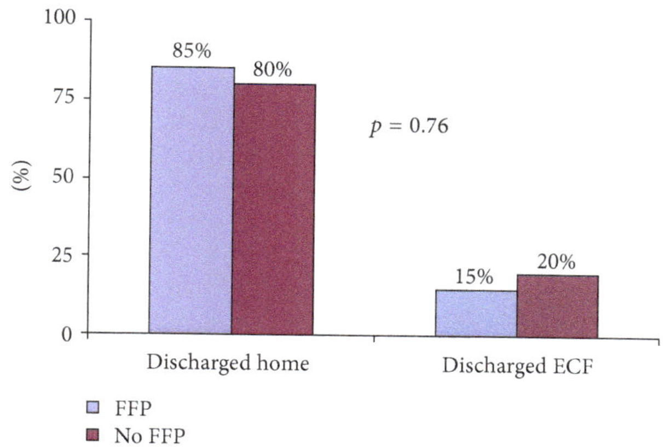


FIGURE 4: Differences in group outcomes did not reach statistical significance. FFP, fresh frozen plasma; ECF, extended care facility.

prompted the discovery of new treatments for HAE [11, 12]. ACE inhibitors decrease bradykinin catabolism, which boosts plasma levels of bradykinin and exacerbates bradykinin-dependent variants of AE [8, 13]. The reported prevalence of AE associated with ACE inhibitors ranges from 0.1% to as high as 6% in some prospective clinical trials [11]. FFP works in bradykinin-induced AE by supplying C1-INH and angiotensin-converting enzyme (ACE) among others to breakdown the accumulated levels of bradykinin.

Only recently (2009) has the US Food and Drug Administration approved other modalities/formulations (plasma-derived human C1-INH, plasma kallikrein inhibitor, C1-INH concentrates, nanofiltered plasma-derived human C1-INH, and bradykinin B2 receptor antagonist) for treating HAE attacks only [10]. Off-label use of some of these agents such as bradykinin B2 receptor antagonist in ACE inhibitors-induced AE has been reported with successful results [14]. However, the cost and availability limit in-hospital usage of these agents.

A large survey of US physicians conducted between October 2009 and February 2010 indicated that strategies for managing HAE vary substantially, with physicians still relying chiefly on supportive therapy for acute attacks. About 75% of physicians in this survey were unfamiliar with new FDA-approved treatments for HAE. Possible barriers for the use of these newly approved agents include cost, insurance restrictions, and practicality of drug delivery (i.e., lack of self-administration programs) [10].

As such, we decided to explore the use of FFP for life-threatening bouts of airway AE, particularly in instances where etiologies were unclear or difficult to ascertain. FFP use in acute attacks has proved beneficial and may be a reasonable option if C1-INH is too costly or unavailable, or in patients refractory to traditional treatment (steroid, antihistamine, and epinephrine) [9]. There is a theoretical risk that FFP can aggravate symptoms of AE but review of literature from 1969–2003 has not revealed any report to demonstrate such risk [15].

Side effects of FFP include alloimmunization, anaphylactic or allergic reaction, infection transmission (viral, Creutzfeldt-Jakob disease), and intravascular volume overload. However, the related risks must be weighed carefully against the danger of a life-threatening airway compromise [16]. Plasma is also available as a solvent/detergent-treated product, which ostensibly lowers the comparative risk of viral transmission, but the data on solvent detergent-treated plasma are scant [17].

FFP dosing for AE has not been studied and generally is administered as in coagulation disorders, infusing 2 units of 200 mL each (10 mL/kg) [16]. If volume overload is an issue, then 10–15 mL per kg body weight is recommended instead, with careful monitoring of volume status and cardiopulmonary function [17].

*4.1. Strengths.* Our study was done in a community hospital, with the majority of the study sample having African-American ethnicity. This has important implications for the generalizability of the study's findings to minority populations. The majority of study participants were being treated with ACE-I for hypertension. None of these patients was found to have another etiology for their AE, suggesting that FFP might be considered in ACE-I induced AE. This is an important finding, due to the broad use of ACE-I for hypertension and other indications. Although the number of patients who received FFP did not reach the study's calculated target to achieve 80% power, we nonetheless achieved statistically significant differences for ICU length of stay, which might have important implications in reducing cost of inpatient stays and risk for iatrogenic complications.

*4.2. Limitations.* The major limitation of this investigation includes its retrospective approach with two related issues.

The first one is the chart review with the following limitations: incomplete or missing data within the medical record, difficulty in interpreting or verifying documented information, and variability in the quality of documentation among health care personnel. The second one is the lack of control over unmeasured variables which can be potential confounders, such as patient level of severity, time limitation, availability of FFP, patient preferences, and treating physician knowledge about available treatment options for AE. We had no valid measures of disease severity.

The effectiveness of FFP as a therapeutic option for AE with airway compromise needs a better, well-controlled design to establish; however by comparing the two groups in the same cohort (cases and controls) in our study we were able to shed the light into statistical significant differences with our measured outcomes. The poor general awareness of available treatment options for AE [10] and the bewildering array of guidelines for AE variants made this study challenging to conduct.

## 5. Conclusions

In patients with acute idiopathic AE and airway compromise, we hypothesized based on our observation that using FFP (versus no FFP) shortened the ICU stay. To our knowledge, this is the first study to explore this relationship. It was our intent to shed light on a widely available, promising intervention that is suitable for use in ED settings, should conventional modalities (steroid, antihistamine, and epinephrine) fail. We also looked to bridge the gap in knowledge of ED physicians and other practitioners who are dealing with such a fairly common and life-threatening condition. A final clinical implication of the study would include simplifying and solidifying the ED practice when managing acute AE and airway compromise. We hope that our study will spur further prospective well-controlled studies on a larger scale to test our hypothesis and to generate treatment guidelines that would address both idiopathic and ACE-I induced AE.

## Conflict of Interests

The authors declare that there is no conflict of interests regarding the publication of this paper.

## Acknowledgment

Thanks are due to Amanda Hendrix for assistance with editing.

## References

[1] V. M. Temiño and R. S. Peebles Jr., "The spectrum and treatment of angioedema," *The American Journal of Medicine*, vol. 121, no. 4, pp. 282–286, 2008.

[2] M. Sánchez-Borges, R. Asero, I. J. Ansotegui et al., "Diagnosis and treatment of urticaria and angioedema: a worldwide perspective," *World Allergy Organization Journal*, vol. 5, no. 11, pp. 125–147, 2012.

[3] M. Mansi, A. Zanichelli, A. Coerezza et al., "Presentation, diagnosis and treatment of angioedema without wheals: a retrospective analysis of a cohort of 1058 patients," *Journal of Internal Medicine*, vol. 277, no. 5, pp. 585–593, 2015.

[4] R. G. Wilkerson, "Angioedema in the emergency department: an evidence-based review," *Emergency Medicine Practice*, vol. 14, no. 11, pp. 1–21, 2012.

[5] J. J. Moellman, J. A. Bernstein, C. Lindsell et al., "A consensus parameter for the evaluation and management of angioedema in the emergency department," *Academic Emergency Medicine*, vol. 21, no. 4, pp. 469–484, 2014.

[6] R. J. Pickering, J. R. Kelly, R. A. Good, and H. Gewurz, "Replacement therapy in hereditary angioedema: successful treatment of two patients with fresh frozen plasma," *The Lancet*, vol. 1, no. 7590, pp. 326–330, 1969.

[7] M. Pekdemir, M. Ersel, E. Aksay, S. Yanturali, A. Akturk, and S. Kiyan, "Effective treatment of hereditary angioedema with fresh frozen plasma in an emergency department," *The Journal of Emergency Medicine*, vol. 33, no. 2, pp. 137–139, 2007.

[8] M. R. Warrier, C. A. Copilevitz, M. S. Dykewicz, and R. G. Slavin, "Fresh frozen plasma in the treatment of resistant angiotensin-converting enzyme inhibitor angioedema," *Annals of Allergy, Asthma and Immunology*, vol. 92, no. 5, pp. 573–575, 2004.

[9] M. Winters, *Clinical Practice Guideline: Initial Evaluation and Management of Patients Presenting with Acute Urticaria or Angioedema*, AAEM, 2006.

[10] M. Riedl, R. G. Gower, and C. A. Chrvala, "Current medical management of hereditary angioedema: results from a large survey of US physicians," *Annals of Allergy, Asthma and Immunology*, vol. 106, no. 4, pp. 316–322.e4, 2011.

[11] T. Caballero, M. Baeza, R. Cabañas et al., "Consensus statement on the diagnosis, management, and treatment of angioedema mediated by bradykinin. Part I. classification, epidemiology, pathophysiology, genetics, clinical symptoms, and diagnosis," *Journal of Investigational Allergology and Clinical Immunology*, vol. 21, no. 5, pp. 333–347, 2011.

[12] A. E. Davis III, "New treatments addressing the pathophysiology of hereditary angioedema," *Clinical and Molecular Allergy*, vol. 6, article 2, 2008.

[13] M. S. Dykewicz, "Cough and angioedema from angiotensin-converting enzyme inhibitors: new insights into mechanisms and management," *Current Opinion in Allergy and Clinical Immunology*, vol. 4, no. 4, pp. 267–270, 2004.

[14] N. H. Crooks, J. Patel, L. Diwakar, and F. G. Smith, "Icatibant in the treatment of angiotensin-converting enzyme inhibitor-induced angioedema," *Case Reports in Critical Care*, vol. 2014, Article ID 864815, 3 pages, 2014.

[15] M. Prematta, J. G. Gibbs, E. L. Pratt, T. R. Stoughton, and T. J. Craig, "Fresh frozen plasma for the treatment of hereditary angioedema," *Annals of Allergy, Asthma & Immunology*, vol. 98, no. 4, pp. 383–388, 2007.

[16] T. Caballero, M. L. Baeza, R. Cabañas et al., "Consensus statement on the diagnosis, management, and treatment of angioedema mediated by bradykinin. Part 2. Treatment, follow-up, and special situations," *Journal of Investigational Allergology and Clinical Immunology*, vol. 21, no. 6, pp. 422–441, 2011.

[17] H. J. Longhurst, "Emergency treatment of acute attacks in hereditary angioedema due to C1 inhibitor deficiency: what is the evidence?" *International Journal of Clinical Practice*, vol. 59, no. 5, pp. 594–599, 2005.

# Permissions

All chapters in this book were first published in EMI, by Hindawi Publishing Corporation; hereby published with permission under the Creative Commons Attribution License or equivalent. Every chapter published in this book has been scrutinized by our experts. Their significance has been extensively debated. The topics covered herein carry significant findings which will fuel the growth of the discipline. They may even be implemented as practical applications or may be referred to as a beginning point for another development.

The contributors of this book come from diverse backgrounds, making this book a truly international effort. This book will bring forth new frontiers with its revolutionizing research information and detailed analysis of the nascent developments around the world.

We would like to thank all the contributing authors for lending their expertise to make the book truly unique. They have played a crucial role in the development of this book. Without their invaluable contributions this book wouldn't have been possible. They have made vital efforts to compile up to date information on the varied aspects of this subject to make this book a valuable addition to the collection of many professionals and students.

This book was conceptualized with the vision of imparting up-to-date information and advanced data in this field. To ensure the same, a matchless editorial board was set up. Every individual on the board went through rigorous rounds of assessment to prove their worth. After which they invested a large part of their time researching and compiling the most relevant data for our readers.

The editorial board has been involved in producing this book since its inception. They have spent rigorous hours researching and exploring the diverse topics which have resulted in the successful publishing of this book. They have passed on their knowledge of decades through this book. To expedite this challenging task, the publisher supported the team at every step. A small team of assistant editors was also appointed to further simplify the editing procedure and attain best results for the readers.

Apart from the editorial board, the designing team has also invested a significant amount of their time in understanding the subject and creating the most relevant covers. They scrutinized every image to scout for the most suitable representation of the subject and create an appropriate cover for the book.

The publishing team has been an ardent support to the editorial, designing and production team. Their endless efforts to recruit the best for this project, has resulted in the accomplishment of this book. They are a veteran in the field of academics and their pool of knowledge is as vast as their experience in printing. Their expertise and guidance has proved useful at every step. Their uncompromising quality standards have made this book an exceptional effort. Their encouragement from time to time has been an inspiration for everyone.

The publisher and the editorial board hope that this book will prove to be a valuable piece of knowledge for researchers, students, practitioners and scholars across the globe.

# List of Contributors

**H. R. Sawe, J. A. Mfinanga and V. Mwafongo**
Muhimbili University of Health and Allied Sciences, Dar es Salaam, Tanzania
Muhimbili National Hospital, Dar es Salaam, Tanzania

**F. H. Ringo**
University of California, San Francisco, CA, USA

**T. A. Reynolds**
Muhimbili National Hospital, Dar es Salaam, Tanzania
University of California, San Francisco, CA, USA

**M. S. Runyon**
Carolinas Medical Center, Charlotte, NC, USA

**Tariq Alam, Yasir Jamil Khattak and Muhammad Anwar**
The Aga Khan University Hospital, Pakistan

**Asif AlamKhan**
Khyber Medical College Peshawar, Pakistan

**İsmail Gülşen**
Yüzüncü Yıl University, School of Medicine, Department of Neurosurgery, Van, Turkey

**Hakan Ak**
Bozok University, School of Medicine, Department of Neurosurgery, Yozgat, Turkey

**Sevdegül Karadaş**
Yüzüncü Yıl University, School of Medicine, Department of Emergency Medicine, Van, Turkey

**İsmail Demır**
Van Regional Training and TeachingHospital, Clinic of Neurosurgery, Van, Turkey

**Mehmet Deniz Bulut**
Yüzüncü YılUniversity, School of Medicine,Department of Radiology, Van, Turkey

**Soner Yaycioğlu**
Adnan Menderes University, School of Medicine, Department of Neurosurgery, Aydın, Turkey

**Valentina Bestetti, Emma E. Fisher, David S. Srivastava, Meret E. Ricklin and Aristomenis K. Exadaktylos**
Department of Emergency Medicine, University Hospital and University of Bern, Freiburgstrasse 16c, 3010 Bern, Switzerland

**Kelli N. O'Laughlin**
Department of Emergency Medicine, Brigham &Women's Hospital, 75 Francis Street, Boston, MA 02115, USA
HarvardMedical School, 25 Shattuck Street, Boston, MA 02115, USA

**Jerome R. Hoffman and Michael I. Zucker**
University of California, Los Angeles (UCLA) David Geffen School of Medicine, 10833 Le Conte Avenue No. 12138, Los Angeles, CA 90095, USA

**Steven Go**
Department of Emergency Medicine, University of Missouri-Kansas City (UMKC) School of Medicine, 2411 Holmes Street, Kansas City, MO 64108, USA

**Gelareh Z. Gabayan**
Greater Los Angeles Veterans Affairs Healthcare System, 11301Wilshire Blvd, Los Angeles, CA 90073, USA
Ronald Reagan UCLA, Emergency Medicine Center, 757Westwood Plaza, Los Angeles, CA 90095, USA
Department of Medicine, University of California, Los Angeles (UCLA), 757Westwood Plaza, Los Angeles, CA 90095, Irvine, USA

**Erum Iqbal**
School of Medicine, University of California, Irvine, 1001 Health Sciences Road, 252 Irvine Hall, Irvine, CA 92697-3950, USA

**Guy Merchant**
UCLA Medical Center, 757Westwood Plaza, Los Angeles, CA 90095, USA

**Roberto A. Lopez-Freeman**
Department of Emergency Medicine, University of Cincinnati, 234 Goodman Street, Cincinnati, OH 45219, USA

**William R. Mower**
University of California, Los Angeles (UCLA) David Geffen School of Medicine, 10833 Le Conte Avenue No. 12138, Los Angeles, CA 90095, USA
Ronald Reagan UCLA, Emergency Medicine Center, 757Westwood Plaza, Los Angeles, CA 90095, USA
Emergency Medicine Center, University of California, Los Angeles (UCLA), 924 Westwood Blvd., Suite 300, Los Angeles, CA 90095, USA

**Colleen Cuca and Magnus Barth**
Ultrasound Regional Network SonoABCD and Frankfurter Institut für Notfallmedizin und Simulationstraining, Fachbereich Medizin der JohannWolfgang Goethe-Universit¨at, Klinikum der JohannWolfgang Goethe-Universität, 60528 Frankfurt am Main, Germany

**Patrick Scheiermann**
Klinik für Anaesthesiologie, Klinikum der Universität München, Campus Grosshadern, 81377 München, Germany

**Dorothea Hempel**
II. Medizinische Klinik und Poliklinik, Universitätsmedizin Mainz, 55131 Mainz, Germany

**Gabriele Via**
Anestesia e Rianimazione I, Fondazione IRCCS, Policlinico San Matteo, 27100 Pavia, Italy

**Armin Seibel**
Ultrasound Regional Network SonoABCD and Frankfurter Institut für Notfallmedizin und Simulationstraining, Fachbereich Medizin der JohannWolfgang Goethe-Universit¨at, Klinikum der JohannWolfgang Goethe-Universität, 60528 Frankfurt am Main, Germany
Klinik für Anästhesiologie, Intensiv- und Notfallmedizin, Diakonie Klinikum Jung Stilling, 57074 Siegen, Germany

**Tim O. Hirche**
Fachbereich Pneumologie, Deutsche Klinik für Diagnostik GmbH, 65191Wiesbaden, Germany

**Felix Walcher**
Ultrasound Regional Network SonoABCD and Frankfurter Institut für Notfallmedizin und Simulationstraining, Fachbereich Medizin der JohannWolfgang Goethe-Universität, Klinikum der JohannWolfgang Goethe-Universität, 60528 Frankfurt am Main, Germany
Klinik für Unfall-, Hand- und Wiederherstellungschirurgie, Klinikum der Johann Wolfgang Goethe-Universität, 60590 Frankfurt am Main, Germany

**Raoul Breitkreutz**
Ultrasound Regional Network SonoABCD and Frankfurter Institut für Notfallmedizin und Simulationstraining, Fachbereich Medizin der JohannWolfgang Goethe-Universität, Klinikum der Johann Wolfgang Goethe-Universität, 60528 Frankfurt am Main, Germany
Zentrale Notaufnahme, Klinikum Frankfurt Höchst, 65929 Frankfurt am Main, Germany

**W. A. M. H. Thijssen**
Catharina Hospital, Michelangelolaan 2, P.O. Box 1350, 5602ZA NB Eindhoven,The Netherlands
IQ Scientific Institute for Quality of Healthcare (IQ Healthcare), Radboud University Nijmegen Medical Centre, IQ P.O. Box 9101, Healthcare 114, 6500HBGLO Nijmegen,The Netherlands
Emergency Department, Catharina Hospital, Eindhoven P.O. Box 1350, 5602ZA NB Eindhoven,The Netherlands

**M. Wijnen-van Houts**
Catharina Hospital, Michelangelolaan 2, P.O. Box 1350, 5602ZA NB Eindhoven,The Netherlands

**J. Koetsenruijter P. Giesen and M.Wensing**
IQ Scientific Institute for Quality of Healthcare (IQ Healthcare), Radboud University Nijmegen Medical Centre, IQ P.O. Box 9101, Healthcare 114, 6500HBGLO Nijmegen,The Netherlands

**Abbasali Ebrahimian**
School of Nursing and Allied Medical Sciences, Semnan University of Medical Sciences, Semnan, Iran
Department of Health Services Management, School of Health Management and Information Sciences, Iran University of Medical Sciences, Tehran, Iran

**Hesam Seyedin**
Department of Health Services Management, School of Health Management and Information Sciences, Iran University of Medical Sciences, Tehran, Iran

**Roohangiz Jamshidi-Orak**
School of Health Management and Information Sciences, Iran University of Medical Sciences, No. 6, Rashid Yasemi Street, Vali-e-asr Avenue, Tehran 1995614111, Iran

**Gholamreza Masoumi**
Emergency Department, 7th Tir Hospital, Iran University of Medical Sciences, Tehran, Iran

**Asheq Rahman Catherine Martin and Rose Chapman**
Monash Health, 135 David Street, Dandenong, VIC 3175, Australia
Australian Catholic University, 115 Victoria Parade, Fitzroy, VIC 3065, Australia

**Andis Graudins**
Monash University, Clayton, VIC 3168, Australia

**Getaw Worku Hassen**
Lutheran Medical Center, Department of Emergency Medicine, Brooklyn, NY 11220, USA
NYMC, Metropolitan Hospital Center, Department of Emergency Medicine, New York, NY 10029, USA

Department of Emergency Medicine, St. George's University School of Medicine, St. George's, Grenada

**Ana Costea, Hossein Kalantari and Roger Chirurgi**
NYMC, Metropolitan Hospital Center, Department of Emergency Medicine, New York, NY 10029, USA

**Bonnie Simmons**
Lutheran Medical Center, Department of Emergency Medicine, Brooklyn, NY 11220, USA
Department of Emergency Medicine, St. George's University School of Medicine, St. George's, Grenada

**Tsion Frew and Anand Swaminathan**
Bellevue Medical Center, Department of Emergency Medicine, New York, NY 10016, USA

**Jason Feliberti**
Department of Internal Medicine, NYU, New York, NY 10016, USA

**Tennyson Smith**
Medgar Evers College, Brooklyn, NY 11225, USA

**Alice Chen and Claire Carrazco**
School of Osteopathic Medicine, A.T. Still University, Mesa, AZ 85206, USA

**Sarah Thompson and Neola Gushway-Henry**
Lutheran Medical Center, Department of Family Practice, Brooklyn, NY 11220, USA

**George Fernaine**
Lutheran Medical Center, Department of Internal Medicine, Brooklyn, NY 11220, USA

**Soheila Talebi**
NYMC, Metropolitan Hospital Center, Department of Internal Medicine, New York, NY 10029, USA

**Sharon Chekijian, Anthony J. Tomassoni, David C. Cone and Federico E. Vaca**
Department of Emergency Medicine, Yale University School of Medicine, 464 Congress Avenue, Suite 260, NewHaven, CT 06519, USA

**Melinda Paul**
Yale University, New Haven, CT 06520, USA

**Vanessa P. Kohl**
Department of Family Medicine,White Memorial Medical Center, Los Angeles, CA 90033, USA

**David M.Walker**
Division of Pediatric Emergency Medicine, Elmhurst Hospital Center, Ichahn School of Medicine at Mount Sinai School, Elmhurst, NY 11373, USA

**Julia Lai-Kwon and Alvin H. Chong**
Department ofMedicine (Dermatology), St. Vincent'sHospital, Melbourne, VIC, Australia

**Tracey J. Weiland and George A. Jelinek**
Emergency Practice Innovation Centre, St. Vincent's Hospital, 41 Victoria Parade Fitzroy, Melbourne, VIC 3065, Australia
Faculty of Medicine Dentistry and Health Sciences,The University of Melbourne, VIC, Australia

**Thana Khawcharoenporn**
Division of Infectious Diseases, Faculty of Medicine,Thammasat University, Pathum Thani 12120, Thailand
Section of Infectious Diseases, Rush University Medical Center, Chicago, IL 60612, USA

**Shawn Vasoo and Kamaljit Singh**
Division of Infectious Diseases, Faculty of Medicine,Thammasat University, Pathum Thani 12120, Thailand

**Hossein Samaei**
Department of Emergency Medicine, St. Vincent's Hospital, Melbourne, VIC 3065, Australia

**Tracey Joy Weiland and George Alexander Jelinek**
Emergency Practice Innovation Centre, St. Vincent's Hospital, Melbourne, VIC 3065, Australia
Department of Medicine, Dentistry and Health Sciences,The University of Melbourne, Melbourne, VIC 3010, Australia

**Stuart Dilley**
Department of Emergency Medicine, St. Vincent's Hospital, Melbourne, VIC 3065, Australia
Department of Medicine, Dentistry and Health Sciences,The University of Melbourne, Melbourne, VIC 3010, Australia

**Kijja Jearwattanakanok**
Department of Surgery, Nakornping Hospital, Chiang Mai 50180,Thailand

**Sirikan Yamada**
Division of Gastrointestinal Surgery and Endnoscopy, Department of Surgery, Faculty of Medicine, Chiang Mai University, Chiang Mai 50200,Thailand

**Watcharin Suntornlimsiri**
Department of Obstetrics & Gynecology, Nakornping Hospital, Chiang Mai 50180,Thailand

**Waratsuda Smuthtai**
Department of Emergency Medicine, Nakornping Hospital, Chiang Mai 50180,Thailand

**Jayanton Patumanond**
Clinical Epidemiology Unit, Clinical Research Center, Faculty of Medicine, Thammasat University, PathumThani 12120,Thailand

**Abbasali Ebrahimian and Hesam Seyedin**
Department of Health Services Management, School of Health Management and Information Sciences, Iran University of Medical Sciences, No. 6, Rashid Yasemi Street, Vali-e-asr Avenue, Tehran 1995614111, Iran

**Roohangiz Jamshidi-Orak**
School of Health Management and Information Sciences, Iran University of Medical Sciences, Tehran, Iran

**Gholamreza Masoumi**
Department of Emergency Medicine, School of Medicine, Iran University of Medical Sciences, Tehran, Iran
Tobias Lindner, Anna Slagman, Arthur Senkin,Martin Möckel and Julia Searle
Division of Emergency Medicine, Charité-Universitätsmedizin Berlin, Campus Virchow Klinikum (CVK), Augustenburger Platz 1, 13353 Berlin, Germany

**W. Frank Peacock and Zubaid Rafique**
Section of Emergency Medicine, Baylor College of Medicine, Ben Taub General Hospital, 1504 Taub Loop, Houston, TX 77030, USA

**Adam J. Singer**
Department of Emergency Medicine, Stony Brook School of Medicine, University Medical Center L4, 100 Nicolls Road, Stony Brook,NY 11794-8350, USA

**Sylvana Papoutsi, LucaMartinolli, Christian Tasso Braun and Aristomenis K. Exadaktylos**
Department of Emergency Medicine, University Hospital and University of Bern, Freiburgstraße 16c, 3010 Bern, Switzerland

**Raoul Breitkreutz**
Emergency Department, Hospital of the City of Frankfurt (Höchst), Gotenstraße 6-8, 65929 Frankfurt am Main, Germany
Emergency Ultrasound Regional Network and the Frankfurt Institute of Emergency Medicine and Simulation Training, JohannWolfgang Goethe University Hospital, Marienburgstraße 5-7, 60528 Frankfurt am Main, Germany

**Marco Campo dell' Orto**
Emergency Ultrasound Regional Network and the Frankfurt Institute of Emergency Medicine and Simulation Training, Johann Wolfgang Goethe University Hospital, Marienburgstraße 5-7, 60528 Frankfurt am Main, Germany
Department of Cardiology, Kerckhoff Klinik Bad Nauheim, Benekestraße 2-8, 61231 Bad Nauheim, Germany

**Christian Hamm**
Department of Cardiology, Kerckhoff Klinik Bad Nauheim, Benekestraße 2-8, 61231 Bad Nauheim, Germany

**Colleen Cuca**
Deptartment of Anaesthesiology and Intensive Care, Hospital zum Heiligen Geist, Lange Straße, 60311 Frankfurt, Germany

**PeterM. Zechner**
Landeskrankenhaus GrazWest, Abteilung für Innere Medizin, G¨ottinger Straße 22, 8020 Graz, Austria

**Tanja Stenger**
Städtisches Klinikum Neunkirchen, Brunnenstraße 20, 66538 Neunkirchen/Saar, Germany
Brainfactory, 66288 Bildstock, Germany

**FelixWalcher**
Trauma Surgery, Johann Wolfgang Goethe University Hospital,Theodor Stern Kai 7, 60590 Frankfurt am Main, Germany

**Florian H. Seeger**
Department of Cardiology, Johann Wolfgang Goethe University Hospital,Theodor Stern Kai 7, 60590 Frankfurt am Main, Germany

**Assaad Sayah, Lisa Kingsley-Rocker and Luis F. Lobon**
Department of Emergency Medicine, Cambridge Health Alliance, 1493 Cambridge Street, Cambridge, MA 02139, USA

**Loni Rogers and Karthik Devarajan**
Tufts University School of Medicine, Boston, MA, USA
Heller School of Social Policy and Management, Brandeis University,Waltham, MA, USA

**Mohamed El Sayad**
Trauma and Orthopaedics,Wishaw General Hospital,Wishaw, UK

**Hussein Noureddine**
Trauma and Orthopaedics, Ninewells Hospital, Dundee, UK

**Amy Sue Biondich and Jeremy David Joslin**
Department of Emergency Medicine, SUNY Upstate Medical University, 550 E. Genesee Street, Suite 103, Syracuse, NY 13202, USA

**Sharonjeet Kaur, Sujit Rajagopalan, Navjot Kaur, Nusrat Shafiq, Promila Pandhi and Samir Malhotra**
Department of Pharmacology, PGIMER, Chandigarh 160012, India

**Ashish Bhalla**
Department of Internal Medicine, PGIMER, Chandigarh 160012, India

**Abdulaziz Alburaih**
Department of Emergency Medicine, University of Maryland Shore Regional Health, Easton, MD, USA

**Ismail Mahmood, Ahmad Zarour, Ibrahim Afifi, Suresh Kumar, Ruben Peralta, Rifat Latifi and Hassan Al-Thani**
Department of Surgery, Section of Trauma Surgery, Hamad General Hospital, P.O. Box 3050, Doha, Qatar

**Zainab Tawfeek**
Department of Emergency, Hamad Medical Corporation, P.O. Box 3050, Doha, Qatar

**Ayman El-Menyar**
Clinical Research, Section of Trauma Surgery, Hamad General Hospital, Doha, Qatar
ClinicalMedicine, Weill Cornell Medical School, P.O. Box 24144,Doha, Qatar
Internal Medicine, Ahmed Maher Teaching Hospital, Cairo, Egypt

**Thomas Carter, Chris Conrad and J. Link Wilson**
Emergency Department, Southern Ohio Medical Center, Portsmouth, OH 45662, USA

**Godwin Dogbey**
CORE Research Office, Ohio University Heritage College of Osteopathic Medicine, Athens, OH 45701, USA

**Christine M. Van Dillen, Matthew R. Tice, Archita D. Patel, David A.Meurer, Joseph A. Tyndall and Marie Carmelle Elie**
Department of Emergency Medicine, University of Florida College of Medicine, Gainesville, FL 32610, USA

**Jonathan J. Shuster**
Department of Health Outcomes and Policy, University of Florida College of Medicine, Gainesville, FL 32610, USA

**Amanda S. Newton**
Faculty of Medicine & Dentistry, University of Alberta, Edmonton Clinic Health Academy (ECHA), 11405-87 Avenue, Room 3-526, Edmonton, AB, Canada T6G 1C9

**Sachin Rathee**
Faculty of Medicine & Dentistry, University of Alberta,WC Mackenzie Health Sciences Centre, Edmonton, AB, Canada T6G 2R7

**Simran Grewal**
Faculty of Medicine & Dentistry, University of Alberta, Edmonton Clinic Health Academy (ECHA), 11405-87 Avenue, Room 3-582B, Edmonton, AB, Canada T6G 1C9

**Nadia Dow**
Faculty of Medicine & Dentistry, University of Alberta, Edmonton Clinic Health Academy (ECHA), 11405-87 Avenue, Room 3-582, Edmonton, AB, Canada T6G 1C9

**Rhonda J. Rosychuk**
Faculty of Medicine & Dentistry, University of Alberta, Edmonton Clinic Health Academy (ECHA), 11405-87 Avenue, Room 3-524, Edmonton, AB, Canada T6G 1C9

**Hnin Khine and Jeffrey R. Avner**
Division of Pediatric Emergency Medicine, Children's Hospital at Montefiore, 3415 Bainbridge Avenue, Bronx, NY 10467, USA
Department of Pediatrics, Albert Einstein College of Medicine, Bronx, NY 10467, USA

**David L. Goldman**
Department of Pediatrics, Albert Einstein College of Medicine, Bronx, NY 10467, USA
Division of Pediatric Infectious Diseases, Children's Hospital at Montefiore, Bronx, NY 10467, USA

**Jeremy D. Joslin**
Department of Emergency Medicine, State University of New York Upstate Medical University, Syracuse, NY, USA

**Jarem B. Lloyd**
Department of Orthopedics and Sports Medicine, St. Luke's University Health Network, Bethlehem, PA, USA

**Nikoli Copeli**
Department of Emergency Medicine, New York Hospital Queens, Flushing, NY, USA

**Derek R. Cooney**
Department of Emergency Medicine, 550 East Genesee St., Syracuse, NY 13210, USA

**P. C. M. Musiitwa, M. Galukand and R.Wangoda**
Department of Surgery, College of Health Sciences, Makerere University, Kampala, Uganda

**S. Bugeza**
Department of Radiology, College of Health Sciences, Makerere University, Kampala, Uganda

**H. Wanzira**
Infectious Diseases Research Collaboration, Makerere University, Kampala, Uganda

**Confidence Alorse Atakro**
University of Cape Coast, Cape Coast, Ghana

**Jerry Paul Ninnoni**
Faculty of Nursing and Midwifery School, University of Cape Coast, Cape Coast, Ghana

**Peter Adatara**
The School of Nursing and Midwifery, University of Health and Allied Sciences, Ho, Ghana

**Janet Gross**
Morehead State University, Morehead, KY, USA
Global Health Services Partnership, US Peace Corps,Washington, DC, USA

**Michael Agbavor**
Volta Regional Hospital, Ho, Ghana

**Ward Patrick**
Department of Critical Care, Dalhousie University, Suite 377, Bethune Building, 1276 South Park Street, Halifax, NS, Canada B3H2Y9

**Robert S. Green**
Department of Critical Care, Dalhousie University, Suite 377, Bethune Building, 1276 South Park Street, Halifax, NS, Canada B3H2Y9
TraumaNova Scotia, Room 1-026B, Centennial Building, 1276 South Park Street, Halifax,NS, Canada B3H2Y9

**Andrew H. Travers and Jan L. Jensen**
Department of Emergency Medicine, Dalhousie University, Division of EMS, 1796 Summer Street, Halifax Infirmary, Suite 355, Halifax,NS, Canada B3H3A7
Emergency Health Service, 239 Brownlow Avenue, Suite 300, Dartmouth, NS, Canada B3B 2B2

**Edward Cain and Samuel G. Campbell and David A. Petrie**
Department of Emergency Medicine, Dalhousie University, Division of EMS, 1796 Summer Street, Halifax Infirmary, Suite 355, Halifax,NS, Canada B3H3A7

**Mete Erdogan**
TraumaNova Scotia, Room 1-026B, Centennial Building, 1276 South Park Street, Halifax,NS, Canada B3H2Y9

**Gredi Patrick**
Performance Excellence, Nova Scotia Health Authority, Halifax, NS, Canada B3H 4R2

**Aya Saeb**
Department of Internal Medicine, St. John Hospital & Medical Center, 22101 Moross Road, Detroit, MI 48236, USA
Geriatric Research Education and Clinical Center (GRECC), VA Ann Arbor Healthcare System, 2215 Fuller Road 11 G, Ann Arbor, MI 48105, USA
Department of Internal Medicine, University of Michigan, 3110 Taubman Center, SPC 5368, 1500 East Medical Center Drive, Ann Arbor, MI 48109, USA

**Karen H. Hagglund**
Department of Internal Medicine, St. John Hospital & Medical Center, 22101 Moross Road, Detroit, MI 48236, USA

**Christine T. Cigolle**
Geriatric Research Education and Clinical Center (GRECC), VA Ann Arbor Healthcare System, 2215 Fuller Road 11 G, Ann Arbor, MI 48105, USA
Department of Internal Medicine, University of Michigan, 3110 Taubman Center, SPC 5368, 1500 East Medical Center Drive, Ann Arbor, MI 48109, USA
Department of Family Medicine, University of Michigan, 1150W. Medical Center Drive, M7300 Med Sci I, SPC 5625, Ann Arbor, MI 48109, USAs

# Index